Improving the Quality of Life for Dementia Patients through Progressive Detection, Treatment, and Care

Jinglong Wu
Okayama University, Japan

A volume in the Advances in Psychology, Mental Health, and Behavioral Studies (APMHBS) Book Series

IGI GLOBAL
DISSEMINATOR OF KNOWLEDGE
www.igi-global.com

Published in the United States of America by
IGI Global
Medical Information Science Reference (an imprint of IGI Global)
701 E. Chocolate Avenue
Hershey PA 17033
Tel: 717-533-8845
Fax: 717-533-8661
E-mail: cust@igi-global.com
Web site: http://www.igi-global.com

Library of Congress Cataloging-in-Publication Data

Names: Wu, Jinglong, 1958- editor.
Title: Improving the quality of life for dementia patients through progressive detection, treatment, and care / Jinglong Wu, editor.
Other titles: Advances in psychology, mental health, and behavioral studies.
Description: Hershey, PA : Medical Information Science Reference, [2017] | Series: Advances in psychology, mental health, and behavioral studies | Includes bibliographical references and index.
Identifiers: LCCN 2016032786| ISBN 9781522509257 (hardcover) | ISBN 9781522509264 (ebook)
Subjects: | MESH: Alzheimer Disease--diagnosis | Alzheimer Disease--therapy | Alzheimer Disease--psychology | Quality of Life | Emotions | Aged
Classification: LCC RC523 | NLM WT 155 | DDC 616.8/31--dc23 LC record available at https://lccn.loc.gov/2016032786

This book is published in the IGI Global book series Advances in Psychology, Mental Health, and Behavioral Studies (APMHBS) (ISSN: pending; eISSN: pending)

British Cataloguing in Publication Data
A Cataloguing in Publication record for this book is available from the British Library.

Advances in Psychology, Mental Health, and Behavioral Studies (APMHBS) Book Series

ISSN: pending
EISSN: pending

Mission

The complexity of the human mind has puzzled researchers and physicians for centuries. While widely studied, the brain still remains largely misunderstood.

The **Advances in Psychology, Mental Health, and Behavioral Studies (APMHBS)** book series presents comprehensive research publications focusing on topics relating to the human psyche, cognition, psychiatric care, mental and developmental disorders, as well as human behavior and interaction. Featuring diverse and innovative research, publications within APMHBS are ideally designed for use by mental health professionals, academicians, researchers, and upper-level students.

Coverage

- Socialization
- Addiction
- Emotional Health
- Anxiety
- Human Behavior
- Cognition
- Personality Disorders
- Substance Abuse
- Trauma & Stress
- Psychiatry

IGI Global is currently accepting manuscripts for publication within this series. To submit a proposal for a volume in this series, please contact our Acquisition Editors at Acquisitions@igi-global.com or visit: http://www.igi-global.com/publish/.

The Advances in Psychology, Mental Health, and Behavioral Studies (APMHBS) Book Series (ISSN pending) is published by IGI Global, 701 E. Chocolate Avenue, Hershey, PA 17033-1240, USA, www.igi-global.com. This series is composed of titles available for purchase individually; each title is edited to be contextually exclusive from any other title within the series. For pricing and ordering information please visit http://www.igi-global.com/book-series/advances-psychology-mental-health-behavioral/110200. Postmaster: Send all address changes to above address.

Titles in this Series

For a list of additional titles in this series, please visit: www.igi-global.com

Police Psychology and Its Growing Impact on Modern Law Enforcement
Cary L. Mitchell (Pepperdine University, USA) and Edrick H. Dorian (Los Angeles Police Department, USA)
Information Science Reference • copyright 2017 • 345pp • H/C (ISBN: 9781522508137) • US $190.00 (our price)

Seduction in Popular Culture, Psychology, and Philosophy
Constantino Martins (Nova University of Lisbon, Portugal) and Manuel Damásio (Lusófona University, Portugal)
Information Science Reference • copyright 2017 • 332pp • H/C (ISBN: 9781522505259) • US $175.00 (our price)

Chronic Mental Illness and the Changing Scope of Intervention Strategies, Diagnosis, and Treatment
Barre Vijaya Prasad (Dharwad Institute of Mental Health and Neurosciences, India)
Medical Information Science Reference • copyright 2017 • 404pp • H/C (ISBN: 9781522505198) • US $220.00 (our price)

Identifying, Treating, and Preventing Childhood Trauma in Rural Communities
Marion Baker (Center of Hope Arizona, USA) Jacqueline Ford (Center of Hope Arizona, USA & Walden University, USA) Brittany Canfield (Center of Hope Arizona, USA & Fielding Graduate University, USA) and Traci Grabb (Arizona's Children Association, USA & Center of Hope Arizona, USA)
Information Science Reference • copyright 2016 • 306pp • H/C (ISBN: 9781522502289) • US $185.00 (our price)

Handbook of Research on Diagnosing, Treating, and Managing Intellectual Disabilities
Rejani Thudalikunnil Gopalan (Gujarat Forensic Sciences University, India)
Information Science Reference • copyright 2016 • 496pp • H/C (ISBN: 9781522500896) • US $210.00 (our price)

Neuroeconomics and the Decision-Making Process
Bryan Christiansen (PryMarke LLC, USA) and Ewa Lechman (Gdansk University of Technology, Poland)
Business Science Reference • copyright 2016 • 354pp • H/C (ISBN: 9781466699892) • US $195.00 (our price)

Table of Contents

Detailed Table of Contents

Touch has been described as the most fundamental means of contact with the world and the most primitive modality among all sensory systems. In the past, the study of emotional communication has focused almost exclusively on facial and vocal channels but has ignored the channel for the sense of touch. However, the latest studies have documented that the sense of touch can convey at least six emotions, and its accuracy rate is comparable to that of facial expressions and vocal communication. Moreover, there is also mounting evidence indicating that the modality of touch encompasses two dimensions, which provide not only its well-recognized discriminative input from glabrous skin to sensory cortex but also an affective input from hairy skin to the insular cortex because a type of low-threshold mechanosensitive receptor that innervates hairy skin has been shown to convey emotions via C fibers. In light of recent advances in our research, this chapter aims to illustrate the cognitive and neural mechanisms that underlie interactions between touch and emotion.

Bimodal audiovisual signals can be detected more quickly and accurately than unimodal visual signals or auditory signals. This beneficial effect is called audiovisual integration. Audiovisual integration has often been described according to the spatial principle, the temporal principle and the inverse effectiveness principle. Inverse effectiveness indicates that the largest audiovisual enhancements are inversely correlated with the strength of the response to unisensory component stimuli; thus, weaker stimuli generate greater enhancement when presented together. In addition, some studies have suggested that the visual contrast feature can modulate audiovisual integration and obtained an inverse relationship between visual contrast

Foreword

It is my great pleasure and honor to be invited to contribute a foreword to the book titled *Improving the Quality of Life for Dementia Patients through Progressive Detection, Treatment, and Care*, written and edited by Mr. Qiong Wu and Prof. Jinglong Wu of Okayama University, Japan.

In recent years, the life of the human beings is getting longer in many countries and regions, owing to the progress of scientific knowledge and clinical technologies in health care and medical treatment. It is, as a matter of course, a big benefit for the human beings. However, it brings about a big threat to the human society, that is, a rapid increase of unhealthy aged population. Especially, increase of the dementia patients is quite remarkable as indicated in Chapter 1: Alzheimer's disease is a typical neurodegenerative disease that affects more than 30% of the population older than 85. In addition, the number of dementia patients in younger generations is also increasing. These indicates the fact that more than a billion people are suffering from dementia! Then, there exist urgent needs to realize effective means for early detection, treatment and also care of dementia patients.

A wide variety of the topics included is one of the remarkable feature of the book. There are included physiological and psychological methods of detecting/caring dementia, various methods of giving

physical/physiological and psychological stimuli for treating/caring dementia patients, and also a method of designing environmental landscape design, etc. A big variety of the authors is another feature of the book. Authors have been invited from Japan, China, Turkey. Canada and Greece.

Thus, the book gives, without any doubt, an excellent reference both to the basic researchers and clinical practitioners in the field.

In order to overcome the increasing difficulties brought about by dementia, it is essentially needed to develop the following ways:

1. Further progress of scientific research on the physiological mechanism, especially from the viewpoint of neural mechanism.

2. Clarification of process of cognitive defects from the viewpoint of psychology and behavioral science.
3. Development of effective means of early detection and practical methods of suppressing progress of neural defects.
4. Organizing an international federation of scientists and practitioners to activate worldwide exchange and cooperation.
5. Constructing financial support system by the central and the local governments to make the advanced medical and technological means enjoyable to all the people.

Yoshikazu Nishikawa
Kyoto University, Japan & Osaka Institute of Technology, Japan

Preface

Dementia is a progressive neurodegenerative disease. Presently, 44.4 million people have developed into such disease in the world, and the number is increasing every year as the aging processing (Department of Economic and Social Affairs Population Division, n.d.). While the diagnosis and treatment of such disease is still in the infant stage, and is the huge challenge of the present society. So many countries recognize the living condition of the dementia people as a significant investigate project, and try their best to develop effective diagnosis and treatment scheme to improve the living condition of the patients. Dementia is a serious loss of cognitive ability in a previously unimpaired person beyond what might be expected from normal aging. Until the end of the nineteenth century, dementia was a much broader clinical concept.

The typical dementia is Alzheimer's disease (AD), and it also includes other types, such as Lewy body dementia, vascular dementia, frontotemporal dementia, progressive supranuclear palsy, corticobasal degeneration, normal pressure hydrocephalus and Creutzfeldt–Jakob disease. This dysfunction can seriously affect the routine life, such as thought, memory, and logic, and this may also grievously change their personality, mood, and behavior. Because the mechanism and the pathology of dementia are still unclear, there is no effective treatment of Dementia. Therefore, early detection is the only method to erase the suffering of the patients.

AD is characterized by the progressive formation of insoluble amyloid plaques and vascular deposits of amyloid beta peptide in the brain. AD patients suffer from a loss of neurons and synapses in the cerebral cortex and certain sub-cortical regions. Numerous researchers in pathophysiology and molecular neurology have focused on the cause of AD in an effort to identify clinical markers, such as the beta-site amyloid precursor protein-cleaving enzyme 1, which can be used to diagnose AD. However, until recently, there were no medical tests capable of conclusively diagnosing AD pre-mortem. The mini-mental state examination (MMSE), a brief, 30-point questionnaire, as well as the clinical dementia rating (CDR), a five-point numeric scale, are the standard tests used to help the physician determine whether a person suffering from memory impairments has AD. Both of these tests include simple questions and problems in a number of areas, such as arithmetic, memory and orientation, used to quantify the severity of dementia symptoms. However, the sensitivity of the MMSE test is approximately 80%, and it has very limited use in screening for patients with mild cognitive impairment (MCI), a major risk factor for the development of AD (Bachman, et al., 1993; MacKenzie, Copp, Shaw, & Goodwin, 1996; McGue & Christensen, 2001; Cacho, et al., 2010).

Recent fMRI studies have used spatial attention tasks to study the different neural substrates activated in adults with AD and in normal age-matched adults. These reports found that the most pronounced differences between the two groups were found in the superior parietal lobule (SPL), which was more highly activated in controls, and the frontal and occipitotemporal (OCT) areas, which showed greater activity in AD patients. Differentiating between default networks in AD and normal age-matched adults is another approach and typically uses independent component analysis. A third kind of study uses functional connectivity MRI and focuses on the identification of hubs within the human cerebral cortex, determining the stability of hubs across subject groups and task states and exploring whether the locations of hubs can be correlated with one component of AD pathology.

In the very early stages of AD, altered cognitive symptoms involve mild impairments in learning, memory, or planning. Several researchers use cognitive tasks, including memory tasks, visuospatial tasks, and language tasks, in order to identify differences in cognitive function between AD patients and normal controls. These studies have convincingly demonstrated that it is possible to use cognitive tasks to detect deficits in AD patients during a preclinical period spanning several years. For instance, some researchers have found high levels of pathological lesions in the primary visual areas and certain visual association areas within the occipito-parieto-temporal junction and posterior cingulate cortex in AD patients.

The application of neuroimaging technology to the study of AD has been steadily increasing over the last two decades. To date, the majority of neuroimaging reports that have contributed to the understanding of the pathophysiology and clinical course of AD have utilized structural magnetic resonance imaging (MRI) and positron emission tomography (PET). In addition, functional MRI (fMRI) has been used as a research tool to study AD since 1999. The fMRI studies of AD have focused on two overlapping objectives: understanding the basic biological mechanisms and pathophysiology of AD and developing an effective diagnostic tool or clinical biomarker. The development of biomarkers via fMRI is anticipated to influence the clinical management of AD in three significant ways: differentiating healthy aging from AD, enhancing diagnostic specificity when evaluating a patient with dementia, and monitoring the biological progression of AD for the purposes of drug development and drug testing.

Language is succinctly defined as a "human system of communication that uses arbitrary signals, such as voice sounds, gestures, or written symbols" ("What Is Language?", n.d.). This system is used to encode and decode information. In the literature on dementia, the presence or absence of language deficits has come to occupy a pivotal position with respect to certain nosological and nosographical issues. Simply using the correct language engenders trust. This is especially true of the language we use when talking about medical issues-particularly AD. Media reports on AD contribute significantly to the public's awareness and knowledge of the condition. Increasing the general understanding of dementia makes seeking diagnosis or support easier for people with concerns about memory loss. The more that other people understand about their experience, the better the quality of life will be for people living with dementia. Language appears to be affected in the early stages of dementia, but the effect is often seen only in selected areas and with significant individual variability. It would appear that impairments in transcribing dictated information and in the pragmatic use of language can be detected early if sensitive tasks are employed. Performance transcribing dictations may indicate a partial lexical knowledge of written words, suggesting that some features of the words' specification in the brain's lexical stores are either absent or inaccessible as a result of brain degeneration.

While the present investigation indicated that some non-invasive cognitive neuroscience technologies can used to prove some available information. For example, via fMRI (functional magnetic resonance imaging) and EEG (Electroencephalogram), alteration of DMN (default mode network) state is connected with Dementia to some degree. Additionally, the behavioral information also can provide evidence for Dementia. All the cues described above can be used as proof of early detection, and healthcare for dementia.

Now, we considered that it is important for diagnosing some mental diseases and healthcare. For example, by using non-invasive fMRI (functional magnetic resonance imaging) and EEG (Electroencephalogram), change of DMN (default mode network) state could be found out and linked to the diagnosis of dementia. On the other hand, by watching the behavioral cognition, abnormal aspect could be considered by the reason of related mental disease. Thus, the early diagnose of mental diseases could be done by using several cognitive neuroscience methods, such as mentioned above, and it is necessary since the data could provide useful advice for healthcare before the arise or at the early state of disease.

Dementia is a serious loss of cognitive ability in a previously unimpaired person beyond what might be expected from normal aging. It may be static, as in the case of a unique global brain injury, or progressive, resulting in long-term decline due to damage or disease in the body. Although dementia is far more common in the geriatric population, it can occur in any stage of adulthood. Similar sets of symptoms due to organic brain syndromes or dysfunction are given different names when they occur before adulthood. Until the end of the nineteenth century, dementia was a much broader clinical concept.

The diseases that can cause dementia include Alzheimer's disease, vascular dementia, Lewy body dementia, frontotemporal dementia, Huntington's disease, and Creutzfeldt-Jakob disease. Doctors have identified other conditions that can cause dementia or dementia-like symptoms, including reactions to medications, metabolic problems and endocrine abnormalities, nutritional deficiencies, infections, poisoning, brain tumors, anoxia or hypoxia, and heart and lung problems.

While there is no cure for dementia, advances have been made toward developing medications that can slow down the process. Cholinesterase inhibitors are often used early in the course of the disease. Cognitive and behavioral interventions may also be appropriate. Educating and providing emotional sup- port to the caregiver are also important. There is some evidence that the regular, moderate consumption of alcohol and a Mediterranean diet may reduce the risk of developing dementia. In addition, a recent study has shown a link between high blood pressure and developing dementia. The studies, published in the *Lancet Neurology Journal* in July 2008, found that medications that lower blood pressure reduced dementia by 13% (Davis, Massman, & Doody, 2003; Kennelly, Lawlor, & Kenny, 2009).

Neurological rehabilitation is often used to reduce physical and cognitive impairments and related disabilities. It has also been shown to increase independence, so patients can participate in daily self-care and other activities to improve their health-related quality of life (QOL). Learning skills after a stroke, a traumatic brain or spinal cord injury or other diseases target the neural networks for movement, sensation, perception, memory, planning, motivation, reward, language, and other aspects of cognition that remain undamaged to compensate for those that were lost.

The rehabilitation of sensory and cognitive functions typically involves retraining neural pathways or training new neural pathways to regain or improve the neurocognitive functioning that has been diminished by disease or traumatic injury.

Speech therapy, occupational therapy and other methods that "exercise" specific brain functions are used. For example, eye-hand coordination exercises may rehabilitate certain motor deficits, while well-structured planning and organizing exercises might help rehabilitate certain frontal lobe "executive functions" following a traumatic blow to the head.

OBJECTIVE OF THE BOOK

The purpose of this book is to bring researchers and practitioners together, including engineers, medical doctors, health professionals, and neuroscientists, informatics and computer scientists. They are engaged in dementia from pathological to healthcare in both theoretical advances and applications of information systems, artificial intelligence, signal processing, electronics and other engineering tools in biomedical areas related to cognitive neuroscience and medicine. Thus, researches can contribute to the survey on the disease principle of dementia and make efforts in order to cure patients.

TARGET AUDIENCE

Academicians, researchers, medical personnel, rehabilitation personnel, care personnel, advanced-level students and technology developers will find this book useful in furthering their research exposure to pertinent topics in assisting in furthering their own research efforts in this field.

ORGANIZATION OF THE BOOK

The book is organized into fourteen chapters. A brief description of each of the chapters follows:

Chapter 1 identifies the early diagnosis of Alzheimer's. The chapter introduced that there is no effective treatment to stop the decline of the cognitive and memory. Only measures we can take are to ease or improve symptoms temporarily. Therefore, it is necessary to diagnosis the disease in the early stage, such as through imaging detection via CT, MRI, PET and MSR, or prediction before the disease (genetic examination). However, literature data have supported the notion that Alzheimer's disease patients show cognitive reserve abilities to some degree. In the future, research perspectives may focus on the cognitive training paradigms in compensatory and restorative strategies.

Chapter 2 focused on the best practice in treatment is to help them maintain a positive view of their lives and balance their emotions, both personally, in terms of keeping their sense of self, and in social environments, where they have to recognize and interact with others. In this way, good environmental landscape design will have an important role to play in improving their quality of life.

Chapter 3 was to determine nutritional status and its influence on their quality of life in Alzheimer's disease (AD) patients with Mini Nutritional Assessment (MNA) and anthropometric measurements. Found that nutrient intake among aged individuals with AD was found unbalanced; a statistically significant correlation between energy / nutrient intake and quality of life also was not detected.

Chapter 4 addressed the problem of the early detection of dementia from two points of view: Detection based on unobtrusive paradigms both in lab and home environments (behavioral monitoring, serious games, home based assisted living applications in telemedicine) and detection based on neuroimaging approaches. The chapter also provides information on setting up ecologically valid home labs for dementia related experiments. Consequently, the aim of this chapter is to provide an overview of a complete methodology of how researchers can possibly detect or predict the onset of dementia through the current state-of-the-art, underline open challenges and illustrate future work in the field.

Chapter 5 summarized a review of studies on bilingualism and dementia, supporting the viewpoint that bilinguals have an advantage in delaying dementia compared with monolinguals.

Chapter 6 introduced the tactile stimulation devices, which can be divided into many categories according to qualities, including their geometric properties, temperature, force, and vibration. Also introduced some devices that can be used to guide clinical diagnosis and treatment. These devices can be used to examine a patient's haptic perception to help the patient's doctors diagnose their illness.

Chapter 7 summarize the empirical evidence for the rehabilitation of individuals with cognitive disorders by using training tasks to enhance specific cognitive functions to combat against cognitive degradation and transfer the benefits to other widely used domains.

Chapter 8 aims to illustrate the cognitive and neural mechanisms that underlie interactions between touch and emotion.

Chapter 9 aims to summarize previous studies and describe the relationship between visual contrast and inverse effectiveness by behavior, ERP and fMRI experimental methods. By summarizing previous studies, we have determined the direction of future work.

Chapter 10 summarizes the current status of research into intention recognition and gives a brief description of the relationship between emotion and intention. We hope to provide more ideas for optimizing human-computer interactions.

Chapter 11 focused on the time cognition of the dementia. Summarizes numerous research studies on the neural networks involved in explicit timing during the measurement of sub-second and supra-second intervals.

Chapter 12 discusses tactile device scan provide the best rehabilitation program for patients. Presents previous fMRI-compatible stimulation devices, including texture stimulation, shape stimulation, vibrotactile stimulation, etc., which involve the hands, face, ears, legs and other parts of the body. Examine the design of the devices in greater detail. Summarize the characteristics of these devices and create an outlook for future fMRI-compatible devices.

Chapter 13 summarizes current visual system equipment and how this equipment can be used to determine how the visual system functions.

Chapter 14 provides a review of humanoid robots and mind control humanoid robots. Information was obtained mainly from journals and conference proceedings on robotics and mind control technology. We primarily focus on providing an overview of commercially available robots and prototype research-stage humanoid robots in addition to mind control humanoid robot systems. First, a history and overview of the humanoid robot is presented. Then, typical mind control humanoid robot systems are described, including the relevant brain-computer interface and the whole control framework. Finally, the remaining research challenges in the field of humanoid robot safety are summarized.

Qiong Wu
Okayama University, Japan

Jinglong Wu
Okayama University, Japan & Beijing Institute of Technology, China

REFERENCES

Bachman, D. L., Wolf, P. A., Linn, R. T., Knoefel, J. E., Cobb, J. L., Belanger, A. J., & D'Agostino, R. B. et al. (1993). Incidence of dementia and probable Alzheimer's disease in a general population: The Framingham study. *Neurology*, *43*(3), 515. doi:10.1212/WNL.43.3_Part_1.515 PMID:8450993

Cacho, J., Benito-León, J., García-García, R., Fernández-Calvo, B., Vicente-Villardón, J. L., & Mitchell, A. J. (2010). Does the combination of the MMSE and clock drawing test (mini-clock) improve the detection of mild Alzheimer's disease and mild cognitive impairment? *Journal of Alzheimer's Disease*, *22*(3), 889–896. PMID:20858951

Davis, R. N., Massman, P. J., & Doody, R. S. (2003). Effects of blood pressure on neuropsychological functioning in Alzheimer's disease. *Archives of Clinical Neuropsychology*, *18*(1), 19–32. doi:10.1093/arclin/18.1.19 PMID:14591475

Department of Economic and Social Affairs Population Division. (n.d.). *2015world population ageing report*. Retrieved from http://www.un.org/en/development/desa/population/publications/pdf /ageing/WPA2015_Report.pdf

Kennelly, S. P., Lawlor, B. A., & Kenny, R. A. (2009). *Blood pressure and dementia: A comprehensive review*. Therapeutic Advances in Neurological Disorders.

MacKenzie, D. M., Copp, P., Shaw, R. J., & Goodwin, G. M. (1996). Brief cognitive screening of the elderly: A comparison of the mini-mental state examination (MMSE), abbreviated mental test (AMT) and mental status questionnaire (MSQ). *Psychological Medicine*, *26*(2), 427–430. doi:10.1017/S0033291700034826 PMID:8685299

McGue, M., & Christensen, K. (2001). The heritability of cognitive functioning in very old adults: Evidence from Danish twins aged 75 years and older. *Psychology and Aging*, *16*(2), 272–280. doi:10.1037/0882-7974.16.2.272 PMID:11405315

What Is Language ? (n.d.). Retrieved from http://grammar.about.com/od/grammarfaq/f/whatislang.htm

Acknowledgment

We are very thankful to everyone who supported us for this book and gave their guidance to complete our thesis work effectively and moreover on time.

We are equally grateful to Dr. Yoshikazu Nishikawa (President, Research Institute for Applied Sciences; Professor Emeritus, Kyoto University and Osaka Institute of Technology), who contribute a foreword to this book.

We also express our deep sense of gratitude to the workbook editor, Miss Janine Haughton (Development Editor, IGI Global) and IGI staff, thanks for taking the time to show us how to complete this book.

Finally, this book was partly supported by a Grant-in-Aid for Scientific Research (A) 25249026, (B) 25303013 and (B) 16K18052, Japan and by the AA Science Platform Program of the Japan Society for the Promotion of Science.

Chapter 1
The Early Diagnosis of Alzheimer's Disease:
From Behavioral to Genetic Study

Yanna Ren
Okayama University, Japan

Weiping Yang
Hubei University, China & Okayama University, Japan

Xiaoyu Tang
Liaoning Normal University, China & Okayama University, Japan

Fengxia Wu
Okayama University, Japan

Satoshi Takahashi
Okayama University, Japan

Jinglong Wu
Okayama University, Japan

ABSTRACT

Alzheimer's disease, a common form of dementia, is a type of neurodegenerative disease that affects more than 30% of the population older than 85. Clinically, it is characterized as memory loss and cognitive decline. Pathologically, its symptoms include cerebral atrophy, amyloid plaques and NFTs. Generally, the life expectancy is no more than nine years after the definite diagnosis, and life expectancy exceeds 14 years in only 3% of patients. Presently, there is no effective treatment to stop the process; the only measures we can take are to ease or improve symptoms temporarily. Therefore, it is necessary to diagnosis the disease in the early stage, such as through imaging detection via CT, MRI, PET and MSR, or prediction before the disease (genetic examination). However, literature data have supported the notion that Alzheimer's disease patients show cognitive reserve abilities to some degree. In the future, research perspectives may focus on the cognitive training paradigms in compensatory and restorative strategies.

DOI: 10.4018/978-1-5225-0925-7.ch001

INTRODUCTION

Alzheimer's disease (AD), also known as just Alzheimer's, is the sixth leading cause of death in the United States and is the fifth leading cause of death in Americans aged 65 or older (Association, 2011). Alzheimer's disease, which is a chronic neurodegenerative disease, accounts for 60 to 70% of dementia cases. It often begins in people over 65 years of age and is an aging-related neurodegenerative disorder (Palop et al., 2003). According to Hebert, in next 40 years, the number of individuals with Alzheimer's disease in the United States will increase dramatically (Hebert et al., 2013). There were approximately 4.5 million people with Alzheimer's disease in 2000, and this number has since reached 5.1 million. This number is expected to reach 5.7 million by 2020, 7.7 million by 2030, 11.0 million by 2040, and 13.2 million by 2050 (Figure 1).

The exact causes that lead to Alzheimer's disease are not yet known. However, many experts have now reached an agreement that, similar to other chronic diseases, Alzheimer's disease likely develops as a result of multiple factors. Changes in the brain include the accumulation of the protein β amyloid outside of the neuron and the accumulation of the protein tau in the neuron (Hebert et al., 2013). In addition, approximately 70% of the risk is believed to be genetic, with many genes usually involved, such as apolipoprotein E- ε4 (APOE ε4). The APOE gene has three common forms, APOE ε2, APOE ε3 and APOE ε4; this gene provides a

Figure 1. Estimated number of people aged 65 and over with AD in the United States

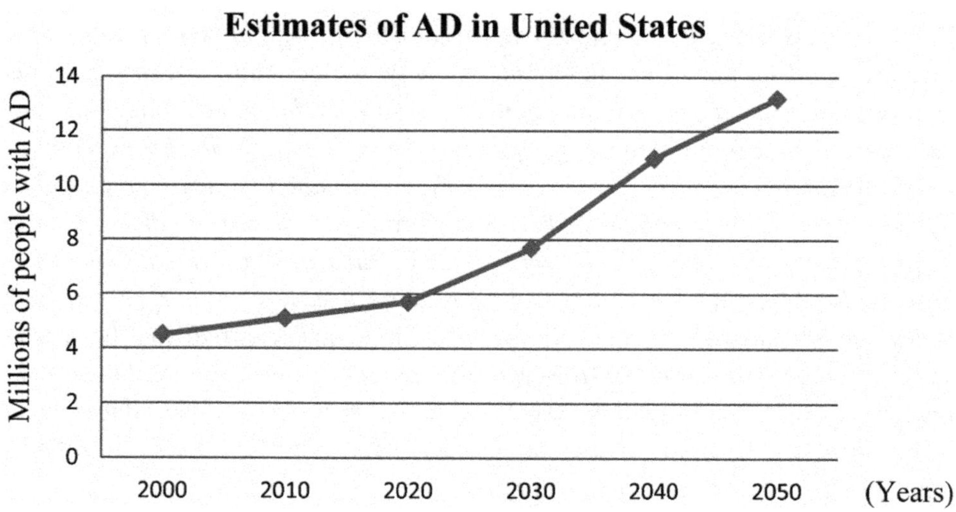

blueprint for one type of transmitter protein that carries cholesterol in the bloodstream. Every individual inherits one form from each of his or her parents. If an individual inherits APOE ε4, their risk of developing Alzheimer's disease is increased. Moreover, those individuals have an increased risk of developing it at an earlier age than those who inherit the APOE ε2 or APOE ε3 genes from their parents. However, those who inherit two APOE ε4 genes have a higher risk. Other risk factors include a history of head injuries, depression, or hypertension (Hebert et al., 2013).

Clinically, in the early stage, the most common symptom is short-term memory problems, which mainly present as the inability to remember recent events. As the disease advances, symptoms can include problems with language, disorientation (including easily getting lost), mood swings, not managing self-care, and behavioral issues. Generally, during long-term memory deficits, episodic memory is the most vulnerable, followed by semantic memory and, finally, procedural memory (Figure 2).

Pathologically, the main characteristics include the following: loss of neurons, neuritic plaques, granular-vacuolar degeneration, abundant amyloid plaques, neurofibrillary tangles (NFTs), and dystrophic neurites containing hyperphosphorylated tau. All of these neuropathological characteristics can be used as diagnostic markers of AD (Crews & Masliah, 2010).

No treatments stop or reverse the progression of AD, although some may temporarily improve symptoms. However, the present neuroscience investigations show that the cognitive deficits of Alzheimer's disease can produce significant functional impairments. Although memory deficits are typically most prominent, impairments in attention, visuospatial functioning, language, reasoning, and executive functioning are common, along with personality changes and behavioral disturbances (Sitzer et al., 2006). The most important measure is early diagnosis and consequent interven-

Figure 2. The sequence of memory impairment in AD

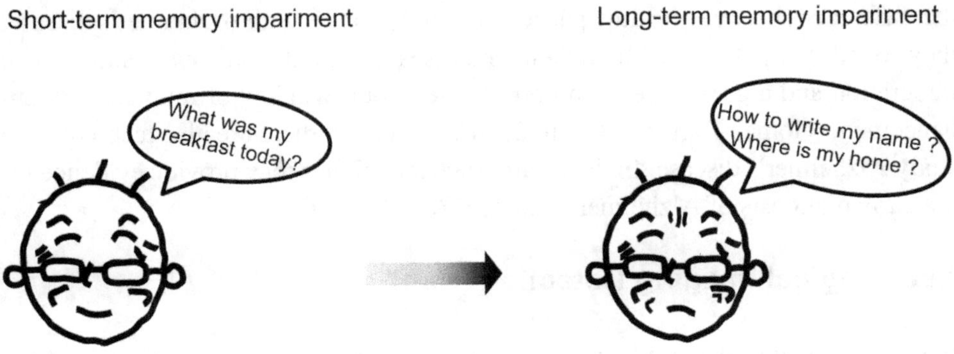

tion. Recently, with the development of investigative techniques for the diagnosis of Alzheimer's disease, neuroimaging, biological markers and genetic examinations increase the probability of the early diagnosis of Alzheimer's disease.

DIAGNOSIS

Alzheimer's disease is a progressive degenerative disorder of insidious onset, characterized by memory loss, confusion, and a variety of cognitive dysfunctions. There is no effective treatment; therefore, the current plan of action is to ensure an accurate diagnosis and delay further development of Alzheimer's disease.

Behavioral Test

The diagnosis of Alzheimer's disease is based on the criteria of the Diagnostic and Statistical Manual of Mental Disorders, 4th edition (DSM-IV-TR) (Association, 2000), and the National Institute of Neurological Disorders and Stroke (NINDS), Alzheimer Disease and Related Disorders (NINCDS-CADRDA) working group (McKhann et al., 1984a). These accepted criteria include two steps. The first step involves a diagnostic process in which there is an initial identification of a dementia syndrome (DSM-IV-TR); the second step involves the application of criteria based on the clinical features of the Alzheimer's disease phenotype. The publication of NINCDS-CADRDA criteria greatly advanced our understanding of the biological basis of Alzheimer's disease in 1984 by the National Institute of Neurological and Communicative Disorders and Stroke and the Alzheimer's Disease and Related Disorders Association (McKhann et al., 1984b). After the detection of the above two steps, the exclusion of dementia caused by other factors is necessary.

In addition, some other methods are currently being developed for the diagnosis of Alzheimer's disease. In 2012, Wu et al. used audiovisual facilitation to compare the differences between healthy participants and patients with Alzheimer's disease; they found that patients with Alzheimer's disease exhibited adequate audiovisual integration and a greater peak and broader temporal window of multisensory enhancement (Gomez-Ramirez & Wu, 2014). Moreover, there are also techniques to study Alzheimer's disease. In the future, such techniques may provide evidence for the early diagnosis of Alzheimer's disease(Ren et al., 2014).

Neurological Imaging Detection

In the last few decades, we have witnessed major advances in research technology in Neuroscience, including Computed Tomography (CT), Magnetic Resonance Imaging (MRI), Positron Emission Tomography (PET), and Electroencephalography (EEG). Compared with diagnostic markers, neuropil threads, abundant amyloid plaques, neurofibrillary tangles (NFTs), and dystrophic neurites containing hyperphosphorylated tau neuroimaging methods maybe provide more precise measures for the diagnosis of Alzheimer's disease.

Computed Tomography, CT

CT was introduced in 1983 and has been an extremely important medical tool for the structural imaging of neurological damage without invasion in living people. The key principle underlying CT is that the density of biological material varies and that the absorption of X-ray radiation is correlated with tissue density. The absorption capacity of neural tissue lies between these extremes. Thus, the software for making CT scans actually provides an image of the differential absorption of the intervening tissue. The typical spatial resolution for CT scanners is approximately 0.5 to 1.0 cm in all directions. Each point on the image reflects an average density of that point and the surrounding 1.0 mm of tissue. Thus, it is impossible to discriminate two objects that are closer than approximately 5 mm.

The initial criteria for a CT scan diagnosis of Alzheimer's disease is the presence of diffuse cerebral atrophy with increased ventricles and enlarged cortical sulci. Several studies have indicated that cerebral atrophy is significantly greater in patients with Alzheimer's disease than in aging adults without Alzheimer's disease. However, this concept was soon challenged because cerebral atrophy can be present in elderly healthy persons, and some patients with dementia may have no cerebral atrophy, particularly in the early stages of Alzheimer's disease. The extent of cerebral atrophy was determined using linear measurements; in particular, the bi-frontal and bi-caudate diameters and the diameters of the third and lateral ventricles. Various measurements were adjusted according to the diameter of the skull to account for normal variation.

To make up for this modification, volumetric investigations of the ventricles were performed. Despite these efforts, it is still difficult to distinguish between findings in a healthy elderly patient and those in a patient with dementia (Bird et al., 1986). Moreover, some clinical studies have indicated that CT results for cerebral atrophy cannot provide sufficient evidence for the diagnosis of Alzheimer's disease alone.

Recent studies have found that the rate of atrophy progression may be an important factor in diagnosing Alzheimer's disease (Jagust et al., 1987). The third and lateral ventricles are significantly larger in patients with Alzheimer's disease than in healthy older subjects (Luxenberg et al., 1987). In addition, the hippocampal sulcus, known as the hippocampal fissure, is a sulcus that separates the dentate gyrus from the subiculum and the CA1 field in the hippocampus. Numerous studies have reported that hippocampal degeneration has a close relationship with Alzheimer's disease and that there is AD-type alteration in the hippocampus. In 1989, researchers examined 175 individuals using a medical and neuropsychological investigation protocol consistent with the US consensus criteria for the clinical assessment of Alzheimer's disease. They found that CT hippocampal fissure dilatation appears to correlate well with post-mortem hippocampal degeneration and that the hippocampal fissure may be a useful radiologic marker for the early stage diagnosis of Alzheimer's disease. Moreover, studies have showed that although the specificity of hippocampal atrophy has not been established, the predictive accuracy of hippocampal degeneration can reach 81% with a specificity of 67% (Bastos-Leite et al., 2006).

Magnetic Resonance Imaging, MRI

In contrast to CT, MRI exploits the magnetic properties of organic tissue. MRI creates a powerful magnetic field, measured in Tesla units. When a person is placed within the magnetic field of the MRI machine, a significant proportion of the protons become oriented in the direction parallel to the magnetic force. Radio waves then pass through the magnetized regions, and as the protons absorb the energy in these waves, their orientation is perturbed in a predictable direction. When the radio waves are turned off, the absorbed energy is dissipated, and the protons rebound toward the orientation of the magnetic field. This synchronized rebound produces energy signals that are picked up by detectors surrounding the head. MRI scans provide a much clearer image of the brain than is possible with CT scans.

Structural MRI can be considered the preferred neuroimaging examination for Alzheimer's disease because it allows the accurate measurement of the three-dimensional (3D) volume of brain structures, particularly the size of the hippocampus and related regions. Studies have shown that hippocampal atrophy detected by structural MRI is a sensitive feature of early Alzheimer's disease (Laakso et al., 1996). Together with CT, structural MRI is the most common method used to diagnose Alzheimer's disease clinically in the cranial capacity (Frisoni et al., 2010).

However, the structural alterations that are always present in the middle and later stages of Alzheimer's disease may not be useful for the diagnosis of early stage disease. According to an AD-related study, the function of the brain begins to decline before cerebral atrophy. Therefore, it is meaningful to make use of functional magnetic resonance imaging (fMRI) for the diagnosis of Alzheimer's disease in the early stage (Gomez-Ramirez & Wu, 2014). fMRI can not only detect the activation of the brain, it can also evaluate the regions and the level of the activation. fMRI is a functional neuroimaging procedure that uses MRI technology to measure the activity of the brain by detecting alterations associated with blood flow (Matthews & Jezzard, 2004). This technique depends on the foundation that cerebral blood flow and neuronal activation are coupled. When an area of the brain is in use, the blood flow to that brain region also increases. According to blood-oxygen-level dependent (BOLD) contrast, the function of the detected region can be evaluated (Logothetis, 2008). Studies have indicated that decreased connectivity between the hippocampus and the visual cortices may indicate reduced integrity of hippocampus-related cortical networks in AD (Wang et al., 2006). Currently, fMRI has been widely used clinically to map functional areas of the brain by checking left-right hemispherical asymmetry in language and memory regions (such as the hippocampus). In addition, a recent study showed that resting-state functional Magnetic Resonance Imaging (rs-MRI) can provide useful evidence for the early diagnosis of Alzheimer's disease (Yamaguchi Shuhei, 2014). rs-MRI is a method of functional brain imaging that can be used to evaluate regional interactions that occur when a subject is not conducting an explicit task (Wang et al., 2006; Onoda & Yamaguchi, 2013).

Positron Emission Tomography, PET

Positron emission tomography is a functional imaging technique that is based on nuclear medicine. Using small amounts of radioactive materials (radiotracers), a camera, and a computer, it can evaluate the function of an organ and tissue at the cellular level (Valk, 2003). The system detects pairs of gamma rays emitted indirectly by the radiotracers, which are introduced into the body by being injected, inhaled or swallowed depending on which organ or tissue is being studied by the PET scan. 3D images of the tracer concentration within the body are then constructed by computer analysis.

Alzheimer's disease is characterized by progressive loss of cognitive function with β-amyloid (Aβ) (Southwick et al., 1996), neurofibrillary tangles (NFTs) and senile plaques (SPs) serving as the pathological hallmarks of this disease (Vickers et al., 2000;Jin et al., 2011). PET in Alzheimer's disease patients has indicated that in the early stage of Alzheimer's disease, the metabolism of the limbic system declines. PET has a sensitivity of 84% and a specificity of 93% for the diagnosis of Alzheimer's disease. In particular, when the biologically active molecule is 18F-fluorodeoxyglucose (18F-FDG), the detection of Alzheimer's disease is based on changes in the glucose metabolic rate; for example, studies have found that the glucose metabolic rates in the temporal and parietal lobes are reduced (Small et al., 2006). Moreover, the abnormal levels of β-amyloid and the tau protein in cerebrospinal fluid (CSF) provide important evidence for the diagnosis of Alzheimer's disease in the early stage. Recently, researchers have used a new compound to diagnose Alzheimer's disease; this compound is known as 18F-FDDNP, and it is bound to the plaques and tangles within the brain that are the characteristic features of Alzheimer's disease. In addition, tracer Pittsburgh Compound-B (PIB) can selectively combine with amyloid β-protein (Zhang et al., 2005). Therefore, positron emission tomography is helpful for the diagnosis of Alzheimer's disease in the early stage.

In 2011, Behrooz and his colleagues reported that a novel series of 11C-labeled imidazo[2,1-b]benzothiazoles (IBTs) were used as tracers for the imaging of cerebral β-amyloid (Aβ) deposits in Alzheimer's disease patients using positron emission tomography (PET); they found that the IBTs were useful PET imaging agents for high-sensitivity detection of Aβ plaques (Yousefi et al., 2011). Additionally, on a limited basis, many other radioactive tracers are used in PET to image the tissue concentrations of other types of molecules of interest. However, one of the disadvantages of PET scanners is their operating cost.

PET scans measure functions of the body, such as oxygen use, blood flow, and sugar (glucose) metabolism. These results can help doctors evaluate the present function of certain organs or tissues. CT imaging uses special x-ray equipment, and in some cases, a contrast material, to produce multiple images of the inside of the body. Then, these images are interpreted by a radiologist on a computer monitor to provide anatomic information for other doctors. Presently, a combination of PET and CT scanners is commonly used. Combined PET/CT scans provide images that pinpoint the anatomic location of abnormal metabolic activity within the body. These combined scans have been shown to provide more accurate diagnosis evidence than the scans separately.

Magnetic Resonance Spectroscopy (^{1}H-MRS)

Magnetic resonance spectroscopy is a non-invasive technique that has been used to measure the concentration of low molecular weight metabolites in-vivo, with a detection threshold of approximately 1 mmol/L (mM) from a volume of interest typically between 1 to 8 cm^3 (Gujar et al., 2005). Detectable brain metabolites, including glutamine (Gln), glutamate (Glu), creatine compounds (Cr), N-acetylaspartate (NAA), choline-containing compounds (Cho) and myo-inositol (mI), have a typical concentration between 1 and 10 mM (Gujar et al., 2005). Although MRS can theoretically be performed in almost any tissue of the human body, the main area of focus has been the brain.

Reduced N-acetylaspartate has been found in Alzheimer's disease, and alterations in the level of N-acetylaspartate or N-acetylaspartate/Cr are the most common findings in patients with Alzheimer's disease (Chantal et al., 2002). Therefore, the use of magnetic resonance spectroscopy in the early diagnosis of Alzheimer's disease has been reported in many studies. N-acetylaspartate has been reported to have poor clinical specificity for Alzheimer's disease, and the ratio of N-acetylaspartate to myo-inositol is significantly different between Alzheimer's disease patients and healthy age-matched controls. The ratio of N-acetylaspartate to myo-inositol in Alzheimer's disease patients is much lower than that in control groups (Killiany et al., 2000).

Genetic Examination

All of the above described neuronal imaging biomarkers are based on pathological changes. However, it will be advantageous if Alzheimer's disease can be predicted before these pathological changes occur. The development of genetic investigations regarding Alzheimer's disease makes this possible. Some Alzheimer's related genes come directly from kindreds, such as the Aβ42 risk factors for Alzheimer's disease. Moreover, it is well known that those who have Down's syndrome, are APOE ε4 allele homozygotes, or who are either amyloid precursor protein (APP) or presenilin (PSEN) mutation carriers have an extremely high risk of developing Alzheimer's disease (Hampel et al., 2010). Previous studies have indicated that in the cerebrospinal fluid (CSF), the concentration of β-amyloid protein decreases, whereas the concentrations of the Tau protein and the phosphorylated Tau protein increase. In addition, genetic examinations are available for individuals who have family members with early onset familial Alzheimer's disease. These genetic screens include testing for PSEN1, PSEN2, APP and APOE mutations (Schellenberg et al., 1992).

MEDICATIONS FOR TREATING ALZHEIMER'S DISEASE

Presently, there is no effective treatment to stop the progression of Alzheimer's disease; however, there are some medicines that can reserve or improve clinical symptoms (Tariot et al., 2004).

Cholinesterase Inhibitors

Since the introduction of the first cholinesterase inhibitor (ChEI) in 1997 (McGleenon et al., 1999), many researchers have begun developing cholinesterase inhibitor drugs. Currently, clinical trials in Japan, Europe, and the USA are evaluating approximately 10 cholinesterase inhibitor drugs, and most of these drugs have already advanced to clinical phases III and IV (Giacobini, 2000). The cholinesterase inhibitors that are currently used in the clinic include Aricept, rivastigmine, Galantamine, and Huperzine. All of these drugs are used to improve the choline system. These drugs have slightly different pharmacological properties; however, all of them work by inhibiting the breakdown of acetylcholine. Acetylcholine is an important neurotransmitter that is associated with memory by blocking the enzyme acetylcholinesterase (Larner, 2010).

N-Methyl-D-Aspartate (NMDA) Receptor Antagonists

N-methyl-D-aspartate (NMDA) receptor antagonists, such as Namenda, help block the activity of the neurotransmitter glutamate by binding to N-methyl-D-aspartate (NMDA) receptors on the surface of brain cells (Olivares et al., 2012). Glutamate plays an important role in learning and memory. If the level of glutamate is too low, cognitive problems develop. If the level is too high, glutamate overstimulates nerve cells, leading to cell death. Moreover, selective NMDA receptor antagonists completely block Aβ1–42 uptake or internalization and the subsequent up-regulation of cathepsin D and activation of microglia in organotypic hippocampal cultures (Danysz & Parsons, 2012).

Additionally, there are some other types of medicine that can improve the symptoms of Alzheimer's disease, such as fibroblast repair factor (bFGF).

REHABILITATION

Patients with Alzheimer's disease may derive some cognitive and functional benefits from cognitive training. In 1996, Hofmann and colleagues used a computer-based cognitive training experiment to evaluate the effect of training on patients with Alzheimer's disease. Their results showed that after three weeks of training (three to four sessions a week), the patients required less help in performing the programs, they became faster, and eight out of ten patients made fewer mistakes (Hofmann et al., 1996). This study suggested that it is possible to improve the cognitive function in patients with Alzheimer's disease.

Presently, there are two main categories of cognitive training strategies: compensatory and restorative strategies (Sitzer et al., 2006). Compensatory strategies mainly teach new ways to perform cognitive tasks by working around cognitive deficit regions (Bäckman, 1996; Bellack et al., 1999; Spaulding et al., 1999; De Vreese et al., 2001; Mahendra, 2001). Compensatory interventions, as described above, may use internal strategies, for example, organizing information by visualizing or categorizing information to be remembered (Bäckman, 1996; Hofmann et al., 1996); focusing on a single task and asking questions and paraphrasing during learning (Mahendra, 2001; Tang et al., 2016); procedural training to teach complex, higher-order cognitively mediated behaviors, such as balancing a checkbook; or external strategies, such as environmental cues, memory notebooks, and calendars (Sitzer et al., 2006).

Restorative strategies attempt to improve functioning in specific domains, with the ultimate goal of returning functioning in those domains to premorbid levels. In actuality, there are many examples in our life. Restorative techniques include drills in which patients engage in repeated attention and memory tasks; errorless learning, which involves preventing mistakes during recall trials (Bäckman, 1996; Mahendra, 2001); spaced retrieval, which requires patients to recall information over longer periods of time; and reminiscence therapy, in which patients discuss remote events to place one's life in perspective (Woods et al., 1992).

CONCLUSION AND FUTURE DIRECTIONS

Because there are not effective measures to stop the symptoms of Alzheimer's disease, the key to combatting this disease is to develop effective prediction or early diagnosis methods. For early diagnosis, the combination of the present imaging techniques may provide a more sensitive biomarker. In addition, to improve the quality of life of patients with Alzheimer's disease, cognitive intervention is necessary.

ACKNOWLEDGMENT

This study was partly supported by the Japan Society for the Promotion of Science (JSPS) Kakenhi, grant numbers 25249026 and 25303013; a Grant-in-Aid for Strategic Research Promotion from Okayama University; the National Natural Science Foundation of China (NSFC61473043); and the National Science Foundation of Hubei University (098379, WY).

REFERENCES

Alzheimer's Association. (2011). 2011 Alzheimer's disease facts and figures. *Alzheimer's & Dementia: The Journal of the Alzheimer's Association, 7*, 208.

American Psychiatric Association. (2000). *Diagnostic criteria from dsM-iV-tr.* American Psychiatric Pub.

Bäckman, L. (1996). Utilizing compensatory task conditions for episodic memory in Alzheimer's disease. *Acta Neurologica Scandinavica, 94*(S165), 109–113. doi:10.1111/j.1600-0404.1996.tb05880.x PMID:8740997

Bastos-Leite, A., Van Waesberghe, J., Oen, A., Van Der Flier, W., Scheltens, P., & Barkhof, F. (2006). Hippocampal sulcus width and cavities: Comparison between patients with Alzheimer disease and nondemented elderly subjects. *American Journal of Neuroradiology, 27*, 2141–2145. PMID:17110684

Bellack, A. S., Gold, J. M., & Buchanan, R. W. (1999). Cognitive rehabilitation for schizophrenia: Problems, prospects, and strategies. *Schizophrenia Bulletin, 25*(2), 257–274. doi:10.1093/oxfordjournals.schbul.a033377 PMID:10416730

Binder, L. I., Guillozet-Bongaarts, A. L., Garcia-Sierra, F., & Berry, R. W. (2005). Tau, tangles, and Alzheimer's disease. *Biochimica et Biophysica Acta (BBA)- Molecular Basis of Disease, 1739*(2-3), 216–223. doi:10.1016/j.bbadis.2004.08.014

Bird, J., Levy, R., & Jacoby, R. J. (1986). Computed tomography in the elderly: Changes over time in a normal population. *The British Journal of Psychiatry, 148*(1), 80–85. doi:10.1192/bjp.148.1.80 PMID:3485462

Chantal, S., Labelle, M., Bouchard, R. W., Braun, C. M., & Boulanger, Y. (2002). Correlation of regional proton magnetic resonance spectroscopic metabolic changes with cognitive deficits in mild Alzheimer disease. *Archives of Neurology, 59*(6), 955–962. doi:10.1001/archneur.59.6.955 PMID:12056931

Crews, L., & Masliah, E. (2010). Molecular mechanisms of neurodegeneration in Alzheimer's disease. *Human Molecular Genetics*. PMID:20413653

Danysz, W., & Parsons, C. G. (2012). Alzheimer's disease, β-amyloid, glutamate, NMDA receptors and memantine–searching for the connections. *British Journal of Pharmacology, 167*(2), 324–352. doi:10.1111/j.1476-5381.2012.02057.x PMID:22646481

De Vreese, L. P., Neri, M., Fioravanti, M., Belloi, L., & Zanetti, O. (2001). Memory rehabilitation in Alzheimer's disease: A review of progress. *International Journal of Geriatric Psychiatry, 16*(8), 794–809. doi:10.1002/gps.428 PMID:11536347

Frisoni, G. B., Fox, N. C., Jack, C. R., Scheltens, P., & Thompson, P. M. (2010). The clinical use of structural MRI in Alzheimer disease. *Nature Reviews. Nephrology, 6*(2), 67–77. doi:10.1038/nrneurol.2009.215 PMID:20139996

Giacobini, E. (2000). Cholinesterase inhibitors stabilize Alzheimer's disease. *Annals of the New York Academy of Sciences, 920*(1), 321–327. doi:10.1111/j.1749-6632.2000.tb06942.x PMID:11193171

Gomez-Ramirez, J., & Wu, J. (2014). Network-based biomarkers in Alzheimer's disease: review and future directions. *Frontiers in Aging Neuroscience, 6*.

Gujar, S. K., Maheshwari, S., Björkman-Burtscher, I., & Sundgren, P. C. (2005). Magnetic resonance spectroscopy. *Journal of Neuro-Ophthalmology, 25*, 217–226. doi:10.1097/01.wno.0000177307.21081.81 PMID:16148633

Hampel, H., Frank, R., Broich, K., Teipel, S. J., Katz, R. G., Hardy, J., & Hoessler, Y. C. et al. (2010). Biomarkers for Alzheimer's disease: Academic, industry and regulatory perspectives. *Nature Reviews. Drug Discovery*, *9*(7), 560–574. doi:10.1038/nrd3115 PMID:20592748

Hebert, L. E., Weuve, J., Scherr, P. A., & Evans, D. A. (2013). Alzheimer disease in the United States (2010–2050) estimated using the 2010 census. *Neurology*, *80*(19), 1778–1783. doi:10.1212/WNL.0b013e31828726f5 PMID:23390181

Hofmann, M., Hock, C., Kühler, A., & Müller-Spahn, F. (1996). Interactive computer-based cognitive training in patients with Alzheimer's disease. *Journal of Psychiatric Research*, *30*(6), 493–501. doi:10.1016/S0022-3956(96)00036-2 PMID:9023793

Jagust, W. J., Budinger, T. F., & Reed, B. R. (1987). The diagnosis of dementia with single photon emission computed tomography. *Archives of Neurology*, *44*(3), 258–262. doi:10.1001/archneur.1987.00520150014011 PMID:3493756

Jin, M., Shepardson, N., Yang, T., Chen, G., Walsh, D., & Selkoe, D. J. (2011). Soluble amyloid β-protein dimers isolated from Alzheimer cortex directly induce Tau hyperphosphorylation and neuritic degeneration. *Proceedings of the National Academy of Sciences of the United States of America*, *108*(14), 5819–5824. doi:10.1073/pnas.1017033108 PMID:21421841

Killiany, R. J., Gomez-Isla, T., Moss, M., Kikinis, R., Sandor, T., Jolesz, F., & Albert, M. S. et al. (2000). Use of structural magnetic resonance imaging to predict who will get Alzheimer's disease. *Annals of Neurology*, *47*(4), 430–439. doi:10.1002/1531-8249(200004)47:4<430::AID-ANA5>3.0.CO;2-I PMID:10762153

Laakso, M., Partanen, K., Riekkinen, P., Lehtovirta, M., Helkala, E.-L., Hallikainen, M., & Soininen, H. et al. (1996). Hippocampal volumes in Alzheimer's disease, Parkinson's disease with and without dementia, and in vascular dementia An MRI study. *Neurology*, *46*(3), 678–681. doi:10.1212/WNL.46.3.678 PMID:8618666

Larner, A. (2010). *Cholinesterase inhibitors: beyond Alzheimer's disease*. Academic Press.

Logothetis, N. K. (2008). What we can do and what we cannot do with fMRI. *Nature*, *453*(7197), 869–878. doi:10.1038/nature06976 PMID:18548064

Luxenberg, J., Haxby, J. V., Creasey, H., Sundaram, M., & Rapoport, S. (1987). Rate of ventricular enlargement in dementia of the Alzheimer type correlates with rate of neuropsychological deterioration. *Neurology*, *37*(7), 1135–1135. doi:10.1212/WNL.37.7.1135 PMID:3496557

Mahendra, N. (n.d.). Direct interventions for improving the performance of individuals with Alzheimer's disease. Seminars in Speech and Language, 291-303.

Matthews, P., & Jezzard, P. (2004). Functional magnetic resonance imaging. *Journal of Neurology, Neurosurgery, and Psychiatry*, *75*, 6–12. PMID:14707297

Mcgleenon, B., Dynan, K., & Passmore, A. (1999). Acetylcholinesterase inhibitors in Alzheimer's disease. *British Journal of Clinical Pharmacology*, *48*(4), 471–480. doi:10.1046/j.1365-2125.1999.00026.x PMID:10583015

Mckhann, G., Drachman, D., Folstein, M., Katzman, R., Price, D., & Stadlan, E. (1984a). Report of the NINCDS-ADRDA work group under the auspices of Department of Health and Human Services task force on Alzheimer's disease. *Neurology*, *34*(7), 939–943. doi:10.1212/WNL.34.7.939 PMID:6610841

Mckhann, G., Drachman, D., Folstein, M., Katzman, R., Price, D., & Stadlan, E. M. (1984b). Clinical diagnosis of Alzheimer's disease Report of the NINCDS-ADRDA Work Group under the auspices of Department of Health and Human Services Task Force on Alzheimer's Disease. *Neurology*, *34*(7), 939–939. doi:10.1212/WNL.34.7.939 PMID:6610841

Olivares, D. K., Deshpande, V., Shi, Y. K., Lahiri, D. H., Greig, N. T., Rogers, J., & Huang, X. (2012). N-Methyl D-Aspartate (NMDA) receptor antagonists and memantine treatment for Alzheimer's disease, vascular dementia and Parkinson's disease. *Current Alzheimer Research*, *9*, 746–758. doi:10.2174/156720512801322564 PMID:21875407

Onoda, K., & Yamaguchi, S. (2013). Small-worldness and modularity of the resting-state functional brain network decrease with aging. *Neuroscience Letters*, *556*, 104–108. doi:10.1016/j.neulet.2013.10.023 PMID:24157850

Palop, J. J., Jones, B., Kekonius, L., Chin, J., Yu, G.-Q., Raber, J., & Mucke, L. et al. (2003). Neuronal depletion of calcium-dependent proteins in the dentate gyrus is tightly linked to Alzheimer's disease-related cognitive deficits. *Proceedings of the National Academy of Sciences of the United States of America*, *100*(16), 9572–9577. doi:10.1073/pnas.1133381100 PMID:12881482

Ren, Y.-N., Yang, W., & Wu, J. (2014). Book Review: The New Handbook of Multisensory Processing. Barry E. Stein, ed. June 2012. The MIT Press. No. of pages 823. ISBN: 987-0-262-01712-1. Neuroscience and Biomedical Engineering, 2, 105-108.

Schellenberg, G. D., Bird, T. D., Wijsman, E. M., Orr, H. T., Anderson, L., Nemens, E., & Alonso, M. E. et al. (1992). Genetic linkage evidence for a familial Alzheimer's disease locus on chromosome 14. *Science*, *258*(5082), 668–671. doi:10.1126/science.1411576 PMID:1411576

Sitzer, D., Twamley, E., & Jeste, D. (2006). Cognitive training in Alzheimer's disease: A meta-analysis of the literature. *Acta Psychiatrica Scandinavica*, *114*(2), 75–90. doi:10.1111/j.1600-0447.2006.00789.x PMID:16836595

Small, G. W., Kepe, V., Ercoli, L. M., Siddarth, P., Bookheimer, S. Y., Miller, K. J., & Vinters, H. V. et al. (2006). PET of brain amyloid and tau in mild cognitive impairment. *The New England Journal of Medicine*, *355*(25), 2652–2663. doi:10.1056/NEJMoa054625 PMID:17182990

Southwick, P. C., Yamagata, S. K., Echols, C. L. Jr, Higson, G. J., Neynaber, S. A., Parson, R. E., & Munroe, W. A. (1996). Assessment of amyloid β protein in cerebrospinal fluid as an aid in the diagnosis of Alzheimer's disease. *Journal of Neurochemistry*, *66*(1), 259–265. doi:10.1046/j.1471-4159.1996.66010259.x PMID:8522962

Spaulding, W. D., Fleming, S. K., Reed, D., Sullivan, M., Storzbach, D., & Lam, M. (1999). Cognitive functioning in schizophrenia: Implications for psychiatric rehabilitation. *Schizophrenia Bulletin*, *25*(2), 275–289. doi:10.1093/oxfordjournals.schbul.a033378 PMID:10416731

Tang, X., Wu, J., & Shen, Y. (2016). The interactions of multisensory integration with endogenous and exogenous attention. *Neuroscience and Biobehavioral Reviews*, *61*, 208–224. doi:10.1016/j.neubiorev.2015.11.002 PMID:26546734

Tariot, P. N., Farlow, M. R., Grossberg, G. T., Graham, S. M., Mcdonald, S., Gergel, I., & Group, M. S. (2004). Memantine treatment in patients with moderate to severe Alzheimer disease already receiving donepezil: A randomized controlled trial. *Journal of the American Medical Association*, *291*(3), 317–324. doi:10.1001/jama.291.3.317 PMID:14734594

Valk, P. E. (2003). *Positron emission tomography: Basic sciences*. Springer Science & Business Media.

Vickers, J. C., Dickson, T. C., Adlard, P. A., Saunders, H. L., King, C. E., & Mccormack, G. (2000). The cause of neuronal degeneration in Alzheimer's disease. *Progress in Neurobiology*, *60*(2), 139–165. doi:10.1016/S0301-0082(99)00023-4 PMID:10639052

Wang, L., Zang, Y., He, Y., Liang, M., Zhang, X., Tian, L., & Li, K. et al. (2006). Changes in hippocampal connectivity in the early stages of Alzheimer's disease: Evidence from resting state fMRI. *NeuroImage*, *31*(2), 496–504. doi:10.1016/j.neuroimage.2005.12.033 PMID:16473024

Woods, B., Portnoy, S., Head, D., & Jones, G. (1992). Reminiscence and life review with persons with dementia: which way forward. *Care Giving in Dementia*, 137-161.

Yamaguchi Shuhei, O. K. (2014). Early diagnosis of dementia by resting-state functional MRI. Higher Brain Function Research (Japan Society for Higher Brain Dysfunction), 34, 9-16.

Yousefi, B.H., Manook, A., Drzezga, A., & Reutern, , B., Schwaiger, M., Wester, H.-J. R., & Henriksen, G. (2011). Synthesis and Evaluation of 11C-labeled Imidazo [2, 1-b] benzothiazoles (IBTs) as PET tracers for Imaging β-Amyloid Plaques in Alzheimer's Disease. *Journal of Medicinal Chemistry*, *54*, 949–956. doi:10.1021/jm101129a PMID:21275403

Zhang, W., Oya, S., Kung, M.-P., Hou, C., Maier, D. L., & Kung, H. F. (2005). F-18 stilbenes as PET imaging agents for detecting β-amyloid plaques in the brain. *Journal of Medicinal Chemistry*, *48*(19), 5980–5988. doi:10.1021/jm050166g PMID:16162001

KEY TERMS AND DEFINITIONS

Amyloid β (Aβ): Aggregation-prone peptide derived from the amyloid precursor protein. The 42 amino acid isoform of the peptide is the main component of plaques in Alzheimer's disease (Hampel et al., 2010).

Amyloid Plaques: The accumulation of amyloid plaques between nerve cells, or neurons in the brain. In the normal brain, such fragments of protein can be broken down, but in patients with Alzheimer's disease, protein fragments accumulate to form hard plaques.

Neurofibrillary Tangles (NFTs): Aggregates of filamentous tau polymers that comprise a portion of the fibrillar pathologies in Alzheimer's disease (AD). Other elements include the neuropil threads and the dystrophic neurites that invade a subset of amyloid plaques (neuritic plaques) (Binder et al., 2005).

Tau Protein: A microtubule-associated protein located in the neuronal axons. Hyperphosphorylated tau is the main component of neurofibrillary tangles in Alzheimer's disease (Hampel et al., 2010).

Chapter 2
Environmental Landscape Design for Alzheimer's

Gökçen Firdevs Yücel
Istanbul Aydın University, Turkey

ABSTRACT

People suffering from Alzheimer's may feel anxious or unsettled as a result of these symptoms – in particular the decrease in their cognitive abilities and in their ability to take into account new information or external stimuli – as well from the effects of their medications. Because of their sensitivity, such individuals find it difficult to keep up a positive attitude and remain emotionally stable for long: they experience mood swings, and are unable to keep their negative emotions in check. For this reason, the best practice in treatment is to help them maintain a positive view of their lives and balance their emotions, both personally, in terms of keeping their sense of self, and in social environments, where they have to recognize and interact with others. In this way, good environmental landscape design will have an important role to play in improving their quality of life.

INTRODUCTION

The disorder known as Alzheimer's disease falls into the general category of dementia, which refers to various symptoms of progressive cognitive deterioration that have an impact on daily life. It is characterized by loss of memory, a decline in cognitive, commmunicative and decision making abilities, loss of orientation in time and space, and an inability to tolerate intense, or even moderate sensory stimuli.

DOI: 10.4018/978-1-5225-0925-7.ch002

As such, it may lead to other neurodegenerative disorders, the inability to function normally; and to behavioral problems, for example, if the environment provides too many stimuli to process, or if the intervention poses a cognitive challenge (Detweiler et al., 2012; Chong & Hermreck, 2011).

In cognitive terms, the progress of the disease may lead to the individual's having confused or fragmented memories, ideas and feelings; these may be accompanied by the frustrations of short-term amnesia, problems in processing or using language, impaired judgment and spatial disorientation. Yet despite these difficulties, Alzheimer's patients are typically able to carry out such functions as walking, gesturing, and responding to environments that are mildly stimulating. Thus older patients may develop a modicum of control and a feeling of familiarity with their environment by exercising their long-term memories, along with engaging in gentle physical activities outdoors (Garcia, 2014).

This places various restrictions on designing environments for individuals with Alzheimer's, because both their specific needs and their daily routines must be taken into account. In the first place, they may be living their lives in particular contexts. Patients in the early stages tend to stay in their own homes, but eventually may require support from friends, family members, or carers. Or they may move from an assisted living apartment to a home providing personal care. Such facilities may or may not have specialized healthcare services, depending on the philosophy of their programs, which should both clarify the purposes of the care and explain how it is related to the physical environment provided (Brawley, 1997).

Indeed, one of the characteristics of people with Alzheimer's is that it becomes more and more difficult for them to relate to their environment. A setting that feels familiar also feels more easily controllable, so patients do not feel the stress or fear associated with a sense of alienation. It is therefore essential that in designing for such people, environments are made to feel more familiar and more like home (Nord, 2004); in addition, there should be recognition of Alzheimer's sufferers as people who wish to be independent, and to keep their self-respect and dignity. The environment should therefore provide familiarity and a feeling of comfort and confidence; for elderly patients, or others with advanced cognitive or perceptual problems, care should also be taken to see that safety is ensured. This is, of course, a rather complex problem.

Depression, stress, and some of the symptoms of Alzheimer's, may be reduced by engaging in activities outdoors (Kuo & Taylor, 2004; Mooney & Nicell, 1992). Alzheimer's sufferers tend to become disoriented more easily in complex environments, where they both lose their way and lose the concept of where they were intending to go or what they were trying to find; they often react to such situations by acting out their frustration and being aggressive. The incidence of such situations can be decreased if information that can help a person move around in an environment is embedded in it in the form of clear paths, markers, and signs (Ziesel, 2003); in some cases, prosthetic aids can be made available at clearly indicated locations to help people orientate themselves. One study has indicated that Alzheimer's patients in care facilities with access to gardens experience fewer negative reactions and less anger than those in environments without access to gardens (Mooney & Nicell, 1992). Gardens are a useful feature in residential environments, as they provide Alzheimer's patients with a sense of tradition and cultural memories, as well as natural images; they are removed from the cold, clinical atmosphere that many longterm care facilities have.

Well-designed outdoor spaces may help to offset some of the behavioral problems of patients as they become weaker and less in control of their environment; and that poorly designed spaces will exacerbate the confusion, disorientation and frustration of the cognitively impaired. Yet it is only recently that healthcare settings for Alzheimer's sufferers have begun to be designed with a focus on the salutary effects of the outdoors, sunlight and fresh air; there is a real need to create spaces responsive to climate that are simple to negotiate, and still provide a wealth of meaningful associations (Brawley, 2002). This simply requires recognition that Alzheimer's sufferers have, besides specific conditions related to the disease, the same basic physical and psychological needs as other people: to have a sense of security, social relations, external stimulation, and to be valued as individuals. Thus the main aims in designing interventions for people with Alzheimer's should be focused on maintaining their dignity and their quality of life (including the experience of nature), and providing comfort.

Symptoms Affect the Design Process

The symptoms of Alzheimer's vary from case to case; they may first appear when an individual is in his or her fifties, but may not be recognized as such until much later, and will eventually affect them in nearly every aspect of life. In general, they may be categorized as cognitive, behavioural and physical.

Cognitive Symptoms

In its early phases, the disease begins to affect an individual's thought processes, memories, and ability to make judgments. The patient finds it difficult to make rational decisions or judgments, to connect visual images with their meanings, and may have problems with visual perception, particularly perceiving depth. He or she becomes less able to learn new things, react to information and follow everyday routines. Language and reasoning skills deteriorate; there is a sense of disorientation in terms of time and space; and the patient has an increasing tendency to forget recent events.

But although people with Alzheimer's do have problems with remembering recent events, they often retain clear long-term memories of past experiences; and these can be stimulated in an outdoor setting – Brawley (1997), for example, suggests this can be done through basic activities like mowing, raking leaves, gardening, or hanging clothes out on a line. An Alzheimer's patient's age is a factor that should also be taken into account in the design process; the landscaping around a facility should reflect the long-term memories of residents: gardens they remember from their childhoods, flowers they remember from earlier times, or plants that were important or meant something personal to them in the past (Dixon, 2002).

Behavioral Symptoms

Various behavioral symptoms are associated with the progression of Alzheimer's. The 1987 National Medical Expenditure Survey found that 59% of cases diagnosed with dementia exhibited symptoms such as wandering aimlessly, hurting themselves or others, dressing inappropriately, extended periods of crying, hoarding, becoming upset, making no effort to avoid danger, stealing, and inappropriate sexual behaviour (U.S. Congress, 1992). Another common symptom is "sundowning," where patients become confused or disturbed when the sun is setting; this is because as the disease progresses, changes in the brain are affected by environmental changes.

In general, patients' defensive or aggressive behavior is the result of fear or confusion caused by their difficulty in understanding their surroundings: they need to distance themselves from environmental situations that may be causing tension or discomfort such as noise or crowds. For this reason, both individual and group situations need to be planned for in designing their environments (Dixon, 2002). Interestingly, garden environments have been shown to generally improve morale, but to have negligible effects on patients' behavior (Mather, Nemecek & Oliver, 1999).

Physical Symptoms

Patients in advanced stages of Alzheimer's, frequently remain quite fit; however, physical changes may include weakened muscles and problems in perceiving depth, so some patients may have a tendency to trip and fall and may require walking support or wheelchairs. In general, outdoor activities such as regular walks can provide structured daily routines and contribute to patients' health and feeling of well-being (Cedervall & Aberg, 2010).

The Benefits of Environmental Design

Studies have shown that Alzheimer's patients' stress and blood pressure levels may be lowered and they may recover faster from illnesses if they can both see and physically experience natural surroundings. For example, patients diagnosed with stroke and dementia have been shown to have better social skills, be more self-confident, and have better mobility and dexterity if they are engaged in working in gardens (Hartig at all., 2003; Kaplan, 1993; Rappe, 2005; Ulrich, 2002, Ulrich at al., 1991). The garden may connect them to experiences, objects, interests or thought processes from before the onset of the disease, and so create a "sense of normality" (Whear at all., 2014). Thus one patient in a study commented:

Resident – "I like it all. The fountain, the fish, the memory boxes – everything. The table and chairs in the sunroom came from my lounge room at home, you know. We all sit around it and talk." (Edwards et al, 2013).

In general, being in or having access to outdoor environments helps stabilize patients' circadian rhythms and sleeping and waking cycles; and has the added benefit, if there is exposure to sunlight, of promoting vitamin D absorption, which is critical for bone strength. Alzheimer's patients should also be able to continue to engage in their previous outdoor activities in a safe and comfortable environment. Being able to see elements of nature, for example, from a window (Figure 1), can have a positive effect on their sense of being comfortable in the setting of their neighborhood, as well on their general sense of well-being (Kaplan, 2001; Traynor, Fernandez & Caldwell, 2013; Bechtel & Churchman, 2003).

LITERATURE REVIEW

Jackson (2005) suggests that older patients feel freer, and less limited by the physical spaces of a room when they can see natural settings and the expanse of the sky, because these refer them back to memories of their personal lives. In this connection, "healing gardens" can be designed for Alzheimer's patients which provide both a comfortable space for physical activities and sensory stimuli that help them recall positive events and feelings (HCNDACRSP 2004; Hartig and Cooper-Marcus 2006). Studies indicate that such gardens help make patients more independent; Zeisel's (2007) research, for example, showed that in a healing garden at an assisted-living facility for Alzheimer's patients in Massachusetts, 36% of the patients would visit the garden of their own accord, and 59% were able to return without assistance (Zeisel, 2007).

Figure 1. Alzheimer' respite center, Temple road, Blackrock, Dublin, Fotography Nick Kane/Joanna Karatzas
Source: Niall McLaughlin Architects Bedford House, 2012

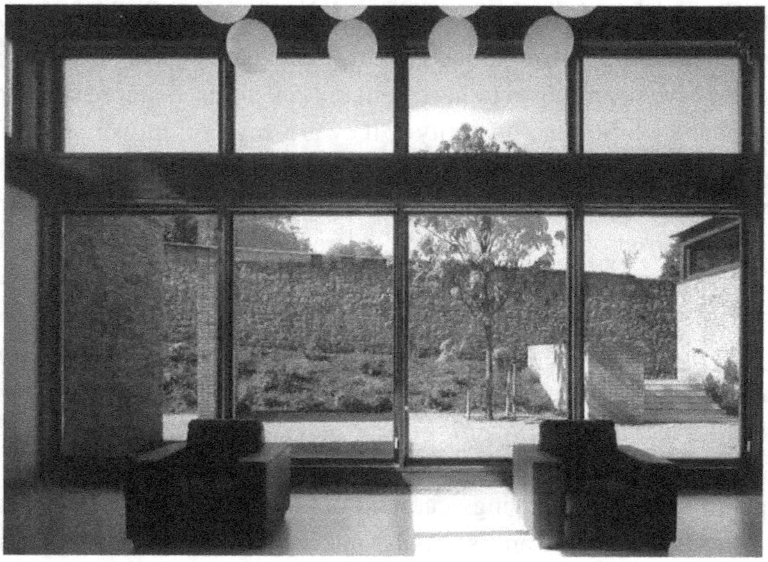

Activities related to horticulture have also been shown to help reduce behavioral issues and problems of insomnia in patients with Alzheimer's or other types of dementia (Cohen-Mansfield & Werner, 1998); a study of green day activities for psychogeriatric patients in several care institutions in the Netherlands suggests that activities of this type help improve quality of life for these patients (Andreoli, 2003). Using plants that vary with the seasons is aesthetically pleasing, and also has a salutary effect on mental activity, maintaining interest and providing a sense of time as well as cues that stimulate memories of past home environments in the elderly (Browne, 1992). Horticultural activities help generate more positive emotions, more of a sense of wellbeing, and decreased agitation, in comparison with other activities (Gigliotti et al., 2004; Lee & Kim, 2007; Bomalaski, 2011); and making use of wander gardens over a year has been found to decrease not only the number of falls recorded among individuals with dementia, but also their "use of high-dosage anti-psychotic medications" (Detweiler et al., 2008, 2009).

In a pilot study of nursing-home residents with dementia conducted over a year, Cornell et al. analyzed the relation of indoor and outdoor activities to these patients' behavior and sleep patterns. In both cases the total amount of sleep increased, but there was a significant increase in the maximum length of sleep, and increased verbalization in those engaged in outdoor activities (Connell, Sanford & Lewis, 2007). And a longitudinal study by Mooney and Nicel (1992) comparing five facilities with and without outside environments showed that over time, the incidence of episodes of violence in patients living in the former decreased, while in the latter they increased.

Various outdoor design solutions have been suggested by Randall et al. (1990), making use of ideas from both nurses and landscape architects. These solutions are intended to supplement other approaches, and to focus on creating safe outdoor environments where Alzheimer's patients can feel comfortable. They therefore take into account specific symptoms of the disease exhibited by patients, including amnesia, apraxia (deterioration of motor skills), frailty, agnosia (problems processing sensory data), disorientation and wandering, eating plants, sundowning, and delusions or hallucinations. (Randall, Burkahrdt & Kutcher, 1990). As we have seen, physical exercise can improve these patients' cognitive abilities; purpose-designed gardens can provide colors, odors and textures that evoke positive feelings and recollections (Elings, 2006); and there is also evidence to suggest that patients in advanced stages of Alzheimer's become calmer in the presence of simulations of nature, such as recordings of birdsong or flowing brooks, or pictures of natural scenes (Whall et al., 1997).

DESIGN

The principles of design that are appropriate for Alzheimer's patients should be based on primordial and basic concepts of healing and well-being, such as feelings of safety and freedom, understanding the surroundings, being aware of social norms and expectations; being able to get away and relax, to see a destination and enjoy the process of approaching it; taking pleasure in nature, the weather and the seasons; and feeling confident and comfortable in acting, accepting failures and celebrating achievements (Volicer & Charette,1999).

Environmental Perceptions

In designing for Alzheimer's patients, the primary aim is to create an environment that accentuates positive and reduces negative stimuli as far as possible. The critical elements are (Figure 2):

- **Color:** A general problem experienced by such patients is distinguishing surfaces, planes, and objects from each other; one consideration must therefore be to provide strong light-dark, textural and color contrasts, which can help them find their way. As these patients often become disorientated and get lost; the use of color can help patients to find their way: floors and areas of a

Figure 2. Design for dementia: A visual snapshot
Source: Willatt, 2011

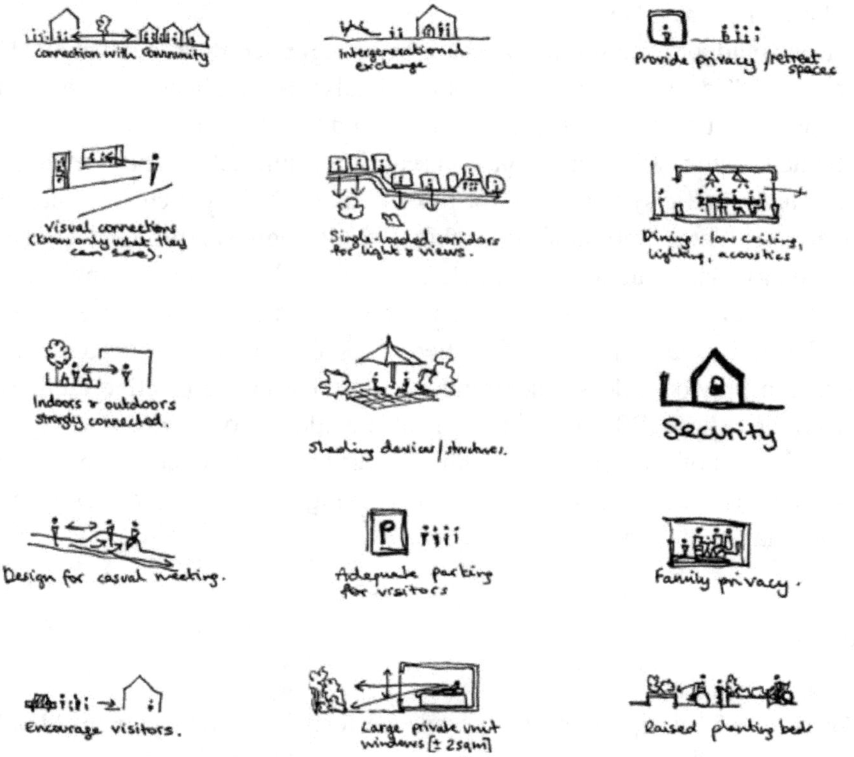
connection with Community
Intergenerational exchange
Provide privacy/retreat spaces
Visual connections (know only what they can see).
Single-loaded corridors for light & views.
Dining: low ceiling, lighting, acoustics
Indoors & outdoors strongly connected.
Shading devices/structures.
Security
Design for casual walking.
Adequate parking for visitors
Family privacy.
Encourage visitors.
Large private unit windows [± 25sqm]
Raised planting beds

space should be color-coded for this purpose (Bissell, 2010); and successful techniques include using colored inlays, varying the flooring material in different areas, and using patterns to provide guidance and facilitate movement.

It should be borne in mind, however, that perception of contrast varies with individuals: aspects of color such as hue, brightness and saturation can be affected by visual disorders, and some patients are unable to distinguish an object from others nearby if they are similar in color; the redder colors of the spectrum appear to be perceived more easily than the blues. Colors used in design should therefore generally be calm and soothing, evoking comfort and a sense of healing; the addition of some bright accents may contribute to a sense of pleasurable excitement and youth.

- **Taste, Smell and Touch:** A roughly circular space can be designed which attracts patients, where they can engage in various activities, including gardening, and enjoy themselves; here they should have the opportunity to touch and smell plants, herbs and flowers, and perhaps pick fruit, if they so choose.

- **Hearing:** One way of providing pleasant auditory experiences is to set up an aviary in the center of the garden; this is a traditional concept, and may may also serve as a visual landmark by which patients can orient themselves (Nord, 2004).
- **Acoustics:** In general, gardens provide a range of pleasant auditory stimuli, such as the sound of wind in the trees or leaves, that can have a soothing and healing effect on Alzheimer's patients.

Location

In designing gardens, care should be taken to ensure that they can adapt to seasonal changes in temperature; a garden with an ideal microclimate in one season may not feel pleasant in another.

In addition, the choice of location and vegetation should take into account the problem of sundowning: patients need to feel that they are in a comfortable and familiar environment, and effort should be made to reduce shadows that might have a frightening effect. For this reason, a garden space at the southeast of the facility's building is recommended, so that the only shadow cast in it by the sun will be that of the recognizable form of the building (Randall, Burkhardt & Kutcher, 1990).

Designing for Other User Groups

Designing an external environment that is appropriate for Alzheimer's patients and suitable for facility staff and visitors as well presents a challenge, but one which is not insurmountable. Research shows that all users can appreciate garden environments that enable relaxation, bring back memories, and encourage and facilitate outdoor activities (Whear at all., 2014); and that all benefit from the stress relief provided by the access and connection to nature facilitated by gardens, window views, and nature-themed artworks (Ulrich & Gilpin, 2003).

Staff

The role of care facilities for Alzheimer's patients is to maintain a pleasant environment, where there is sufficient space for activities, areas where residents can get away from stress, and where staff can take a break. Staff should be able to modify the environment as the need arises; and they should be able to surveil and monitor the entire area from a distance, so as to minimize the need to accompany patients, and instead enable them to use it as independently as possible.

Family and Visitors

Staff should also ensure that the care provided is of a high standard, and that the environment provides patients with a feeling of home, where they can have privacy as well as a normal social life and engage with visitors and family.

Design Elements

Exit Control

Alzheimer's patients often forget how to return to their homes, because they lack the ability to maintain and negotiate cognitive maps; for this reason, they should always be accompanied when they leave home. As a protective and preventive measure, exit doors that lead out into broader public areas should be controlled, and signals that tell staff they have been opened should be discreet – for example, doorbell chimes may be used, rather than harsh alarm sounds that would clash with the ambience. Less noticeable exits and more discreet signal systems will be less disturbing, and enable residents to feel less confined and more free and independent within the safety of their environment (Ziesel, 2003).

Enclosing Walls

Enclosed areas have the effect of creating a refuge for Alzheimer's patients. Well-designed walled or fenced-off spaces open up interior spaces by allowing views of the outside: a courtyard, for example, can offers views that change during the day and with night lighting, and also vary according to seasonal or weather conditions; perceiving these changes is especially valuable for patients whose capacity for recalling events is reduced. The enclosed space is safe and provides a sense of privacy; and in addition, looking out at a natural environment can provide a pleasant and aesthetic experience (Wells, 2014).

Walking Paths

For the elderly, an active lifestyle helps to maintain the functions of the brain, and it may also delay the advancement of Alzheimer's (Rolland, Abellan van Kan & Vellas, 2008). One symptom of the disease is for a patient to wander in search of something, although without knowing exactly what that thing is. This may pose a problem in facilities without suitable spaces for wandering in; so a pathway, if it is designed to be interesting and leads somewhere, may help turn this activity into the physical exercise of walking (Figure 3). The pathway does not have to take the form of a circular track; instead, it can be created simply by connecting corridors and common spaces leading in a particular direction, and interest can be maintained by ensuring that it has visible goals that can be reached at strategic points, such as pictures, plants, or a new view (Volicer & Charette, 1999). Pathways should have a minimum width of 90cm so they are safe for patients to use on their own or with walkers or wheelchairs. A feature at the end, such as the entrance to a garden, a social area or a hearth can serve as a destination that can be achieved and make the wandering meaningful (Ziesel, 2003).

Steps and Ramps

Sloping gardens may require steps or ramps. For ease of use, steps should be level and regular, with a minimum tread of 28cm and a maximum height of 15cm. Flights larger than eight steps should have level rest areas at least 150cm deep. Ramps should have a maximum gradient of 1:20, and should ideally have rest areas every 10 meters (Harris, Dines & Brown, 1998).

Handrails

Some patients may need handrails for support when using outdoor areas; they help the patient balance and move, and also reduce patients' fear of falling. Handrails should not prevent patients from interacting with the vegetation; they should always be comfortable to hold, and also suitable for patients who have difficulties using their hands because of arthritis (Figure 4).

Figure 3. Possibilities for pathway designs
Source: Cave & Brown, 1992

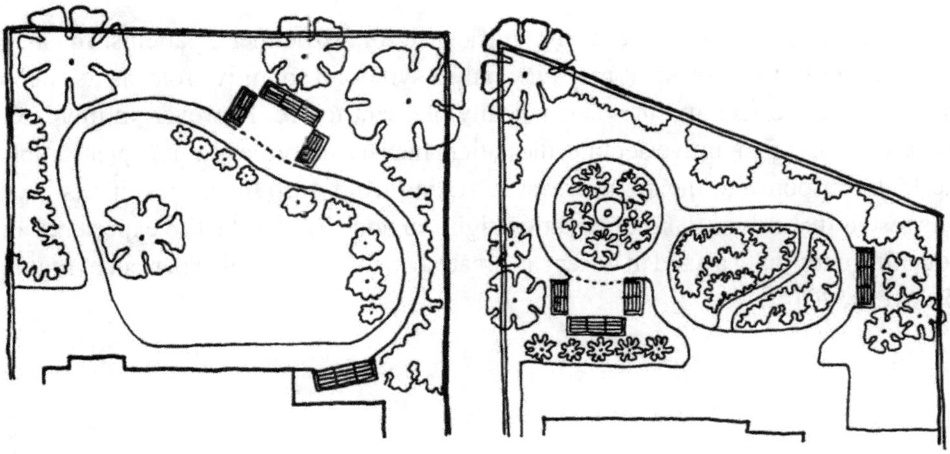

Figure 4. The Lodge at Broadmead, Victoria, BC, Canada
Source: Marcus, 2005

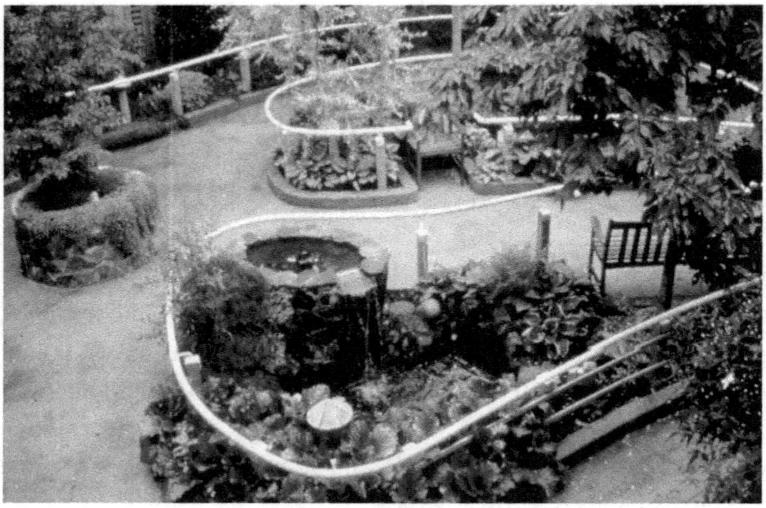

Paving

For outdoor areas, paved surfaces are the most suitable; they should have fine texture, help resist slipping, and not create a glare when reflecting light (this is an important consideration for older patients); and there should also be enough space for walkers and wheelchairs to pass. The aesthetics of paved surfaces plays a significant role in shaping the emotional response to a space, so their color, texture and other characteristics should be taken into account in the design process (Wells, 2014).

Water

Water features can have particular significance for Alzheimer's patients. In early, mild phases of the disease, it may play only a symbolic cognitive role, as its sound has a calming effect and it is aesthetically pleasant to see. However, in more advanced stages of cognitive decline, the patient may have a pre-cognitive, pleasurable aesthetic response to the sight of water, arising from deep memories; it has been suggested that this may be of genetic origin. In addition, the tactile experience of touching or dipping a hand in water can create a positive physical experience (Figure 5) (Wells, 2014).

Figure 5. Shallow reflective pools or bublers pose have the least risk for Alzheimer's
Source: PRP Landscape, 2013

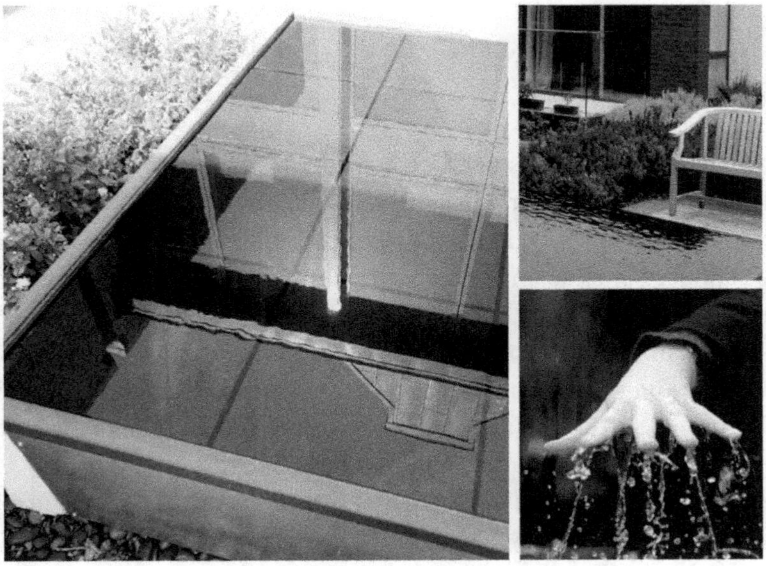

Mount or Hill

Hills may also have therapeutic value as visual elements in gardens designed for Alzheimer's patients. Hills should be subtle, with a low gradient, and as different configurations of space, should help to define the flat and level areas of a garden. If they are near a seating area, hills may serve as metaphors of both places of refuge and areas to wander in.

Sitting Areas

Garden furniture for Alzheimer's patients should be designed so it is heavy and stable; a seating height of 45cm is recommended. There should be alternative types of seating areas at various places: one important area is on the way out from the building into the garden; others should be situated near entrances, areas where activities are done, on routes that patients typically take, and also in quiet, private areas. (Cohen & Weisman, 1991).

Artwork

Studies on patients being treated for psychiatric problems as well as others not undergoing such treatment have shown that their being exposed to abstract art causes negative emotions and stress, and may lead to aggressive behavior. For this reason, artworks used should be representational in character (Ulrich, Bogren & Lundin, 2012).

Planting

Different types of vegetation should be considered when designing outdoor areas for Alzheimer's patients. Elderly patients may slip on fallen leaves, so the most appropriate choices would be non-deciduous plants, and plants whose fallen leaves will not be slippery or slide on walking surfaces. Trees and bushes give a structure to a garden, and the movement of tree branches and leaves can express aspects of climate such as the strength of the wind, and attract patients' interest. Choosing vegetation, including flowering plants, that show seasonal changes in color, will continually provide a diverse and interesting environment; plants that are visited by insects, birds and other animals will add to the interest.

Patients may be stimulated to recall past memories in gardens featuring herbs, vegetables and traditional flowers; such elements have pleasurable and calming effects (Wright, 2014). Care should be taken, however, that non-toxic plants are used, since patients in the advanced stages of Alzheimer's often put things in their mouths. Herbs such as lavender and other aromatic plants release their odor when they are touched (Kennard, 2006); and research has shown that olfactory stimulation, such as the scent of flowers, can have an immediate positive effect on the psychological state of people patients in the advanced stages of Alzheimer's (Witucki & Ïwibell, 1997).

Patients have easy access to plants which are in elevated planters or containers that can be moved; this enables them to interact by seeing, touching or smelling the plants (Figure 6). The "elevated garden" is especially useful for people who cannot bend easily or are confined to a wheelchair. Containers should be set about 6-85cm above the ground, and to make access easier, the arms of chairs or wheelchairs should be able to fit under them (Dixon, 2002).

Wayfinding

Depending on how advanced the symptoms of dementia are, a patient may have difficulties with short-term memory recall. This often leads to problems in direction-finding, because memories of paths or routes travelled recently may be forgotten. Because of this, design for people with dementia should emphasize "wayfinding." Research shows that these individuals perform poorly in wayfinding tasks even in spaces they are familiar with, but do pay the same attention as those who are not affected by the disorder, to similar architectural features and wayfinding features

Figure 6. Portland Memory Garden, Portland, OR
Source: ERIN Research Inc., 2010

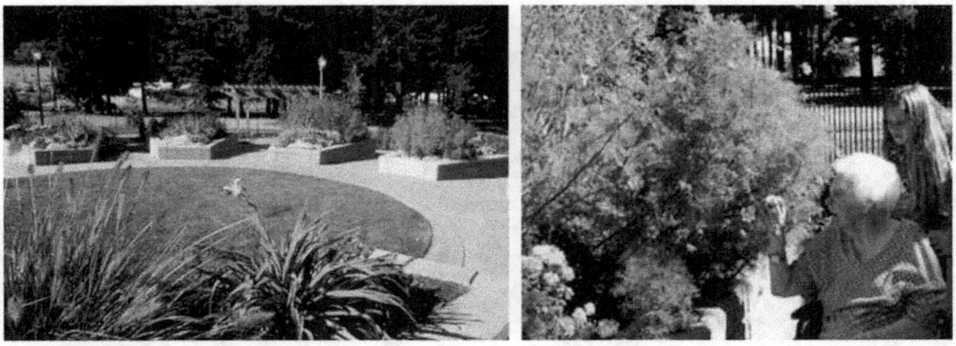

such as signage (Sheehan, Burton & Lynne, 2006). Athough some care facilities for patients with impaired memory focus on other factors, it seems clear that wayfinding should be prioritized as the most important aim in designing environments for Alzheimer's patients (Bissell, 2010). Outdoor areas in particular should have clear points of reference and landmarks – flowerbeds, water features, sculptures, etc. – so the patients can locate themselves (Nord, 2004).

Signage

Signs help patients to orient themselves, and indicate their present location as well as possible destinations that can serve as meaningful goals (Clayton, 2012). The fonts used on signs should be simple, large, and contrasted with the background, so as to be read clearly, particularly by older patients whose eyesight may be weak.

Lighting

Gardens should be accessible to patients as much as possible, and lighting makes them available in the evenings (Figure 7). Good lighting makes patients feel safer, and since they can see others, this creates an informal interaction which also helps staff to monitor other patients (McBride, 1999). Lighting can also be used for effect or to dramatize certain features of the garden so they are visible both from the garden and inside the building (Dixon, 2002). Typical problems encountered with lighting are either that there is not enough, so the surroundings become even darker; that it is uneven, so it creates shadows that may be frightening; that it may be too strong, so it creates a glare; or that it is insufficent to provide safety and security in transition areas (Brawley, 2001).

Figure 7. Illuminated outdoor areas are particularly important for residents experiencing acute sensitivity to sunlight
Source: PRP Landscape, 2013

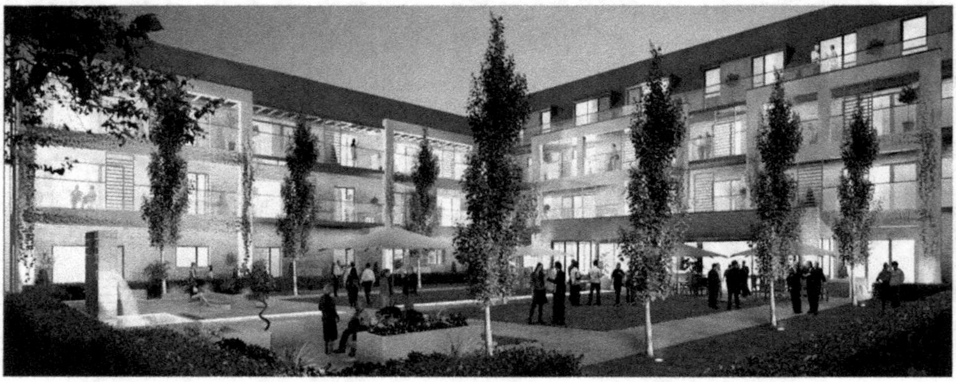

Personal Places

Patients in Alzheimer's care facilities see a lot of each other, so they need spaces where they can be on their own, away from social pressure; in this respect they are no different from anyone else. For this purpose, individual spaces can be made available in the garden (Ziesel, 2003).

Social Space

While time alone is a necessary requirement for Alzheimer's patients, social interaction is no less important, as it contributes to well-being and helps individuals to function in daily life; it is thus crucial that patients interact with others, be it other patients, or staff, or relatives (Figure 8) (Dixon, 2002). Thus two or more common spaces should be available where patients can alleviate the boredom and agitation that might result from their being alone (Ziesel, 2003). Engaging in outdoor physical activities with others contributes to psychosocial well-being, and also encourages commitment to these activities. There are various possibilities for social spaces: these may be intimate areas for two people, or areas where groups of different sizes can meet. Clusters of tables and chairs encourage spontaneous interactions; a chair by a window with a view of a bird feeder, for example, can motivate a patient to engage in bird watching (Alzheimer's Association, 2007).

Figure 8. Movable seating for converstaion
Source: Marcus, 2008

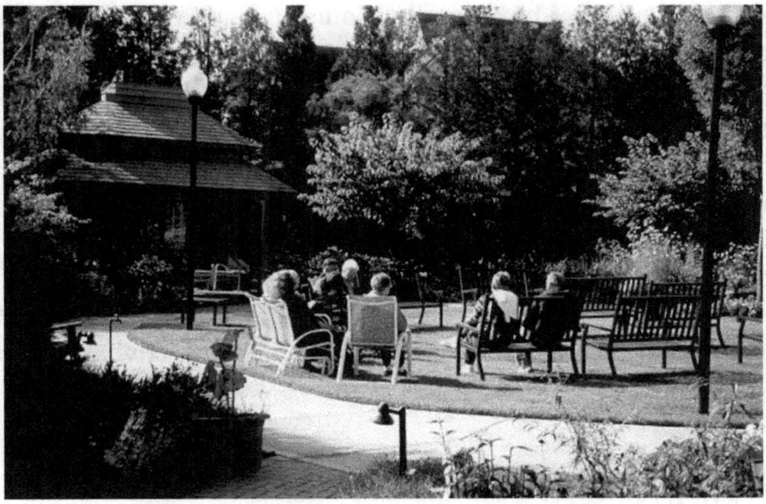

Healing Gardens

The ideal Alzheimer's care facility would have a safe outdoor area next to the residential building; however, in practice this is not always the case, although the importance of such a feature is unquestionable. As these patients live from day to day, the freedom of being outside and relaxing is an essential part of life; but the healing garden, beyond this, serves therapeutic functions and as a refuge.

Potential Risks in the Alzheimer's Garden

Designers of gardens for Alzheimer's patients should follow principles that maximize their benefit to the patients, and also take into account potential risks or dangers that may be encountered.

For example, for patients who tend to put flowers and other plant material or soil in their mouths, types of activities other than gardening should be considered. In selecting vegetation for the garden, it should be remembered that many bulbs and plants, like the philodendron or, for instance, the leaves of the tomato plant, are toxic; and chemical pesticides are used on plants sold by garden centers. If ingested, particularly by the elderly, these may affect their health or cause problems if they interact with medications. Organically grown plants would thus seem to be the safest option.

In terms of the environment to be created, potential hazards include rough, uneven or slippery surfaces; glare produced by the materials used; patients' experiencing problems of balance caused by visually confusing patterns and dark colors; and unsafe transitions between different areas (Brawley, 2001). In addition to these risks of falling, patients may also incur injury when using gardening tools that are not adapted to their safety needs. Patients in advanced stages of Alzheimer's will forget to care for their adopted plants, so for practical reasons, the personal "pet plant" may have to be abandoned in favor of a community garden.

Finally, exposure to too much sunlight or heat can negatively affect elderly patients and others taking some medications; and dehydration may also be a problem. It should therefore be ensured that shaded and sitting areas are available, that patients have readily acccessible drinking water, and that activities in the garden are monitored constantly (Bruce, 2014).

CONCLUSION

Well-designed landscaped gardens can meet many of the needs of Alzheimer's patients; these include design elements such as unobtrusive monitoring systems; handrails, ramps, steps and rest areas; a simple looped pathway, clear signage, and landmark features to facilitate way-finding; lighting elements to accentuate landscape features and encourage use of the garden throughout the day; dark or tinted walking surfaces that do not create glare and are not slippery; non-toxic and accessible vegetation that evokes pleasant memories, other vegetation that evokes seasonal changes and attracts fauna; and seating and recreational areas that provide opportunities for both solitude and socialization.

For Alzheimer's patients there are significant therapeutic benefits to be gained from such purpose-designed environmental landscapes, which also help reduce the load of staff at care facilities. Such landscapes provide calming views and experiences of nature, help lower stress and tension, offer opportunities for exercise and physical activity, stimulate patients to remember positive events and situations, create opportunities and spaces both for escaping or having time alone and for socialization; and in contrast to the stress of clinical spaces, give patients a feeling of safety, security and control in a familiar setting (Ulrich at all., 2004). A well-designed outdoor environment has a positive effect on these patients' thought processes and behaviors; it enables them to live actively and independently, and maintain their sense of wellbeing and quality of life.

REFERENCES

Alzheimer Association. (2007). *Activity-Based Care*. Chicago: Alzheimer's Association. Retrieved June 2015, http://www.alz.org/professionals_and_researchers_activity_based_care.asp

Andreoli, P. J. H. (2003). *Monitoring evaluatie en kennisverzameling: pilotproject: senioren actief in groenkamers*. Amsterdam: Woonzorg Nederland.

Bechtel, R. B., & Churchman, A. (2003). *Handbook of Environmental Psychology*. John Wiley & Sons.

Bissell, K. (2010). *Designing for those with dementia using the principle of wayfinding* (Senior Thesis). Retrieved June 2015, http://muir.wrlc.org/bitstream/handle/10994/77/Final%20Thesis%20by%20Kelly%20Bissell.pdf?sequence=1

Bomalaski, M. N. (2011). Horticultural therapy for persons with severe dementia. *Journal of Investigative Medicine*, *59*(1), 208–209.

Brawley, E. (2001). Environmental design for Alzheimer's disease: A quality of life issue. *Aging & Mental Health*, *5*(sup1), 79–83. doi:10.1080/713650005 PMID:11513503

Brawley, E. (2002). Therapeutic Gardens for Individuals with Alzheimer's Disease. *Alzheimer's Care Quarterly*, *3*(1), 7–11.

Browne, C. (1992). The role of nature for the promotion of wellbeing of the elderly. In D. Relf (Ed.), *The role of horticulture in human wellbeing and social development: A national symposium* (pp. 75–79). Portland, OR: Timber Press.

Bruce, H. (2014). *Gardening activities can help enrich the quality of life for those with Alzheimer's, and their caregivers*. Retrieved June 2015, http://horttherapywithhankbruce.weebly.com/alzheimers-with-a-green-thumb.html

Cave, A., & Brown, J. (1992). *Planning and Design Guide for Community Based Day Care Centres*. Alzheimer's Disease Society.

Cedervall, Y., & Aberg, A. C. (2010). Physical activity and implications on well-being in mild Alzheimer's disease: A qualitative case study on two men with dementia and their spouses. *Physiotherapy Theory and Practice*, *26*(4), 226–239. doi:10.3109/09593980903423012 PMID:20397857

Chong, W. K. O., & Hermreck, C. (2011). *ICSDC 2011: Integrating Sustainability Practices in the Construction Industry*. American Society of Civil Engineers.

Clayton, S. D. (2012). *The Oxford Handbook of Environmental and Conservation Psychology (Oxford Library of Psychology)*. Oxford University Press. doi:10.1093/oxfordhb/9780199733026.001.0001

Cohen, U., & Weisman, G. D. (1991). *Holding on to Home Designing Environments for people with Dementia*. Baltimore, MD: The John Hopkins University press.

Cohen-Mansfield, J., & Werner, P. (1998). Visits to an outdoor garden: impact on behaviour and mood of nursing home residents who pace. In B. J. Vellas & L. J. Fitten (Eds.), *Research and practice in Alzheimer's disease* (pp. 419–436). New York: Springer Publishing Company.

Connell, B. R., Sanford, J. A., & Lewis, D. (2007). Therapeutic effects of an outdoor activity program on nursing home residents with dementia. In S. Rodiek & B. Schwarz (Eds.), *Outdoor Environments for People with Dementia*. Haworth Press. doi:10.1300/J081v21n03_10

Detweiler, M. B., Murphy, P. F., Kim, K. Y., Myers, L. C., & Ashiai, A. (2009). Scheduled medications and falls in dementia patients utilizing a wander garden. *American Journal of Alzheimer's Disease and Other Dementias*, *24*(4), 322–332. doi:10.1177/1533317509334036 PMID:19366885

Detweiler, M. B., Murphy, P. F., Myers, L. C., & Kim, K. Y. (2008). Does a wander garden influence inappropriate behaviors in dementia residents? *American Journal of Alzheimer's Disease and Other Dementias*, *23*(1), 31–45. doi:10.1177/1533317507309799 PMID:18276956

Dixon, C. J. M. (2002). A Return to the garden: Design Criteria for Therapeutic Exterior Environments for People with Alzheimer Disease. (Master's Thesis). University of Manitoba, Winnipeg, Manitoba, Canada.

Edwards, C. A., McDonnell, C., & Merl, H. (2013). An evaluation of a therapeutic garden's influence on the quality of life of aged care residents with dementia. *Dementia (London)*, *12*(4), 494–510. doi:10.1177/1471301211435188 PMID:24336957

Elings, M. (2006). People-plant interaction: the physiological, psychological and sociological effects of plants on people. In Farming for Health. Green-Care Farming Across Europe and the United States of America. Springer. doi:10.1007/1-4020-4541-7_4

ERIN Research Inc. (2010). *Landscape architecture and public welfare*. Council of Landscape Architectural Registration Boards. Retrieved June 2015, https://www.clarb.org/CLARBDocuments/PublicWelfareFINAL.pdf

Garcia, C. (2014). *The Benefits of Memory Gardens at Nursing Homes*. Retrieved June 2015, http://studio-sprout.com/files/The-Benefits-of-Memory-Gardens-at-Nursing-Homes.pdf

Gigliotti, C. M., Jarrott, S. E., & Yorgason, J. (2004). Harvesting health: Effects of three types of horticultural therapy activities for persons with dementia. *Dementia (London)*, *3*(2), 161–180. doi:10.1177/1471301204042335

Grove, K. (2012). *Gardens for People with Dementia*. Retrieved June 2015, http://www.kimgrove-gardendesigner.co.uk/resources/Gardens%20for%20People%20with%20Dementia%20-%20A%20Guide%20to%20Make%20Them%20Safe%20and%20Suitable%20-%202013.pdf

Harris, C. W., Dines, N. T., & Brown, K. D. (1998). *Time-Saver Standards for Landscape Architecture*. McGraw-Hill Education.

Hartig, T., & Cooper-Marcus, C. (2006). Healing Gardens: Places for nature in health care. *Lancet*, *368*, 36–37. doi:10.1016/S0140-6736(06)69920-0

Hartig, T., Evans, G. W., Jamner, L. D., Davis, D. S., & Garling, T. (2003). Tracking restoration in natural and urban field settings. *Journal of Environmental Psychology*, *23*(2), 109–123. doi:10.1016/S0272-4944(02)00109-3

Health Council of the Netherlands and Dutch Advisory Council for Research on Spatial Planning Nature and the Environment (HCNDACRSP). (2004). *Nature and Health. The influence of nature on social, psychological and physical wellbeing*. Health Council of the Netherlands and RMNO.

Jackson, S. (2005). The Potential on the Door step: The Importance of Gardens in the Psychological Well-being of Older People. *Journal of Therapeutic Horticulture*, *16*, 29–36.

Kaplan, R. (1993). The role of nature in the context of the workplace. *Landscape and Urban Planning*, *26*(1-4), 193–201. doi:10.1016/0169-2046(93)90016-7

Kaplan, R. (2001). The nature of the view from home: Psychological benefits. *Environment and Behavior*, *33*(4), 507–542. doi:10.1177/00139160121973115

Kennard, C. (2006). *The Alzheimer's Garden Plan*. Retrieved June 2015, http://alzheimers.about.com/od/familyandfriends/a/garden_design.htm

Kuo, F.E. & Taylor, A.F. (2004). A Potential Natural Treatment for Attention-Deficit/Hyperactivity Disorder: Evidence from a National Study. *American Journal of Public Health, 94*(9), 1580.

Landscape, P. R. P. (2013). *Landscape Design for Dementia, Factsheet 35*. Care-Housing Learning & Improvement Network Press. Retrieved June 2015, http://www.housinglin.org.uk/_library/Resources/Housing/Support_materials/Factsheets/HLIN_Factsheet35_Landscape.pdf

Lee, Y., & Kim, S. (2008). Effects of indoor gardening on sleep, agitation, and cognition in dementia patients: A pilot study. *International Journal of Geriatric Psychiatry*, *23*(5), 485–489. doi:10.1002/gps.1920 PMID:17918774

Marcus, C. C. (2005). *Healing Gardens in Hospitals*. Retrieved June 2015, http://www.umcg.nl/SiteCollectionDocuments/UMCG/C1_Cooper_Marcus.ppt.pdf

Marcus, C.C. (2008). Garden of the Family Life Center, Grand Rapids, Michigan. *Journal of Housing For the Elderly Publication*, 285-304.

Mather, J. A., Nemecek, D., & Oliver, K. (1999). The effect of a walled garden on behavior of individuals with Alzheimer's. *American Journal of Alzheimer's Disease*, *12*(6), 252–257. doi:10.1177/153331759701200603

Mooney, P., & Nicel, P. L. (1992). The Importance of Exterior Environment for Alzheimer Residents: Effective Care and Risk Management. *Healthcare Management Forum*, *5*(2), 23–29. doi:10.1016/S0840-4704(10)61202-1 PMID:10171068

Niall McLaughlin Architects Bedford House. (2012). *The Alzheimer's Respite Centre*. Retrieved June 2015, http://www.niallmclaughlin.com/wp-content/uploads/2014/07/AAIAwards2010-reduced.pdf

Nord, R. D. (2004). *Architecture for alzheimer disease*. Alinea Editrice Press.

Randall, P., Burkhardt, S. J., & Kutcher, J. (1990). Exterior space for patients with Alzheimer's disease and related disorders. *American Journal of Alzheimer's Care and Related Disorders & Research*, *5*(4), 31–37. doi:10.1177/153331759000500408

Rappe, E. (2005). *The Influence of a Green Environment and Horticultural Activities on the Subjective Well-Being of the Elderly Living in Long-Term Care*. University of Helsinki, Department of Applied Biology.

Rolland, Y., Abellan van Kan, G., & Vellas, B. (2008). Physical activity and Alzheimer's disease: From prevention to therapeutic perspectives. *Journal of the American Medical Directors Association*, *9*(6), 390–405. doi:10.1016/j.jamda.2008.02.007 PMID:18585641

Schwarz, B., & Rodiek, S. (2007). Introduction: Outdoor Environments for People with Dementia. In Outdoor Environments for People with Dementia (pp. 3-13). Routledge.

Sheehan, B., Burton, E. J., & Mitchell, L. (2006). Outdoor wayfinding in dementia. *Dementia (London), 5*(2), 271–281. doi:10.1177/1471301206062254

Terry, H. & Cooper Marcus, C. (2006). Healing Gardens – Places for Nature in Health Care. *The Lancet, 368.*

Traynor, V., Fernandez, R., & Caldwell, K. (2013). The effects of spending time outdoors in daylight on the psychosocial wellbeing of older people and family carers: a comprehensive systematic review protocol. *JBI Database of Systematic Reviews & Implementation Reports, 11*(9), 36-55. Retrieved June 2015, http://ro.uow.edu.au/cgi/viewcontent.cgi?article=2184&context=smhpapers

Ulrich, R., & Gilpin, L. (2003). Healing arts – nutrition for the soul. In P. M. Charmel, S. B. Frampton, & L. Gilpin (Eds.), *Putting Patients First—Designing and Practicing Patient-Centered Care* (pp. 117–146). San Francisco: Jossey-Bass.

Ulrich, R., Zimring, C., Quan, X., Joseph, A., & Choudhary, R. (2004). *The Role of the Physical Environment in the Hospital of the 21st Century: A Once-in-a-Lifetime Opportunity.* Report to The Center for Health Design for the Designing the 21st Century Hospital Project. Retrieved June 2015 http://www.healthdesign.org/chd/research/role-physical-environment-hospital-21st-century

Ulrich, R. S. (2002). Health Benefits of Gardens in Hospitals. In *Plants for People,Proceedings of the International Exhibition Floriade.*

Ulrich, R. S., Bogren, L., & Lundin, S. (2012). Toward a design theory for reducing aggression in psychiatric facilities. In Conference Arch 12: Architecture, Research, Care, Health. Gothenburg: Chalmers Institute of Technology.

Ulrich, R. S., Simons, R. F., Losito, B. D., Fiorito, E., Miles, M. A., & Zelson, M. (1991). Stress recovery during exposure to natural and urban environments. *Journal ofEnvironmental Psychology, 11*(3), 201–230. doi:10.1016/S0272-4944(05)80184-7

Volicer, L., & Charette, L. B. (1999). *Enhancing the Quality of Life in Advanced Dementia.* Routledge.

Wells, S. E. (2014). Horticultural Therapy and the Older Adult Population. *Activities, Adaptation & Aging, 22*(1-3).

Whall, A. L., Black, M. E., Groh, C. J., Yankou, D. J., Kupferschmid, B. J. & Foster, N. L. (1997, September/October). The Effect of Natural Environments Upon Agitation and Aggression in Late Stage Dementia patients. *American Journal of Alzheimer Disease,* 216-220.

Whear, R., Coon, J. T., Bethel, A., Abbott, R., Stein, K., & Garside, R. (2014). What Is the Impact of Using Outdoor Spaces Such as Gardens on the Physical and Mental Well-Being of Those with Dementia? A Systematic Review of Quantitative and Qualitative Evidence. *Journal of the American Medical Directors Association.* Retrieved June 2015, http://www.sciencedirect.com/science/article/pii/S1525861014003399

Willat, J. (2011). Design as Therapy: Facilitating the lives of those with Alzheimer's disease through environmental design, Revista AUS, núm. 9 (pp. 4–9). Valdivia, Chile: Universidad Austral de Chile. Retrieved from http://www.redalyc.org/articulo.oa?id=281722876002

Witucki, J. M., & Twibell, R. S. (1997). The Effect of Sensory Stimulation Activities on the Psychological Well Being of Patients with Advanced Alzheimer's Disease. *American Journal of Alzheimer's Disease*, *2*(1), 10–15. doi:10.1177/153331759701200103

Wright, J. (2014). *Garden therapy for those with special needs.* Retrieved June 2015, http://www.thegardener.co.za/kb/article.php?id=996

Zeisel, J. (2007). Creating a Therapeutic Garden That Works for People Living with Alzheimer's. *Journal of Housing for the Elderly, 21*(12), 13-33.

Ziesel, J. (2003). Marketing therapeutic environments for Alzheimer' s care. *Journal of Architectural and Planning Research*, *20*(1), 75–86.

ADDITIONAL READING

Arditi, A. (2005). Enhancing the visual environment for older and visually impaired persons. *Alzheimer's Care Quarterly.* Oct-Dec, 6(4), pp. 294-299.

Brawley, E. C. (2006). *Design Innovations for Aging and Alzheimer's: Creating Caring Environments*. Hoboken, NJ: Wiley.

Chalfont, G., & Rodiek, S. (2005). Building edge: An ecological approach to research and design of environments for people with dementia. *Alzheimer's Care Quarterly: Environmental Innovations in Care*, *6*(4), 341–348.

Hoglund, J. D., & Ledewitz, S. D. (1999). Designing to meet the needs of people with Alzheimer's disease. IN: Schwarz, B.; Brent, R., eds. Aging, autonomy, and architecture: advances in assisted living, pp. 229-259, Baltimore, MD: Johns Hopkins University Press.

Kaplan, R., & Kaplan, S. et al.. (1998). *With People in Mind: Design and Management of Everyday Nature.* Washington, DC: Island Press.

Kaplan, S., & Kaplan, R. (2003). Health, supportive environments, and the reasonable person model. *American Journal of Public Health*, *93*(9), 1484–1489. doi:10.2105/AJPH.93.9.1484 PMID:12948967

Lawton, M. P. (2001). Physical environment of the person with Alzheimer's disease. *Aging & Mental Health*, *5*(1), 56–64. doi:10.1080/713650004 PMID:11513499

Rodiek, S., Lee, C., & Nejati, A. (2014). You Can't Get There From Here: Reaching the Outdoors in Senior Housing. *Journal of Housing for the Elderly*, *28*(1), 63–84. doi:10.1080/02763893.2013.858093

Sugiyama, T., & Thompson, C. W. (2007). Outdoor environments, activity and the well-being of older people: Conceptualising environmental support. *Environment & Planning*, *39*(8), 1943–1960. doi:10.1068/a38226

KEY TERMS AND DEFINITIONS

Alzheimer's Disease: A degenerative disease of the brain that causes people to forget things, including the people in their lives, and which eventually leads to death.

Behavioral Measure: Overt actions and reactions that are observed and recorded, exclusive of self-reported behavior.

Environment Landscape: The physical and interpersonal surroundings landscape that can affect mood and behavior in people with Alzheimer's.

Environmental Perception: The way in which an individual perceives the environment; the process of evaluating and storing information received about the environment.

Chapter 3
Evaluation of the Relationship between Nutritional Status and Quality of Life among Nursing Home Residents with Alzheimer's Disease

Alev Keser
Ankara University, Turkey

Filiz Yildirim
Ankara University, Turkey

ABSTRACT

The purpose of this study was to determine nutritional status and its influence on their quality of life in Alzheimer's disease (AD) patients with Mini Nutritional Assessment (MNA) and anthropometric measurements. This study was conducted with 57 Alzheimer type dementia patients between the ages of 52 and 89 who live in nursing homes in Ankara/Turkey. In this study, it was found that the 57.9% of the AD patients were at risk of malnutrition, and that 19.3% were malnourished. Malnutrition risk rises as the length of stay increases ($p< .05$). A significant correlation between body weight and quality of life as well as one between calf circumference and quality of life was detected ($p< .05$). In this study, nutrient intake among aged individuals with AD was found unbalanced; a statistically significant correlation between energy / nutrient intake and quality of life also was not detected.

DOI: 10.4018/978-1-5225-0925-7.ch003

INTRODUCTION

It is estimated that each year, 4.6 million new cases of dementia were predicted (one new case every 7 seconds), with numbers affected nearly doubling every 20 years to reach 81.1 million by 2040 (Ferri et al., 2005). As the most common cause of neurodegenerative dementia in the elderly population Alzheimer's disease (AD) is a growing health issue and one of the leading causes of death among elderly people (Gillette-Guyonnet et al.,2000; Gurvit, 2004). Two-thirds of all dementia cases are caused by AD, which affects roughly 10% of the elderly. This prevalence increases with age, and reaches 45% among those over 85 years (Gurvit, 2004). In Turkey, the epidemiological data on Alzheimer's disease is not sufficient; however, a relevant study indicates that the AD prevalence among those over 70 years is 11% (Gurvit et al., 2008).

In the present day, quality of life is one of the most important factors considered in the treatment of Alzheimer's disease (Akyar & Akdemir, 2009). On the other hand, it is particularly difficult to define quality of life for these patients due to cognitive, physical, emotional and social factors that are specific to this disease. Moreover, it is not always possible to determine the life quality of Alzheimer's patients using their own assessments since they may lack sufficient cognitive skills (Akyar & Akdemir, 2009; Akpinar & Kucukguclu, 2012). Assessing quality of life using subjective and objective indicators is associated with cognitive and behavioral disorders and, frequently, with nutritional disorders (Gillette-Guyonnet et al.,2000). Hyperphagia, hyporexia, sweet cravings, choice of food, refusal and severe feeding difficulties are prevalent eating patterns (Gillette-Guyonnet, Lauque & Ousset, 2005). Weight loss is also frequent, increasing the risk of complications, especially reduced muscle mass, a loss of autonomy, and an increased risk of falls, decubitus ulcers, and systemic infection. All of these increase the burden of the disease and reduce AD patients' quality of life (Gillette-Guyonnet et al., 2000; Gillette-Guyonnet, Lauque & Ousset, 2005). Various mechanisms may be responsible for weight loss. It may be due to physical changes (e.g., impaired taste and smell functions, reduced appetite due to a decline in endogenous opioids, and increased satiety due to increased sensitivity to cholecystokinin), neuropsychiatric disorders associated with the disease (e.g., memory loss, disorientation, mood disorders, indifference, and impaired judgment), a change in autonomy and dietary habits, or changes in neurotransmitter concentrations (e.g., Neuropeptide Y and norepinephrine) (Knupfer & Spiege, 1986; Spaccavento et al., 2009). Weight loss worsens as the disease progresses and itis considered a predictor of patient mortality (Gillette-Guyonnet, Lauque & Ousset, 2005). Spaccavento et al. (2009) investigated the role of nutritional status on cognitive, functional and neuropsychiatric deficits in patients with AD. They found that patients at risk of malnutrition showed greater impairment, both in simple and instrumental activities of daily living and a more severe ideomotor praxis deficit than well-nourished patients. Neuropsychiatric symptoms (such as hallucinations, apathy, aberrant motor behavior and nocturnal disturbances) were more severe in patients at risk of malnutrition. Therefore, an intervention strategy that can prevent or slow the complications of this disease would have important public health benefits (Nourhashemi et al., 2000). It is critical that malnutrition is detected at an early stage since it is very difficult to reconfigure nutrition habits, especially for patients with dementia (Garry & Vellas, 1996).

Studies in the relevant literature indicate that 60% of AD patients in nursing homes are either malnourished or at risk of malnutrition (Elia, Jones & Russell, 2008). Thus, individuals at nursing homes should be examined regularly for malnutrition. Awareness about the influence of malnutrition on the quality of life should be raised. This requires that malnutrition risk and its clinical outcomes be researched with a variety of populations. Therefore, this study used the Mini Nutritional Assessment (MNA) andanthropometric measurements to determine AD patients' nutritional status and its influence on their quality of life.

Purpose of the Research

The main purpose of this research was to examine the relationship between nutritional status and quality of life among nursing home residents with Alzheimer's disease. It was also aimed following objectives in order to accomplish the main purpose:

- Finding out the nutritional status of the aged individuals with Alzheimer's through anthropometric measures and MNA,
- Determining the amount of the energy and nutrient intakes by a 3-day re-cording of food consumption and evaluating their meeting of Recommended Dietary Allowances (RDA),
- Determining the quality of life of aged individuals with Alzheimer's through Caregivers' Reports on Patients' Quality of Life scale,
- Examining the relationship between the energy intake and quality of life among aged individuals with Alzheimer's.

METHODS

Study Group

This cross-sectional study was conducted with 57 (22 male, 35 female) Alzheimer type dementia patients between the ages of 52 and 89 (76.0±9.84) who live in nursing homes in Turkey's capital city, Ankara, between January 2014 and April

2014. The World Health Organization regards people in the age range 45-59 years as "middle aged", 60-74 as "elderly", 75-89 as "old" and over 90 as "very old" (53). According to this, 8.8% (5 patients) of the participants are middle aged, 31.6% (18 patients) are elderly, and 59.6% (34 patients) are old. Patients who had only lived in nursing homes for less than one year and bedridden patients were excluded in this research. 61.4% of the participants had been staying at nursing homes for 1-2 years, 24.6% of them for 3-4 years and 14.0% of them for 5 and more years. Data were obtained by surveying professional care providers about their patients. In Ankara, there are many nursing homes and elderly care facilities belonging to the public, private owners, associations, foundations and local governments. The patients of two private nursing homes whose owners agreed to participate were included in the study. Before giving the survey to the patients' professional care providers who agreed to participate voluntarily in this study, they were asked to sign a consent form in accord with the Helsinki declaration.

Study Protocol

The participants were enrolled by a dietician and an academic specialist in the field of social work. In the study, authors made appointments with the nursing homes in advance in order to reach each individual. Thus, the authors, who organised the date, the time, and the place of meetings suggested by the institutions/organizations, had the opportunity for a face to face meeting with each professional care providers. In order not to disturb the patients in their living space (their own rooms), authors paid utmost attention during the interviews. Additionally, in advance, after the care providers were informed about the aim of the study and that it was conducted for academic purposes, they were specifically assured that any information that could reveal their identity would not be shared. Afterwards, information about all the patients who participated in the study (age, sex, disease, duration in nursing homes) was collected from their primary caregivers. The Mini Nutritional Assessment (MNA), and anthropometric measurements (weight, height, body mass index, mid-upper arm circumference, calf circumference, waist/hips ratio) were used to evaluate the nutritional status of the each patient. The body weights of AD patients wearing minimal clothing were measured to the nearest 0.5 kg with a portable scale. Height to the nearest 0.1 cm was measured with a fiber-glass tape. Body mass index (BMI) was calculated as weight (kg)/height (m^2). Mid-upper arm circumference (MUAC) were measured in standing position, the calf circumference (CC) was measured in a supine position, using a fiber–glass tape and recorded to the nearest 0.1 cm. All measurements were obtained as described by Lee and Nieman(2003). The BMI is a widely used and generally accepted measure of nutritional status. However, in the elderly, the BMI should be interpreted with caution because of change in body composition (Wellman & Kamp, 2008). Although there has not been an agreement on the best cut-off points for the elderly, BMI categories, that is, the underweight ($\leq$18.5 kg/m^2), normal weight (18.6-24.9 kg/m^2), overweight (25.0-29.9 kg/m^2) and those with obesity ($\geq$30 kg/m^2) were taken as parameters (31). MUAC measures were evaluated compared with 18-74 years of age NCHS Percentile values. According to this, < 5th percentile was regarded as under nutrition (malnutrition) (Frisancho, 1999).Dietary assessment was accomplished as follows for a period of 3 consecutive days. The caregivers kept a food diary recording of everything the patients ate or drank. Portion size was expressed in household units such as cups, ounces, or pieces. The ingredients of mixed dishes were specified. Serving sizes were estimated either by product name, the place of food consumption, standard weights of food items or from the portion size that was determined from a picture booklet of 120 food photographs (Rakıcıoglu et al., 2009). A dietician, who also calculated the energy and nutritional values of the enteral supplements they consumed from their labels, collected and inspected these nutritional surveys. The results were analyzed using BeBİS 6.1 software (the Nutrition Information System), which is based on several international and national food composition tables. The energy and nutrients intakes of the participants were compared to the Recommended Dietary Allowances (RDA). Consuming ±33% of the recommended amount was considered adequate. Consuming less than ±33% of the recommended amount was considered insufficient, and more than ± 33% of the recommended amount were considered overconsumption (RDA, 1989).

Measurements

MNA, Caregivers' Reports on Patients' Quality of Life (C-PQOL) and personal information form were used to collect data in this research.

MNA

The MNA is a sensitive tool for nutritional screening and assessment of the elderly and provides a multidimensional assessment of the patient. Different sections of MNA assess different components of nutritional status:

1. MNA-1 = anthropometric measurements (4 items), including weight and height to calculate body mass index (BMI), arm and calf circumferences, and weight loss (score: 0–8 points);
2. MNA-2 = general assessment (6 items), including residential status, psychological problems, mobility, medications, and skin ulcers (score: 0–9 points);

3. MNA-3 = assessment of dietetic habits (6 items), including number of meals, food and fluid intake, and autonomy of feeding (score: 0–9 points);
4. MNA-4 = subjective assessment (2 items), including self-perception quality of health and nutrition (score: 0–4 points).

Each item has a numerical value and contributes to the final score, which has a maximum of 30 points. The MNA score is used to classify subjects as well nourished (score above 23.5), at risk for malnutrition (score of 17–23.5), or malnourished (score less than 17), according to the original cut-off point of the MNA full test (Guigoz, 2006; Vellas et al., 1999).

Caregivers' Reports on Patients' Quality of Life (C-PQOL)

Caregivers' reports on patients' quality of life was adapted for Turkish use by Akpinar and Kucukguçlu (2012).

Akpinar and Kucukguçlu (2012) performed the reliability and validity analyses of the (C-PQOL) that this study used. The scale was translated and retranslated from the translation to verify its linguistic validity. Expert opinions were solicited to ensure the validity of its content (Kendall's W=.223, p=.095). The C-PQOL had an internal consistency reliability coefficient, or Cronbach's alpha, of 0.77, and its interclass correlation coefficient was 0.72. Akpinar and Kucukguclu (2012) adapted the C-PQOL for use in Turkey. They also showed that it was a reliable and valid C-PQOL measure for Turkish patients.

The necessary permission was obtained from Akpinar, one of the authors of the scale (Akpinar & Kucukguclu, 2012). C-PQOL consists of 13 items concerning physical health, energy, mood, living situation, memory, family, marriage, friends, you as a whole, ability to do chores, ability to do things for fun, money, and life as a whole. C-PQOL is a likert-type scale and scored from 1 (poor) to 4 (excellent). Score range of the scale is 13-52. It takes 5 minutes in total with caregivers to answer this scale concerning the quality of life of patients. Quality of life improves as scores on the scale increase.

Personal Information Form

Socio-demographic variables included sex, age, length of stay in nursing homes in order to obtain certain information about the participants. These variables were selected according to the literature and their potential effects on the nutritional status and quality of life.

Sex was coded as:

1. Male
2. Female

Age was grouped into three groups:

1. 45-59
2. 60-74
3. 75-89

Length of stay in nursing homes was coded as:

1. 1-2 years
2. 3-4 years
3. 5 and over

Statistical Analyses

Data were analyzed using the SPSS statistical software package. Continuous variables were described using means, and standard deviations. Frequencies and percentages were used as descriptive statistics for categorical variables. Normal distributions were evaluated using the single sample Shapiro-Wilk test. When the hypothesis of normality was not met, nonparametric Mann-Whitney U tests were used. Chi-square test was used in the analysis of categorical data. Pearson Chi-square test could not be implemented where more than 20% of the expected counts were less than 5 in cells and they were tested through Monte Carlo simulation. Mean intakes of energy and nutrient were compared with RDA reference values and analyzed for significant differences using one-sample t tests. To evaluate relations among variables, Spearman's Rank Correlation Coefficient was used. A statistically significant p level was set at .05.

Results

Table 1 shows the patient characteristics at inclusion according to nutritional status. While 22.8% of the patients were well nourished, 57.9% were at risk of malnutrition, and 19.3% were malnourished. Nutritional status of male were better comparing to those of female ($p<.05$). All groups were similar in age and score of quality of life. It was found that those who were at risk of malnutrition (2.8 ± 1.4) had been staying in the nursing home longer than those who were well nourished (1.7 ± 0.6) ($p<.05$). Mean BMI was greater than the normal range (18.6-24.9) in well nourished

Table 1. Comparison of patient characteristics by nutritional status

Baseline Parameters	MNA Score at Baseline				
	All patients (n:57)	**>23.5 mean±SD (n:13)**	**23.5-17 mean±SD (n:33)**	**<17 mean±SD (n:11)**	**p**
n (%)	100.0	22.8	57.9	19.3	
Sex (Male/ Female) (%)	100.0	40.9/11.4	45.5/65.7	13.6/22.9	p**=.035
Mean Age (years), SD	76.0±9.8	73.0±11.0	76.7±9.1	77.4±10.6	p>.05
Mean Length of Stay in Nursing Homes (years), SD	2.4±1.3	1.7±0.6[a]	2.8±1.4 [a']	2.1±1.2	p= .015
Mean BMI (kg/ m^2), SD	24.5±4.6	25.8±3.8 [a]	25.0±4.6[b]	21.7±4.7[a',b']	p [a,a']= .011 p [b,b']=.021
Mean MNA, SD	19.7±4.5	25.1±1.0 [a]	19.9±1.9[a',b]	12.5±2.5[a',b']	p [a,a']= .000 p [b,b']=.000
Mean score of C-PQOL, SD	24.9±4.7	26.0±5.8	25.0±4.5	23.3±3.8	p>.05

* [a,a'], [b,b'] $p<.05$ Mann-Whitney U testi for continuous variables

** χ^2-test for categorical variables.

and risk of malnutrition groups. The MNA mean scores were significantly different among three groups ($p<.05$).

The anthropometric measures of AD patients are given in Table 2. The BMI mean were found 23.9±4.2 kg/m^2 for male and 25.0±4.9 kg/m^2 for female. The waist circumference measures of male and female were 90.1±14.7 cm and 87.6±11.1 cm respectively. The mean ratio for waist/hip was the same(0.9±0.1cm). MUAC mean measured for male and female 26.4±3.7 cm and 25.5±5.7 cm respectively. Calf circumference mean was 31.2±4.2 cm for male and 30.1±4.3 cm for female. As the results of the anthropometric measures for male and female, no statistically significance was found ($p>.05$) except for body weight ($p<.05$). When the MNA scores were examined, it was determined that male's scores (21.2±4.47) were higher than those of female (18.8±4.37) ($p<.05$). No significant statistical difference was observed between quality of life scores between male and female.

Distribution of body weight and disease risk status of the AD patients according to some anthropometric measures is given in Table 3. It was found that majority of the male and female were normal according to BMI (54.5% and 60.0%, respectively), both were also in normal group in terms of metabolic diseases according to waist circumference (54.5% and 40.0%, respectively). While the percentage of

Table 2. Anthropometric measurements, MNA and quality of life scores by sex

Baseline Parameters	Sex		
	Male (22)	Female (35)	p[a]
Mean body weight (kg), SD	67.8±13.5	57.4±13.2	p=.007
Mean BMI (kg/m^2), SD	23.9±4.2	25.0±4.9	p=.313
Mean waist circumference (cm), SD	90.1±14.7	87.6±11.1	p=.718
Mean waist/hips ratio, SD	0.9±0.1	0.9±0.1	p=.305
Mean mid-upper arm circumference, SD	26.4±3.7	25.5±5.7	p=.130
Mean calf circumference (cm), SD	31.2±4.2	30.1±4.3	p=.224
Mean score of MNA, SD	21.2±4.47	18.8±4.37	p=.033
Mean Score of quality of life, SD	25.8±5.6	24.4±4.0	p=.532

[a]Mann-Whitney U testi for continuous variables and χ^2-test for categorical variables.

women whom abdominal obesity was observed was 94.3% according to waist/hip ratio, majority of the men (77.3%) were found to be normal,. According to mid-upper arm circumferences, 45.5% of the male and 34.3% of the female were found to be below the 5 percentile.

Correlation between quality of life and some parameters is illustrated in Table 4. As can be seen, a negative correlation was found between sexes, length of stay in the nursing home and the quality of life (p>.05). Only the correlation between body weight, calf circumference and quality of life was found statistically significant (p<.05).

In Table 5, the status of meeting the requirements of AD patients by their daily intake of energy and nutrient is shown. Intake of energy (91.2%) and protein (87.7%) in AD patients was found adequate (67-133), fat (47.4%) excess (133<). However, intakes of carbohydrates (49.1%), dietary fiber (42.1%), vitamin B_1 (49.1%), potassium (63.2%), calcium (52.6%), magnesium (43.9%), and iron (82.5%) were found inadequate (<67). Especially mean intake of potassium and iron weresignificantly lower than RDA (p<.05). On the other hand, mean intake of vitamins E and C were significantly higher than RDA (p<.05).

DISCUSSION

The quality of life of patients with Alzheimer's disease is influenced by nutritional status along with medical, social and psychological factors. Nutritional problems, especially weight loss, are frequent clinical findings in patients with AD (Seth, 1994).

Table 3. Body weight and disease risk status distribution of the AD patients according to some anthropometric measures

Anthropometric Measures			Male		Female		P*
			n	%	n	%	
Classification of BMI	BMI (kg/m^2)						
Underweight	<18.5		1	4.5	1	2.9	χ^2=7.619 p=.040
Normal weight	18.5-24.9		12	54.5	21	60.0	
Overweight	25.0-29.9		8	36.5	4	11.4	
Obesity	≥30.0		1	4.5	9	25.7	
	Waist Circumference (cm)						
Disease risk	Male	Female					
Normal	<94	<80	12	54.5	14	40.0	χ^2=1.525 p=.466
Risk	≥94	≥80	4	18.2	6	17.1	
High risk	≥102	≥88	6	27.3	15	42.9	
	Waist/Hip Ratio (cm)						
Disease risk /obesity type	Male	Female					
Normal	<1.0	<0.80	17	77.3	2	5.7	χ^2=31.128 p=.000
Abdominal obesity	≥1.0	≥0.80	5	22.7	33	94.3	
Nutritional status	MUAC (Percentile)						
Malnutrition	<5		10	45.5	12	34.3	χ^2=0.712 p=.805
Risk of malnutrition	≥5-<25		8	36.4	12	34.3	
Normal	≥25-<75		3	13.6	9	25.7	
Overweight	≥75-<95		1	4.5	1	2.9	
Obesity	>95		-	-	1	2.9	

*Monte Carlo simulation was used as statistical analysis when more than 20% of the expected counts were less than 5 in cells.

Weight loss is always a great concern for the clinical practitioner because it is an indicator of protein and energy malnutrition in the elderly and a predictor of mortality (White, Pieper & Schmader, 1998). For this reason, the nutritional status of the elderly with under-nutrition sensitivity should be monitored regularly via scanning tests and anthropometric measures in order to prevent malnutrition. (Beck, Holst & Rasmussen, 2008). In this study, nutritional status of the elderly with AD staying in nursing homes was examined through MNA and some anthropometric measures.

In this research, it was found that the majority of the patients with AD (57.9%) were at risk of malnutrition, and that 19.3% were malnourished. These rates are considerably higher than rates found in the other countries, with prevalence of

Table 4. Spearman rank correlation coefficients for Quality of life (r)

Measurements	C-PQOL
Age (year)	0.011 (p=.938)
Sex	-0.084 (p=.0537)
Duration in Nursing Homes (year)	-0.246 (p=.066)
Body weight (kg)	0.289 (p=.029)*
BMI (kg/m^2)	0.243 (p=.069)
Waist circumference (cm)	0.203 (p=.131)
Waist/hips ratio (cm)	0.074 (p=.586)
Mid-upper arm circumference (cm)	0.226 (p=.091)
Calf circumference (cm)	0.340 (p=.010)*
MNA	0.239 (p=.073)
Energy consumption (kkal)	0.079 (p=.562)

*p<.05 indicate correlation between Quality of Life with Spearman rank correlation coefficient.

Table 5. Energy and nutrient intake of Alzheimer's patients not meeting and excess meeting RDA (%)

	Intake M(SD)	<67	67-133	133<	Intake, %RDA M(SD)
Energy (kkal)	1723.6±442.5	7.0	91.2	1.8	89.4±21.5
Protein (g)	55.2±14.1	10.5	87.7	1.8	97.3±23.3
Fat (g)	81.2±21.1	3.5	49.1	47.4	124.8±31.1
Carbohydrate (g)	188.9±66.4	49.1	49.1	1.8	68.6±22.5
Fiber (g)	18.8±4.9	42.1	57.9	-	63.1±16.9
Vitamin A (μg)	1060.5±593.3	10.5	56.1	33.3	132.2±73.3
Vitamin E (mg)	33.4±10.3	3.5	-	96.5	280.1±85.5*
Vitamin B_1 (mg)	0.7±0.2	49.1	50.9	-	71.2±21.5
Vitamin B_2 (mg)	1.2±0.5	17.5	56.1	26.3	104.6±44.1
Vitamin B_6 (mg)	1.3±0.3	7.0	68.4	24.6	113.3±29.3
Folat (mcg)	387.2±167.7	26.3	52.6	21.1	97.1±41.8
Vitamin C (mg)	181.9±86.2	7.0	28.1	64.9	179.7±90.4*
Sodium (mg)	1855.1±1323.6	40.4	52.6	7.0	84.4±38.9
Potassium (mg)	2146.5±618.1	63.2	36.8	-	61.8±17.2**
Calcium (mg)	811.6±467.9	52.6	26.3	21.1	81.7±46.2
Magnesium (mg)	214.9±56.2	43.9	56.1	-	69.4±16.8
Phosphor (mg)	964.4±287.6	-	50.9	49.1	138.1±39.9
Iron (mg)	5.9±1.9	82.5	17.5	-	55.0±13.6**
Zinc (mg)	7.1±1.9	8.8	73.7	17.5	103.4±26.8

*Mean intake significantly higher than RDA, p<.05, **Mean intake significantly lower than RDA, p<.05

malnourished 0.0-4.3 (Cuervo et al., 2009; Droogsma et al., 2013; Spaccavento et al., 2009), and different at risk of 14.1-79.5 (Cuervo et al., 2009; Droogsma et al., 2013; Guérin et al., 2005; Spaccavento et al., 2009; Vellas et al., 2005). In contrast with this, in the study of Khan et al. (2013), malnutrition ratio among AD patients were found higher (62%) while risk of malnutrition ratio was found lower (38%) than this study. Despite different prevalence, all these data show that there is a high prevalence of (risk of) malnutrition among AD patients. The differences in prevalence may be explained by variations in size and demographic characteristics of the research population. In addition, the facility differences between nursing homes, such as having special care units that may result in better clinical outcomes (Aukner, Eide & Iversen, 2013; Luo et al., 2010; Nobili et al., 2008) may have been effective on the occurrence of such different results. Finally, as one of the limitations in this study, the progression of the disease, which varied from one year (Ousset et al., 2008; Spaccavento et al., 2009) to five years (Gillioz et al., 2009), could be the reason for the variation seen in the prevalence. When a cross sex comparison is made, MNA scores of male are higher than those of female ($p<.05$,Table 2) where (risk of) malnutrition is more common among female (Table 1). This outcome could have been expected taking into account that female present higher under-nutrition prevalence than male (Cuervo et al., 2009; Kucukerdonmez et al., 2005; Vellas et al., 2005). It is already known that age is one of the indicators of the total MNA score and that it is in a negative correlation with MNA score (Cuervo et al., 2008; Sanlier & Yabanci, 2006). For this reason, as the age increases, MNA scores are expected to decrease. Considering that, although this study seems to be in accord with literature, the variation between values of mean ages is insignificant (Table 1). The fact that majority (59.6%) of the AD patients who participated the survey were placed in "old" category can explain the situation. Additionally, meanage for female (77.4±8.7 years) being higher than that of male (73.8±11.1 years) (data not show) may be one of the reasons why female's MNA scores were lower.

Although the exact mechanism of weight loss in AD patients has not been clarified, many hypothesis have been proposed including brain degeneration eliciting impairment of olfaction and taste, inadequate dietary intake, backhanded malabsorption of the nutrition, increased rate of energy expenditure, biological disturbances, atrophy of the part of the cerebral cortex and the presence of comorbid medical illness (Aukner, Eide & Iversen, 2013; Gillette-Guyonnet et al., 2000; Wang et al., 2004). Weight loss and malnutrition in the AD patients have serious negative health consequences, and it often leads to reduced quality of life (Aukner, Eide & Iversen, 2013; Gillette-Guyonnet et al., 2000). Although, in this study, the mean quality of life scores (26.0±5.8) of the well nourished AD patients were higher than those in malnutrition risk group (25.0±4.5) and malnourished group (23.3±3.8), the variation did not show a statistical significance (Table 1). This may have resulted from the fact that the assessment was based on the observations of caregivers. Moreover, including AD patients in different stages in the study, this group's being a fragile group and the inadequate number of participants in the study sample may have been the reasons why the correlation between quality of life and malnutrition could not be established in the study. When the quality of life scores are compared by sexes, it was seen that female and male had similar quality of life scores (Table 2). In other words, any significant correlation between quality of life and sex was not observed (Table 4). In Winter et al. (2011) conducted on patients with Alzheimer dementia, there was no association between quality of life and sex. In current research, age was not associated with quality of life (Table 4). This finding is consistent with previous literature (Chan et al., 2011; Lucas-Carrasco et al., 2010).

Similar toVellas et al (2005) and Spaccavento et al (2009) studies, in this study as well, as BMI decreases, risk of malnutrition and malnutrition status increases (Table 1). On the other hand, it can be seen that obesity (25.7%) among female and overweight (36.5%) among male are common according to BMI (Table 3), and that male have the mean BMI as 23.9±4.2 kg/m^2 whereas female have an mean of 25.0±4.90 kg/m^2 (Table 2). They may have been overweight or obese before the development of AD. Some studies show that a raised BMI in middle age can be associated with a higher risk of dementia (Kivipelto et al., 2005; Whitmer et al., 2005), and one research showed that in patients with AD, a worse psycho-functional status was associated with obesity (Saragat et al., 2012). In the Cuervo et al (2009) study, BMI is higher among female (28.1± 5.0) with AD patients compared to male (27.7± 4.1), as well. Cuervo et al (2009) and Droogsma et al (2013) found mean BMI of the individuals with AD higher than current study. The reason for this difference may be attributed to the fact that in the other study (Cuervo et al., 2009), individual's height and weight measures were taken self reportedly or that they were newly diagnosed AD (Droogsma et al., 2013). In fact, it is known that weight loss will occur as the stage of the disease increases (Goes et al., 2015). The relation between BMI and quality of life has been investigated in previous studies of elderly people, finding impaired quality of life in both obese and underweight individuals, with the highest quality of life in individuals of the BMI category 20–24.9 kg/m^2 (Groessl et al., 2004; Yan et al., 2004). In a cross-sectional population survey including 1.632 men and 1.654 women aged 65 to 87 years, it was found a significant reduction in quality of life with an increasing risk of malnutrition, and this was more pronounced in men than in women (Kvamme et al., 2011). In the present research, the mean quality of life score of those with an ideal weight (26.7±5.64) was higher than that of those who were overweight and obese (23.7±3.74), and the difference was statistically significant ($p<.05$, data not show). Furthermore, it was found that there was a positive correlation between body weight and quality of life and that this correlation was statistically significant (Table 4). Quality of life in obese individuals may be impaired by associated comorbid conditions, especially pain (Fontaine & Barofsky, 2001).

It is thought, in fact, that it will not be so correct to consider BMI solely in the evaluation of nutritional status since some physical qualities change with aging. For instance, height decreases as a result of vertebral compression. An accurate height measure may be difficult in those unable to stand up straight, the bed bound, those with spinal deformations such as a dowager's hump, and those with osteoporosis. For this reason, in this study, one of the reasons of high BMI despite high (risk of) malnutrition prevalence may be the measurement of height lower due to deformations emerging with aging. Moreover, since MNA tests have been lately inquiring information such as weight losses and food intake as well as present BMI values (Vellas et al, 1999; Guigoz, 2006), even a patient with high BMI might be under the risk of malnutrition or already malnourished. BMI based on questionable heights are inaccurate. Clinical judgment is needed for accuracy. Recent research showed that CC was the best, followed by MUAC and then BMI in predicting the nutritional status and health conditions. CC and MUAC were also more effective than BMI in predicting 12-month follow-up mortality (Tsai, Lai & Chang, 2012). Mid-arm circumference and CC reflect subcutaneous fat and body muscle mass and are influenced by both energy balance and local muscle activity such as arm movement and walking activity. MUAC and CC can decrease in size during functional decline or long-term inactivity even with adequate nutritional intake (Tsai, Lai & Chang, 2012). A calf circumference of <31 cm has been shown to correlate with muscle-related disability and self-reported physical function in elderly men and women (Loreck, Chimakurthi & Steinle, 2012). In this study, mean MUAC and calf circumference measures of both male and female were found similar (Table 2). It can be put forward that nutritional status of the AD patients examined in this study were not adequate according to MUAC and CC, therefore, that their muscle masses were not maintained and that compared to the AD patients examined in some other studies (Goes et al., 2015; Kucukerdonmez et al., 2006; Lecheta et al., 2015; Pivi et al., 2011; Taylor, Albanese & Stewart, 2012), they are in worse condition. Additionally, it was determined that the majority of both female and male AD patients were already malnourished according to MUAC ($<5^{th}$ p, Male: 45.5%, Female: 34.3%) or at malnutrition risk (≥5-<25, Male:36.4%, Female: 34.3%); however, a significant variation was not observed between sexes (Table 3). Although the number of overweight male and obese female are high in this study, lower MUAC and CC values give rise to the thought of sarcopenic obesity. The excess weight and decreased muscle mass together exponentially compound to further decrease in physical activity, which in turn accelerates sarcopenia. Lower physical activity may explain the muscle mass loss, being overweight and obese according to MUAC percentile values and CC measures. That is because maintaining muscle mass is strongly related with physical activity (Landi et al., 2012). On the other hand, an extremely sedentary lifestyle in obese persons is a major detractor from quality of life (Wellman & Kamp, 2008). These mentioned factors may also explain the reason why there was a significant positive correlation between CC and quality of life (Table 4). In this respect, while nutritional therapies in nursing homes are planned, individual-tailored nutrition strategies and physical activities should be considered.

Waist circumference and waist/hip ratio are risk signifiers for chronic diseases and metabolic complications. Waist circumference over 102 cm for men and over 88 cm for women is an indicator for high risk and excessive adiposity (Klein et al., 2007). Women with 0.8 and over waist/hip ratio and men with 1.0 and over waist/hip ratio are accepted as abdominal obese (de Portugal et al., 1997). In this study, although waist circumferences for both female and male were found similar (Table 2), it was determined that the majority of the female (42.9%) and 27.3% of the male were in high risk group in terms of metabolic diseases according to their waist circumference measures. The mean waist circumference value of the AD patients were lower compared to a cross-sectional study conducted with 15.022 participants with 65 and over age group from 7 different countries (Taylor, Albanese & Stewart, 2012) but higher when compared to Kucukerdonmez et al. study (2006). Waist/hip ratio measures indicated that a majority of the women (94.3%) were abdominal obese and that most of the male (77.3%) were normal ($p< .001$) (Table 3). It can be observed that aged women examined in this study undergo abdominal adiposity and are under high risk of chronic diseases according to waist circumference and waist/hip ratios values. In the research (So, 2014) conducted to explore the impact of differential degrees of obesity on health-related quality of life (HRQL) by sex in the Korean elderly, it was found that whereas higher WC quintiles impaired mobility, usual activities, and caused pain/discomfort in women, the fourth WC quintile improved usual activities in men. It was also revealed that after adjustment, only the women of the highest WC quintile reported impaired mobility. As a conclusion, it was stated that extreme obesity worsens mobility and comorbidity in combination with obesity worsening health-related quality of life in elderly women. In this study, any statistical correlation was not found between waist circumference, waist/hip ratio and quality of life (Table 4). According to various anthropometric measures (BMI, waist circumference, waist/hip ratio), it can be observed that among female AD patients participated in this study, obesity ratio was higher than that of male (Table 3). It can be maintained that this stems from less physical activity among female, increased adiposity after menopause, more pronounced height loss among female due to menopause and decrease in the bone mineral density and the fact that increased BMI after middle ages becomes stable earlier among male than female. Due to malnutrition occurrence according to MUAC as well as overweight, obesity and abdominal obesity being common after various anthropometric measures among AD patients, many parameters are strongly suggested to be used including biochemical parameters while evaluating body weight and disease risk status of the aged individuals.

It was observed in this study that length of stay in nursing homes also had an effect on nutritional status. It was determined that comparing to well nourished ones (1.7±0.6 years), those under malnutrition risk (2.8±1.4 years, $p<.05$) and those already malnourished (2.1±1.2 years) had been in the homes longer (Table 1). Higher (risk of) malnutrition among those who stay in the homes longer has been reported by various studies (Kuzu-Kurban et al., 2010; Vellas et al., 2005). This fact gives rise to the opinion that as the length of stay increases, prevalence of malnutrition will also increase among the AD patients examined in this study. Hence, it is important to obtain an accurate nutritional assessment at an early stage of AD to ensure that the dietary needs of each patient are supplied and thus avoid the occurrence of unwanted weight loss. Especially frequent snacks, nutrient-dense foods, and nutrition supplements are needed to combat weight loss. Likewise, behavior modification and the use of altered food choices can improve quality of life (Remig & Weeden, 2008).When the relationship between the length of stay in nursing homes and quality of life was examined, a negative correlation was observed although it was not statistically significant (Table 4). Khader (2011), conducted to assess the quality of life (QOL) as perceived by 140 selected elderly people living in 3 public nursing homes in Jordan, showed also that length of stay in the nursing home was negatively associated with quality of life. Furthermore, in the research (Khader, 2011), it was found that elder people staying in the nursing home 3 years and less had higher quality of life scores. Taking into consideration that daily activities are an important factor that affects quality of life (Low & Molzahn, 2007; Paskulin & Molzahn, 2007), the fact that participants had AD; therefore, were unable to joint leisure activities at nursing homes may be attributed to why this correlation was not found statistically significant in this study.

Food and nutrition is another factor that contributes to quality of life. Adequate and balanced diet play a profound role in leading a quality life. Inadequate nutrient intake may hasten loss of muscle mass and strength, which can have a negative effect on performing activities of daily life (Wellman & Kamp, 2008). A constant change in nutritional habits is generally thought to be related with AD. In the later phases of the disease, anorexia may emerge and support the related weight loss. Possible causes can be given as physical changes such as, worsened taste and smell functions, decreased appetite related to a decline in endogenous opioids, and increased satiety related to an increase in sensitivity to cholecystokinin, neuropsychiatric disorders related to the disease such as, memory loss, disorientation, mood disorders, indifference, and impaired judgment, a change in autonomy and dietary behaviours, or changes in neurotransmitter concentrations such as, neuropeptide Y and norepinephrine (Gillette-Guyonnet et al., 2000). Inadequate and/or imbalanced energy and nutrient intake may occur in such cases. In fact, each factor, nutritional status or food consumption related to nutrition, plays an important role in quality of life of the elderly (Kvamme et al., 2011). Regarding energy intake, 91.2% of the patients presented adequate consumption, according to the RDA. While these results support some of the previously çonducted studies (Winograd et al., 1991; Kucukerdonmez et al, 2006), compared to Lecheta et al (2015), energy and protein intake in most AD patients was inadequate. Since energy expenditures were not inquired in this study, an outcome could not be reached regarding the relationship between the (risk of) malnutrition and energy balances, highly observed among these patients. However, regarding their BMI, it can be estimated that their physical activities are low. It has been suggested that patients with AD may lose weight even though they have a positive energy balance (Dvorak & Poehlman, 1998). In this context, these data corroborate other authors that show that weight reduction can be found in patients with AD in spite of their adequate energy intake (Gillette-Guyonnet et al., 2000; Goes et al., 2014; White et al., 2004). It is not known exactly what causes weight loss in patients with AD, however, as explained previously, several hypotheses have been proposed to explain this phenomenon, such as Mesial Temporal Cortex (CTM) atrophy, which is involved with diet; increased energy needs; and organic disorders (Aukner, Eide & Iversen, 2013; Gillette-Guyonnet et al., 2000; Wang et al., 2004). Reviewing literature, any study looking into the relationship between energy intakes of the individuals with AD and quality of life could not be detected. Nor, in this study, could a relationship between energy intakes of the individuals with AD and quality of life be observed. Mostly adequate energy intake among the elderly may be the reason. In addition to low energy intake in old ages, declining in daily growth hormone secretion by 29-70% may lead to sarcopenia (Corpas, Harman & Blackman, 1993). Sarcopenia is an entity which is associated with functional decline, disability, falls and mortality. Despite many underlying factors in its aetiology,resistance training and nutrition is the only treatment yet known of sarcopenia (Tasoglu & Ozgirgin, 2013). Considering the relationship between low energy intake and sarcopenia, it is thought that there could be an indirect relationship between low energy intake and life quality.

As for individual's macronutrient intakes, it was determined that protein intakes of the majority (87.7%) were adequate, fat intakes were high (47.4%), and carbohydrate intakes were low (49.1%) (Table 5). Moreover, 13.4±2.8% of the energy was taken from protein, 42.2±6.1% of it from fat and 44.2±7.3% of it from carbohydrates (data not shown). Depending on this, it can be claimed that macronutrient intakes were imbalanced. For this reason, keeping the energy content, better rearrangement of the dietary pattern (carbohydrate, protein, fat distribution), decreasing fat content while increasing carbohydrate content with the condition of emphasising complex carbohydrate contents in the menus offered to this patient group can be suggested as a necessity. That is because of the fact that not only adequate protein intake and maintaining nitrogen balance for the AD patients who are at the risk of (malnutrition) are important for bodily functions, cognitive functions and immune system (Volkert & Sieber, 2011; Suominen et al., 2015), but also when the carbohydrates do not meet the majority (55-60%) of the energy needs, proteins taken by diet will be used as fuel primarilyto meet energy demand as well (Gallagher, 2012). In addition to this, it should be paid attention to the fact that fat content of diet should be between 25-30%, and over-restrictions should also be avoided within the framework of healthy diet principles. That is also because severe restriction of dietary fats alters taste, texture, and enjoyment of food, which can affect overall diet, weight, and quality of life negatively (Wellman & Kamp, 2008).

It also stood out in this study that 42.1% of the individuals did not consume adequate fiber (Table 5). Current recommendations are for the consumption of approximately 24 to 38 g of dietary fiber per day from fruits, vegetables, legumes, seeds, and whole grains for (1) maintaining the health of the cells lining the colon, (2) preventing excessive intracolonic pressure, (3) preventing constipation, and (4) maintaining a stable and healthful microbial population (Beyer, 2012). Low fiber intakes among AD patients in this study may be attributed to inadequate fruit and vegetable intakes.

The nutrient intakes of older AD persons tend to decrease over time (Shatenstein, Kergoat & Reid, 2007). On the other hand, the patients' food intake was found to be similar throughout the different stages of the disease (Goes et al, 2015). In this research, a high percentage of patients presented an inadequate intake of some micronutrients (Table 5). A majority of the participants indicated inadequate calcium and iron consumption similar to those in Lecheta et.al. (2015) study. However, calcium intake is very important for maintaining bone mineral density and lowering blood pressure (Gallagher, 2012). Main and between-meals should include dairy products which are rich in calcium and patients should be monitored for consumption. Similarly, an adequate iron intake is essential for the normal function of the immune system. Iron deficiencies result in changes in the immune response (Gallagher, 2012). The subcommittee recommends the same amount of iron RDA for elderly women and men as 10 mg/day (RDA, 1989). Since changes in iron metabolism occur in Alzheimer disease (Gallagher, 2012), amount of iron intake within diet should be paid attention, not to be consumed either less or more. What is more, it was also observed that intakes of antioxidants such as vitamin A, C, and E, known as useful at decreasing oxidative stress which plays an important role on Alzheimer's pathology, were over RDA recommendations. This outcome is surprising as it does not corroborate the other study results (Goes et al., 2014; Lecheta et al., 2015). The high amount of intakes of this group of nutrient among AD patients in this study may be ascribed to enteral nutrition support rather than oral intake. According to Lecheta et.al. (2015), on the other hand, the higher percentage of patients with adequate intake of vitamin A, vitamin C and calcium in severe stage of dementia may be due to the fact that their diets are more often chosen by caregivers, who probably select food of better nutritional quality. It is important to monitor the consumption of these substances since they can act as neuroprotective factors, preventing or slowing the progress of AD (Goes et al., 2014).

The prevailing factors in dementia and Alzheimer's disease are micronutrient and macronutrient deficiency, and it is a fact that undernourishment causes profound outcomes for health, quality of life and survival. Even though, with its many complex-structured causes, loss of body weight is regarded as expected result of the condition, it still needs intervention (Pirince et al., 2014). When adequate energy and balanced nutrient intake among AD patients or the frail elderly is not provided, simple preventative measures such as food supplementation can be effective in stopping and reversing progressive weight loss (Gray-Donald, Payette & Boutier, 1995). Likewise, in Laugueet al. (2004), it was established that 3 months after enteral nutrition therapy of AD patients 65 and over years of age at malnutrition risk, energy and protein intakes significantly improved, resulting in a significant increase in weight and fat free mass. One study of AD patients found that oral nutritional supplementation was more effective compared to nutrition education in improving nutritional status (Pivi et al., 2011). Therefore, it is better for patients with Alzheimer's disease live in special care units since these patients usually have deteriorating eating disorders and health professionals in this field can give them specialized care there. Gillette-Guyonnet et al. (2000) indicated that >40% of AD patients lost significant amounts of weight despite living at home. However, problems with feeding AD patients are related not only to the quantity, but also to the quality of foods consumed (Greenwood et al., 2005). In general, the AD patients who participated in this research seemed to consume enough energy and macronutrients. Still, most of them did not consume adequate quantities of thiamine, which plays a major role in energy metabolism, and other essential nutrients (potassium, calcium, magnesium, phosphorus and iron). This revealed that their diet patterns were sufficient, yet imbalanced. For all these reasons, the diets of individuals with Alzheimer's disease should be prepared by dieticians to ensure that they get sufficient, well-balanced nutrition, that they do not lose weight, that they have a reduced risk of malnutrition and that associated complications are either prevented or mitigated. The nursing homes where data of this research were collected did not employ any dieticians.

It could be argued that measuring quality of life is just as important as measuring severity and progression of the disease, symptom response, cognition, behavioral disturbance and activities of daily living when assessing the effects of the disease and intervention in dementia (Walker, Salek & Bayer, 1998). This research aimed to determine the quality of life of patients with AD staying in private nursing homes based on the assessments of those who gave primary care to these patients. Although the research did not find a significant correlation between quality of life and the consumption of energy and nutrients, it has a significant outcome that the mean quality of life scores of those with an ideal weight were higher than those of the overweight and obese participants. This shows that ideal weight, an important indicator of nutritional status of AD patients, is correlated with quality of life. Although there are studies of nutritional status (Faxen-Irving, 2002; Goes, 2015) and of quality of life (Kuzu-Kurban et al., 2010) in the relevant literature, there are few studies on the correlation between nutritional status and the quality of life (De Sousa & do Amaral, 2014).

SOLUTIONS AND RECOMMENDATIONS

One of the most important results of this study was the high malnutrition and the risk of malnutrition prevalence and imbalanced nutrientsintake among AD patients. In this context, it should be especially highlighted that in the process of the disease, diet influences the nutritional and clinical course of patients and thus, nutritional intervention should be early, appropriate and carried out by qualified dieticians. Early detection of poor nutritional status, and its causes, is crucial for adequate intervention to prevent or diminish the adverse outcomes. Regular scanning and evaluation for the nutritional status of the elderly AD patients, who are sensitive to inadequate nutrition is an essential necessity. However, although the significance in the monitoring the nutritional status is well understood, there have yet been no regulations regarding this at nursing homes in Turkey. It is suggestible that dieticians be employed at nursing homes in order that general and medical nutrition needs of the elderly can be understood better. This is because dieticians are common elements in the teams that will implement algorithms designed to prevent, identify and cure malnutrition among the elderly. Moreover, it is also that they also take place in the core of interdisciplinary team (geriatrists, nurses, dieticians, social workers, psychologists, physiotherapists, occupational therapists) that carry out comprehensive geriatric evaluations. For this reason, so as to prevent and treat malnutrition at nursing homes, it is a necessity that nutrition support teams including dieticians be established, and regular in-service training programs be given in order that the quality of workers in health and nutrition services improved. There have also been various studies claiming that some training programs aiming at caregivers of AD patients may lead to a positive influence on AD patients, improving their body weight, cognitive qualities (Riviere et al., 2001), nutritional and immune status

(Pivi et al., 2011) and lower the risk of malnutrition (Salva et al., 2011) in older individuals with dementia.

On the other hand, compliance of AD patients with the treatment, and supporting families of the patients (if any) in the process psychosocially are crucial to ease the treatment process and make it more effective in shorter period. Furthermore, in order that the members of the professional team working with these patients could evaluate disease related risk factors and outcomes in a more holistic point of view, the significance of micro, mezzo and macro level interventions are obvious. It should be kept in mind that social workers occupy an important place in such intervention processes

FUTURE RESEARCH DIRECTIONS

The research also had limitations as in almost research studies. One limitation of this research was that the sample contained only 57 older patients with AD living in nursing homes in Ankara/Turkey. In this research, this was because owners of other nursing homes except for owners of two private nursing homes in Ankara didn't give permission to conduct the research and the sample was limited to 57 older people with AD from two nursing homes giving permission to carry out the research.

Another limitation of the research was that information about older patients with AD was collected from their primary caregivers because they lacked sufficient cognitive skills. Therefore, data about nutritional status and quality of life of 57 aged individuals in the scope of the study were limited by the answers taken from their primary caregivers. At this point, it is believed that a remake of the study with a larger sample will provide enough evidence-based information for the improvement in the health of aged AD patients and for the treatment of the disease.

Additionally, this study aiming at determining the relationship between nutritional status/nutrientintake and quality of life of AD patients is important as it contributes to fill the gap present in literature in Turkey. In this study, no significant correlation between quality of life and the consumption of energy and nutrients was observed. However, it determined a significant correlation between body weight/calf circumference and quality of life among aged AD patients. In this research, the indicators for their quality of life was evaluated in the scope of 13 items concerning physical health, energy, mood, living situation, memory, family, marriage, friends, you as a whole, ability to do chores, ability to do things for fun, money, and life as a whole. Yet, it should be stated that quality of life for AD patients aged individuals is a multidimensional concept including these subjective and objective indicators and that quality of life of the participants of this study might have been affected by different factors influencing quality of life (stage of disease, stay in special unit care etc.) apart from these indicators. For this reason, it can be suggested to the future scholars to focus especially on unmet care needs for the treatments of aged AD patients staying at nursing homes. That is because not addressing those needs may cause not only the emergence of new problem areas for dementia patients such as new needs, behavioural symptoms, psychological problems such as anxiety and depression (Kovach et al. 2005), but also increase the work load of the caregivers as well as increased risk of mortality among such patients (Gaugler et al., 2005). In this sense, it can be put forward that planning studies aiming at determining unmet care needs of the dementia patients has a profound significance for their treatments.

Most studies on patients with Alzheimer's type dementia focus on cognition. These patients will, however, in time, present other complications of the illness such as nutritional problems. These problems with the nutritional status, weight loss, inadequate, and imbalanced intake of nutrients observed in the patients with AD, highlight the importance of nutritional care and interventions regarding mealtime difficulties, an aspect relevant to the clinical nursing practice with AD patients. In this context, there is a necessity for raising awareness on nutrition education and for longitudinal studies indicating effects of regular training on the prognosis of the disease and nutritional status of the patients. It is not yet well established in these studies whether weight loss and inadequate nourishment in dementia patients brings about more accelerated progression of the disease,disability, institutionalization and death, or itis just an indicator of natural process of the disease. Observing the effects of nutritional interventions in people with dementia may solve the problem via in randomised controlled attempts. Yet, nutritional interventions will be the most beneficial if they slow down the progression of the disease and increase the quality of life

CONCLUSION

As a result, in this study, the ratios of the ones at risk of malnutrition and those already malnourished among AD patients were found quite high. However, it was also found that majority of the patients were normal according to BMI, in normal group in terms of metabolic diseases according to waist circumference, and below 5th. percentile according to mid-upper arm circumferences. When the relationship between nutritional status indicators and quality of life was examined only body weight and calf circumference were found significantly correlated with quality of life. The mean quality of life score of those with ideal weight was higher than overweight and obese individuals and it was found significant statistically. It was also found that the length of stay in nursing homes had an effect on quality of life. In addition, it was reached in the conclusion that AD patients were fed inadequate and imbalanced.

REFERENCES

Akpinar, B., & Kucukguclu, O. (2012). The validity and reliability of the Turkish version of the quality of life scale for patients with Alzheimer's disease (QOL-AD). *Journal of the Neurological Sciences*, *29*(3), 554–565.

Akyar, I., & Akdemir, N. (2009). Alzheimer hastalarına bakım verenlerin yaşadıkları güçlükler[strains of caregivers of Alzheimer patients]. *Sağlık Bilimleri Fakültesi Hemşirelik Dergisi*, *16*(3), 32–49.

Aukner, C., Eide, H. D., & Iversen, P. O. (2013). Nutritional status among older residents with dementia in open versus special care units in municipal nursing homes: An observational study. *BMC Geriatrics*, *13*(1), 26–32. doi:10.1186/1471-2318-13-26 PMID:23496975

Beck, A. M., Holst, M., & Rasmussen, H. H. (2008). Efficacy of the Mini Nutritional Assessment to predict the risk of developing malnutrition or adverse health outcomes for old people. *e-SPEN, the European e-Journal of Clinical Nutrition and Metabolism*, *3*(3), e102-e107.

Beyer, P. L. (2012). Intake: Digestion, absorption, transport, and excretion of nutrients. In L. K. Mahan, S. Escott-Stump, & J. L. Raymond (Eds.), *Krause's food & the nutrition care process* (pp. 1–18). Elsevier Health Sciences.

Chan, I. W. P., Chu, L. W., Lee, P. W., Li, S. W., & Yu, K. K. (2011). Effects of cognitive function and depressive mood on the quality of life in Chinese Alzheimer's disease patients in Hong Kong. *Geriatrics & Gerontology International*, *11*(1), 69–76. doi:10.1111/j.1447-0594.2010.00643.x PMID:20738410

Corpas, E., Harman, S. M., & Blackman, M. R. (1993). Human growth hormone and human aging. *Endocrine Reviews*, *14*(1), 20–39. doi:10.1210/edrv-14-1-20 PMID:8491152

Cuervo, M., Ansorena, D., García, A., Astiasaran, I., & Martinez, J. A. (2008). Food consumption analysis in spanish elderly based upon the mini nutritional assessment test. *Annals of Nutrition & Metabolism*, *52*(4), 299–307. doi:10.1159/000151483 PMID:18714147

Cuervo, M., Ansorena, D., Martínez-González, M. A., García, A., Astiasarán, I., & Martínez, J. A. (2009). Impact of global and subjective mini nutritional assessment (MNA) questions on the evaluation of the nutritional status: The role of gender and age. *Archives of Gerontology and Geriatrics*, *49*(1), 69–73. doi:10.1016/j.archger.2008.05.003 PMID:18573549

de Portugal, A. J., de Portugal, F., Rivera, B. L., Chimpén, R. V., González, S. M. F., & Sánchez, R. A. Waist/hip ratio and vascular risk factors in obese and not obese individuals. Anales de Medicina Interna, 14(1), 3-8.

de Sousa, O. L. V., & do Amaral, T. F. (2014). LB014-MON: Quality of life and nutritional status in moderate Alzheimer's disease patients. *Clinical Nutrition (Edinburgh, Lothian)*, *33*(1), S256. doi:10.1016/S0261-5614(14)50672-3

Droogsma, E., Van Asselt, D. Z. B., Scholzel-Dorenbos, C. J. M., Van Steijn, J. H. M., Van Walderveen, P. E., & Van Der Hooft, C. S. (2013). Nutritional status of community-dwelling elderly with newly diagnosed Alzheimer's disease: Prevalence of malnutrition and the relation of various factors to nutritional status. *The Journal of Nutrition, Health & Aging*, *17*(7), 606–610. doi:10.1007/s12603-013-0032-9 PMID:23933871

Dvorak, R. V., & Poehlman, E. T. (1998). Appendicular skeletal muscle mass, physical activity, and cognitive status in patients with Alzheimer's disease. *Neurology*, *51*(5), 1386–1390. doi:10.1212/WNL.51.5.1386 PMID:9818865

Elia, M., Jones, B., & Russell, C. (2008). Malnutrition in various care settings in the UK: The 2007 nutrition screening week survey. *Clinical Medicine*, *8*(4), 364–365. doi:10.7861/clinmedicine.8-4-364 PMID:18724599

Faxen-Irving, G., Andren-Olsson, B., Geijerstam, A. A., Basun, H., & Cederholm, T. (2002). Original Communications-The effect of nutritional intervention in elderly subjects residing in group-living for the demented. *European Journal of Clinical Nutrition*, *56*(3), 221–227. doi:10.1038/sj.ejcn.1601304 PMID:11960297

Ferri, C. P., Prince, M., Brayne, C., Brodaty, H., Fratiglioni, L., Ganguli, M., & Scazufca, M. et al. (2005). Global prevalence of dementia: A Delphi consensus study. *Lancet*, *366*(9503), 2112–2117. doi:10.1016/S0140-6736(05)67889-0 PMID:16360788

Fontaine, K. R., & Barofsky, I. (2001). Obesity and health-related quality of life. *Obesity Reviews*, *2*(3), 173–182. doi:10.1046/j.1467-789x.2001.00032.x PMID:12120102

Frisancho, A. R. (1999). *Anthropometric standards for the assesment of growth and nutritional status*. The University of Michigan Press.

Gallagher, M. L. (2012). Intake: The nutrients and their metabolism. In L. K. Mahan, S. Escott-Stump, & J. L. Raymond (Eds.), *Krause's food & the nutrition care process* (pp. 32–128). Elsevier Health Sciences.

Garry, P. J., & Vellas, B. J. (1996). Aging and nutrition. In E. E. Ziegler & L. J. Filer Jr., (Eds.), *Present knowledge in nutrition* (pp. 414–419). Washington, DC: ILSI Press.

Gaugler, J. E., Kane, R. L., Kane, R. A., & Newcomer, R. (2005). Unmet care needs and key outcomes in dementia. *Journal of the American Geriatrics Society*, *53*(12), 2098–2105. doi:10.1111/j.1532-5415.2005.00495.x PMID:16398893

Gillette-Guyonnet, S., Lauque, S., & Ousset, P. J. (2005). Nutrition and Alzheimer's disease. *Psychologie & Neuropsychiatrie du Vieillissement*, *3*, S35–S41. PMID:15899603

Gillette-Guyonnet, S., Nourhashémi, F., Andrieu, S., de Glisezinski, I., Ousset, P. J., Rivière, D., & Vellas, B. (2000). Weight loss in Alzheimer disease. *The American Journal of Clinical Nutrition*, *71*(2), 637s–642s. PMID:10681272

Gillioz, A. S., Villars, H., Voisin, T., Cortes, F., Gillette-Guyonnet, S., Andrieu, S., & Vellas, B. (2009). Spared and impaired abilities in community-dwelling patients entering the severe stage of Alzheimer's disease. *Dementia and Geriatric Cognitive Disorders*, *28*(5), 412–417. doi:10.1159/000255635 PMID:19907179

Goes, V. F., Horst, J. A. E., Paganini, J. C. D. A., da Silva, W. C. F. N., Khalil, N. M., & Bonini, J. S. (2015). Nutritional status and food intake of Brazilian patients at various stages of Alzheimer's disease: A cross-sectional study. *Revista de Ciências Farmacêuticas Básica e Aplicada*, *35*(2), 211–215.

Goes, V. F., Mello-Carpes, P. B., Oliveira, L. O. D., Hack, J., Magro, M., & Bonini, J. S. (2014). Evaluation of dysphagia risk, nutritional status and caloric intake in elderly patients with Alzheimer's. *Revista Latino-Americana de Enfermagem*, *22*(2), 317–324. doi:10.1590/0104-1169.3252.2418 PMID:26107841

Gray-Donald, K., Payette, H., & Boutier, V. (1995). Randomized clinical trial of nutritional supplementation shows little effect on functional status among free-living frail elderly. *The Journal of Nutrition*, *125*(12), 2965–2971. PMID:7500174

Greenwood, C. E., Tam, C., Chan, M., Young, K. W., Binns, M. A., & Van Reekum, R. (2005). Behavioral disturbances, not cognitive deterioration, are associated with altered food selection in seniors with Alzheimer's disease. *The Journals of Gerontology. Series A, Biological Sciences and Medical Sciences*, *60*(4), 499–505. doi:10.1093/gerona/60.4.499 PMID:15933391

Groessl, E. J., Kaplan, R. M., Barrett-Connor, E., & Ganiats, T. G. (2004). Body mass index and quality of well-being in a community of older adults. *American Journal of Preventive Medicine*, *26*(2), 126–129. doi:10.1016/j.amepre.2003.10.007 PMID:14751323

Guérin, O., Andrieu, S., Schneider, S. M., Milano, M., Boulahssass, R., Brocker, P., & Vellas, B. (2005). Different modes of weight loss in Alzheimer disease: A prospective study of 395 patients. *The American Journal of Clinical Nutrition*, *82*(2), 435–441. PMID:16087990

Guigoz, Y. (2006). The Mini Nutritional Assessment (MNA) review of the literature-what does it tell us? *The Journal of Nutrition, Health & Aging*, *10*(6), 466–485. PMID:17183419

Gurvit, H., Emre, M., Tinaz, S., Bilgic, B., Hanagasi, H., Sahin, H., & Harmanci, H. (2008). The prevalence of dementia in an urban Turkish population. *American Journal of Alzheimer's Disease and Other Dementias*, *23*(1), 67–76. doi:10.1177/1533317507310570 PMID:18276959

Gurvit, H. I. (2004). Demans sendromu. [Dementia syndrome]. In S. Z. Bahar & A. E. Öge (Eds.), *Alzheimer hastalığı ve Alzheimer dışı Demanslar* [Alzheimer's disease and non-Alzheimer's dementias] (pp. 367–415). İstanbul: Nobel Tıp Kitabevleri. (in Turkish)

Khader, F. (2011). Quality of life in the nursing homes in Jordan: Perspectives of residents. *Care Management Journals*, *12*(4), 149–162. doi:10.1891/1521-0987.12.4.169 PMID:23214238

Khan, F., Risheh, N. A. A., Al-Neghaimshi, H. S., Alhomaidhi, N. A., Siddiqui, A. A., Al-Muammar, M. N., & Adewole, A. H. (2013). Assessment of nutritional status of alzheimer patients in Riyadh, Saudi Arabia. *International Journal of Health Sciences and Research*, *3*(4), 1–10.

Kivipelto, M., Ngandu, T., Fratiglioni, L., Viitanen, M., Kåreholt, I., Winblad, B., & Nissinen, A. (2005). Obesity and vascular risk factors at midlife and the risk of dementia and Alzheimer disease. *Archives of Neurology*, *62*(10), 1556–1560. doi:10.1001/archneur.62.10.1556 PMID:16216938

Klein, S., Allison, D. B., Heymsfield, S. B., Kelley, D. E., Leibel, R. L., Nonas, C., & Kahn, R. (2007). Waist circumference and cardiometabolic risk: a consensus statement from shaping America's health: Association for weight management and obesity prevention; NAASO, the Obesity Society; the American Society for Nutrition; and the American Diabetes Association. *The American Journal of Clinical Nutrition*, *85*(5), 1197–1202. PMID:17490953

Knupfer, L., & Spiegel, R. (1986). Differences in olfactory test performance between normal aged, Alzheimer and vascular type dementia individuals. *International Journal of Geriatric Psychiatry*, *1*(1), 3–14. doi:10.1002/gps.930010103

Kovach, C. R., Noonan, P. E., Schlidt, A. M., & Wells, T. (2005). A model of consequences of need-driven, dementia-compromised behavior. *Journal of Nursing Scholarship*, *37*(2), 134–140. doi:10.1111/j.1547-5069.2005.00025_1.x PMID:15960057

Kucukerdonmez, O., Koksal, E., Rakicioglu, N., & Pekcan, G. (2005). Assessment and evaluation of the nutritional status of the elderly using 2 different instruments. *Saudi Medical Journal*, *26*(10), 1611–1616. PMID:16228066

Kucukerdonmez, O., Rakıcıoglu, N., Eroglu, E., Portakal, O., & Ayaz, S. (2006). Alzheimer tipi senil demanslı hastalarda beslenme durumunun değerlendirilmesi[The determination of nutritional status of patients with Alzheimer type senil dementia]. *Beslenme ve Diyet Dergisi*, *34*(1), 11–22.

Kuzu-Kurban, N., Zencir, M., Kartal, A., & Şahiner, T. (2010). Alzheimer hastal ığıolanveolmayanyaşlıbireylerinyaşamkalitesivedepresyondüzeylerininkarşılaştırı lması[Comparison of quality of life and depression levels of elderly persons with Alzheimer's disease and not]. *Yaşlı Sorunları Arastırma Dergisi*, *1*, 34–43.

Kvamme, J. M., Olsen, J. A., Florholmen, J., & Jacobsen, B. K. (2011). Risk of malnutrition and health-related quality of life in community-living elderly men and women: The Tromsø study. *Quality of Life Research: An International Journal of Quality of Life Aspects of Treatment, Care and Rehabilitation*, *20*(4), 575–582. doi:10.1007/s11136-010-9788-0 PMID:21076942

Landi, F., Liperoti, R., Fusco, D., Mastropaolo, S., Quattrociocchi, D., Proia, A., & Onder, G. (2012). Prevalence and risk factors of sarcopenia among nursing home older residents. *The Journals of Gerontology. Series A, Biological Sciences and Medical Sciences*, *67*(1), 48–55. doi:10.1093/gerona/glr035 PMID:21393423

Lauque, S., Arnaud-Battandier, F., Gillette, S., Plaze, J. M., Andrieu, S., Cantet, C., & Vellas, B. (2004). Improvement of weight and fat-free mass with oral nutritional supplementation in patients with Alzheimer's disease at risk of malnutrition: A prospective randomized study. *Journal of the American Geriatrics Society*, *52*(10), 1702–1707. doi:10.1111/j.1532-5415.2004.52464.x PMID:15450048

Lecheta, D. R., Schieferdecker, M. M., de Mello, A. P., Berkenbrock, I., Neto, J. C., & Maluf, E. P. (2015). Dietary inadequacies in the elderly with Alzhimer's disease followed at the reference health center for elderly care in Curitiba-Brazil. *Journal of Aging Clinical Practice*, *4*(2), 85–91.

Lee, R. D., & Nieman, D. C. (2003). Assessment of the hospitalized patient. In R. D. Lee & D. C. Nieman (Eds.), *Nutritional Assessment* (pp. 216–250). New York: McGraw Hill.

Loreck, E., Chimakurthi, R., & Steinle, N. I. (2012). Nutritional assessment of the geriatric patient: A comprehensive approach toward evaluating and managing nutrition. *Clinical Geriatrics*, *20*(4), 20–26.

Low, G., & Molzahn, A. E. (2007). Predictors of quality of life in old age: A cross-validation study. *Research in Nursing & Health*, *30*(2), 141–150. doi:10.1002/nur.20178 PMID:17380515

Lucas-Carrasco, R., Lamping, D. L., Banerjee, S., Rejas, J., Smith, S. C., & Gómez-Benito, J. (2010). Validation of the Spanish version of the DEMQOL system. *International Psychogeriatrics*, *22*(04), 589–597. doi:10.1017/S1041610210000207 PMID:20447322

Luo, H., Fang, X., Liao, Y., Elliott, A., & Zhang, X. (2010). Associations of special care units and outcomes of residents with dementia: 2004 national nursing home survey. *The Gerontologist*, *50*(4), 509–518. doi:10.1093/geront/gnq035 PMID:20462932

Nobili, A., Piana, I., Balossi, L., Pasina, L., Matucci, M., Tarantola, M., & Tettamanti, M. (2008). Alzheimer special care units compared with traditional nursing home for dementia care: Are there differences at admission and in clinical outcomes? *Alzheimer Disease and Associated Disorders*, *22*(4), 352–361. doi:10.1097/WAD.0b013e31818207d0 PMID:18978601

Nourhashemi, F., Ousset, P. J., Guyonnet, S., Andrieu, S., Rolland, Y., Adoue, D. & Albarède, J. L. (2000). *La Revue de medecine interne/fondee... par la Societe nationale francaise de medecine interne* [Alzheimer's disease: from pathology to preventive methods?]. Academic Press. (in French)

Ousset, P. J., Nourhashemi, F., Reynish, E., & Vellas, B. (2008). Nutritional status is associated with disease progression in very mild Alzheimer disease. *Alzheimer Disease and Associated Disorders*, *22*(1), 66–71. doi:10.1097/WAD.0b013e31815a9dbb PMID:18317249

Paskulin, L. M. G., & Molzahn, A. (2007). Quality of life of older adults in Canada and Brazil. *Western Journal of Nursing Research*, *29*(1), 10–26. doi:10.1177/0193945906292550 PMID:17228059

Pivi, G. A., da Silva, R. V., Juliano, Y., Novo, N. F., Okamoto, I. H., Brant, C. Q., & Bertolucci, P. H. (2011). A prospective study of nutrition education and oral nutritional supplementation in patients with Alzheimer's disease. *Nutrition Journal*, *10*(98), 1–6. PMID:21943331

Prince, M., Albanese, E., Guerchet, M., & Prina, M. (2014). Nutrition and dementia. A review of available research. London: Alzheimer's Disease International (ADI).

Rakıcıoglu, N., Tek, N., Ayaz, A., & Pekcan, G. (2009). Yemek ve besin fotoğraf kataloğu: Ölçü ve miktarlar. Ankara: Ata Ofset Matbaacılık. (in Turkish)

RDA/Recommended Dietary Allowances. (1989). Subcommittee on the tenth edition of the RDAs food and nutrition board commission on life sciences.Washington, DC: National Academy Press.

Remig, V. M., & Weeden, A. (2008). Medical nutrition therapy for neurologic disorders. In L. K. Mahan & S. E. Stump (Eds.), *Krause's food and nutrition therapy* (pp. 923–955). Toronto: Saunders Elsevier.

Riviere, S., Gillette-Guvonnet, S., Voisin, T., Reynish, E., Andrieu, S., Lauque, S., & Micas, M. (2001). A nutritional education program could prevent weight loss and slow cognitive decline in Alzheimer's disease. *The Journal of Nutrition, Health & Aging*, *5*(4), 295–299. PMID:11753499

Salva, A., Andrieu, S., Fernandez, E., Schiffrin, E. J., Moulin, J., Decarli, B., & Vellas, B. (2011). Health and nutrition promotion program for patients with dementia (NutriAlz): Cluster randomized trial. *The Journal of Nutrition, Health & Aging*, *15*(10), 822–830. doi:10.1007/s12603-011-0363-3 PMID:22159768

Sanlier, N., & Yabanci, N. (2006). Mini nutritional assessment in the elderly: Living alone, with family, a nursing home in Turkey. *Nutrition & Food Science*, *36*(1), 50–58. doi:10.1108/00346650610642197

Saragat, B., Buffa, R., Mereu, E., Succa, V., Cabras, S., Mereu, R. M., & Marini, E. (2012). Nutritional and psycho-functional status in elderly patients with Alzheimer's disease. *The Journal of Nutrition, Health & Aging*, *16*(3), 231–236. doi:10.1007/s12603-011-0347-3 and PubMed

Seth, R. V. (1994). Review: Weight loss in Alzheimer's disease. *International Journal of Geriatric Psychiatry*, *9*(8), 605–610. doi:10.1002/gps.930090803

Shatenstein, B., Kergoat, M. J., & Reid, I. (2007). Poor nutrient intakes during 1-year follow-up with community-dwelling older adults with early-stage Alzheimer dementia compared to cognitively intact matched controls. *Journal of the American Dietetic Association*, *107*(12), 2091–2099. doi:10.1016/j.jada.2007.09.008 PMID:18060894

Skeet, M. (1983). *Protecting the health of the elderly*. Retrieved 10 March, 2015, from http://whqlibdoc.who.int/euro/phie/WHO_PHIE_18_(part1).pdf

So, E. S. (2014). Waist Circumference and health-related quality of life by sex in the Korean elderly. *Journal of Aging and Health*, *26*(6), 887–899. doi:10.1177/0898264314531618 PMID:24788716

Spaccavento, S., Del Prete, M., Craca, A., & Fiore, P. (2009). Influence of nutritional status on cognitive, functional and neuropsychiatric deficits in Alzheimer's disease. *Archives of Gerontology and Geriatrics*, *48*(3), 356–360. doi:10.1016/j.archger.2008.03.002 PMID:18448178

Suominen, M. H., Puranen, T. M., Jyväkorpi, S. K., Eloniemi-Sulkava, U., Kautiainen, H., Siljamäki-Ojansuu, U., & Pitkalä, K. H. (2015). Nutritional guidance improves nutrient intake and quality of life, and may prevent falls in aged persons with Alzheimer disease living with a spouse (NuAD Trial). *The Journal of Nutrition, Health & Aging*, 1–7. PMID:26482691

Tasoglu, O., & Ozgirgin, N. (2013). Sarkopeni[Sarcopenia]. *Türkiye Fiziksel Tıp ve Rehabilitasyon Dergisi*, *6*(4), 9–15.

Taylor, C. L., Albanese, E., & Stewart, R. (2012). The association of dementia with upper arm and waist circumference in seven low-and middle-income countries: The 10/66 cross-sectional surveys. *The Journals of Gerontology. Series A, Biological Sciences and Medical Sciences*, *67*(8), 897–904. doi:10.1093/gerona/glr244 PMID:22389465

Tsai, A. C. H., Lai, M. C., & Chang, T. L. (2012). Mid-arm and calf circumferences (MAC and CC) are better than body mass index (BMI) in predicting health status and mortality risk in institutionalized elderly Taiwanese. *Archives of Gerontology and Geriatrics*, *54*(3), 443–447. doi:10.1016/j.archger.2011.05.015 PMID:21663980

Vellas, B., Guigoz, Y., Garry, P. J., Nourhashemi, F., Bennahum, D., Lauque, S., & Albarede, J. L. (1999). The Mini Nutritional Assessment (MNA) and its use in grading the nutritional state of elderly patients. *Nutrition (Burbank, Los Angeles County, Calif.)*, *15*(2), 116–122. doi:10.1016/S0899-9007(98)00171-3 PMID:9990575

Vellas, B., Lauque, S., Gillette-Guyonnet, S., Andrieu, S., Cortes, F., & Nourhashemi, F. et al.. (2005). Impact of nutritional status on the evolution of Alzheimer's disease and on response to acetylcholinesterase inhibitor treatment. *The Journal of Nutrition, 9*(2), 75–80. PMID:15791349

Volkert, D., & Sieber, C. C. (2011). Protein requirements in the elderly. *International Journal for Vitamin and Nutrition Research, 81*(2), 109–119. doi:10.1024/0300-9831/a000061 PMID:22139561

Walker, M. D., Salek, S. S., & Bayer, A. J. (1998). A review of quality of life in Alzheimer's disease. *PharmacoEconomics, 14*(5), 499–530. doi:10.2165/00019053-199814050-00004 PMID:10344915

Wang, P. N., Yang, C. L., Lin, K. N., Chen, W. T., Chwang, L. C., & Liu, H. C. (2004). Weight loss, nutritional status and physical activity in patients with Alzheimer's disease. *Journal of Neurology, 251*(3), 314–320. doi:10.1007/s00415-004-0316-4 PMID:15015012

Wellman, N. S., & Kamp, B. J. (2008). Nutrition in aging. In L. K. Mahan & S. E. Stump (Eds.), *Krause's food and nutrition therapy* (pp. 286–297). Toronto: Saunders Elsevier.

White, H., Pieper, C., & Schmader, K. (1998). The association of weight change in Alzheimer's disease with severity of disease and mortality: A longitudinal analysis. *Journal of the American Geriatrics Society, 46*(10), 1223–1227. doi:10.1111/j.1532-5415.1998.tb04537.x PMID:9777903

White, H. K., McConnell, E. S., Bales, C. W., & Kuchibhatla, M. (2004). A 6-month observational study of the relationship between weight loss and behavioral symptoms in institutionalized Alzheimer's disease subjects. *Journal of the American Medical Directors Association, 5*(2), 89–97. doi:10.1016/S1525-8610(04)70061-4 PMID:14984619

Whitmer, R. A., Gunderson, E. P., Barrett-Connor, E., Quesenberry, C. P. Jr, & Yaffe, K. (2005). Obesity in middle age and future risk of dementia: A 27 year longitudinal population based study. *British Medical Journal, 330*(7504), 1360. doi:10.1136/bmj.38446.466238.E0 PMID:15863436

Winograd, C. H., Jacobson, D. H., Butterfield, G. E., Cragen, E., Edler, L. A., Taylor, B. S., & Yesavage, J. A. (1991). Nutritional intake in patients with senile dementia of the Alzheimer type. *Alzheimer Disease and Associated Disorders, 5*(3), 173–180. doi:10.1097/00002093-199100530-00003 PMID:1772637

Winter, Y., Korchounov, A., Zhukova, T. V., & Bertschi, N. E. (2011). Depression in elderly patients with Alzheimer dementia or vascular dementia and its influence on their quality of life. *Journal of Neurosciences in Rural Practice*, *2*(1), 27. doi:10.4103/0976-3147.80087 PMID:21716831

Yan, L. L., Daviglus, M. L., Liu, K., Pirzada, A., Garside, D. B., Schiffer, L., & Greenland, P. (2004). BMI and health-related quality of life in adults 65 years and older. *Obesity Research*, *12*(1), 69–76. doi:10.1038/oby.2004.10 PMID:14742844

KEY TERMS AND DEFINITIONS

Alzheimer Disease: An irreversible and progressive brain disorder considered to be among the most common of deficits.

Health: Refers to state of complete physical, mental, economic, political and social well-being and not merely the absence of disease or disability.

Malnutrition: Malnutrition is the condition that develops when the body does not get the right amount of the energy and macro-micronutrients it needs to maintain healthy tissues and organ function.

Nursing Home: A convalescence place for especially aged individuals with mobility and feeding restrictions and for those with a chronic illness or disability.

Nutritional Status: The condition of the body in those respects influenced by the diet; the state of the body with respect to each nutrient and to the overall state of the body weight and condition.

Nutritional Support: Nutritional support is therapy for people who cannot get enough nourishment by eating or drinking to prevent malnutrition and to protect them from the consequences.

Quality of Life: An important measure used to evaulate objective and subjective indicators of the life.

Chapter 4
Early Detection of Dementia: Advances, Challenges, and Future Prospects

Stefanos Xefteris
Aristotle University of Thessaloniki, Greece

Charis Styliadis
Aristotle University of Thessaloniki, Greece

Evdokimos Konstantinidis
Aristotle University of Thessaloniki, Greece

Evangelos Paraskevopoulos
Aristotle University of Thessaloniki, Greece

Antonis S. Billis
Aristotle University of Thessaloniki, Greece

Panagiotis Emmanouil Kartsidis
Aristotle University of Thessaloniki, Greece

Panagiotis Antoniou
Aristotle University of Thessaloniki, Greece

Christos A. Frantzidis
Aristotle University of Thessaloniki, Greece

Panagiotis Bamidis
Aristotle University of Thessaloniki, Greece

ABSTRACT

Early detection and prediction of dementia through unobtrusive techniques or obtrusive tests is still in exploratory status and despite the increase of interest in recent years, many challenges remain open in designing methodologies that can accurately predict its onset. This chapter addresses the problem of the early detection

DOI: 10.4018/978-1-5225-0925-7.ch004

of dementia from two points of view: Detection based on unobtrusive paradigms both in lab and home environments (behavioral monitoring, serious games, home based assisted living applications in telemedicine) and detection based on neuroimaging approaches. The chapter also provides information on setting up ecologically valid home labs for dementia related experiments. Consequently, the aim of this chapter is to provide an overview of a complete methodology of how researchers can possibly detect or predict the onset of dementia through the current state-of-the-art, underline open challenges and illustrate future work in the field.

INTRODUCTION

Chronic illnesses impose a great burden on the lives of citizens worldwide. In modern health-care, decentralisation, de-hospitalization and self-management of diseases at home are crucial factors for improving the every-day life of the patients and the people close to them. People in general tend to dislike obtrusive monitoring on their daily activities, so the challenge for home care solutions is to implement systems that provide clinicians with adequate and concise information on their patients' health status while at the same time be unobtrusive and easy to use (Golle & Partridge, 2009; Röcker, Hinske, & Magerkurth, 2007). Based on sets of multimodal monitoring parameters and measuring scales feeding reconfigurable event detection mechanisms used for risk assessment and analysis, AAL systems aim to early detect symptoms that predict decline, avoid emergencies and secondary effects and, ultimately, prolong the period that patients can remain safely cared at home. In this chapter the authors aim at providing a description of current trends in context-aware ambient monitoring for the early detection of dementia and prediction of deterioration, as well as provide a background for minimally obtrusive neuroimaging approaches on prediction of dementia.

BACKGROUND

The current applied paradigm for dementia, revolves around patients in the later stages of the disease, where the patient is beyond the stage of the application of delaying/preventive measures. This follows as a result of the delay in seeking care from the majority of patients and caregivers, until the disease has progressed (Boise, Morgan, Kaye, & Camicioli, 1999). There is a gap in the clinical paradigm which does not include the need for the application of methodologies for early detection of dementia, at the onset of the very first symptoms. This is further exacerbated by the fact that most physicians delay providing a diagnosis as they perceive dementia as a "terminal" disease without adequate remedial ways of treatment. These factors put together, severely compromise healthcare quality for such patients and also deprive them of the chance to face their disease at its early stages where much can be done, directly impacting overall patient care.

Our current understanding of dementia and the underlying mechanisms is that the disorder may well begin one or two decades before symptoms appear (Reiman et al., 2012). Dementia itself is identified as a late stage in the pathological development of neurodegenerative disorders. In the recent years, there has been a clear shift towards addressing the disease at its earlier pathological stages, but still the main focus of clinical practice falls on the later stages, with most diagnoses after the moderate or even severe stage. On the other hand, there is a rising trend to turn our focus on earlier detection of dementia, seeking prodromal, MCI or even completely healthy subjects to volunteer at experimental protocols for the early detection of dementia. Here we discern a huge impediment: Although we are in need of patient populations at the very early stages of dementia, to begin constructively developing better and more efficient detection paradigms and thus enabling clinical research in the race for better treatments, most patients are diagnosed very late. These facts may contribute to delayed or undetected cognitive decline or even false diagnosis among primary care providers (Borson et al., 2013; McCormick et al., 1994).

In the race for early detection of dementia, much can be said and more can be assumed or predicted. Following the rising trend of multidisciplinary practices in many scientific fields, thus early detection of dementia is now moving away from pure clinical practice and clinical instruments and moving towards a holistic approach (Flicker, 1999; Hughes, Robinson, & Volicer, 2005). Making use of machine learning techniques, supporting multimodal data, ranging from biomarkers to behavioral metrics and from social activity to serious games, detection of so far invisible patterns of signs of dementia is now probable, in the near future.

Of course, despite the many advances, there is still a multitude of open problems that need to be addressed. These problems range from the mundane, yet fundamental lack of preclinical or even MCI subjects that are willing to participate in long-term trials, to the organization of experimental trials on home-based or home-like environments for monitoring as well as the more technical need for robust pattern recognition algorithms and decision support mechanisms to fully make use of the not-that-available data.

In 2015, there are over 34 million later stage patients worldwide and the current paradigm must undergo a severe shift towards another direction. By the time of the diagnosis, subjects have mostly declined to the point where they lack the mental capacity to play a role in their care and most certainly are beyond the point of providing useful data to the research community. Moreover, over 50% of patients with dementia go undiagnosed by their primary care provider (Boise et al., 1999; Bradford, Kunik, Schulz, Williams, & Singh, 2009; Kotagal et al., 2015).

Dementia care should and must shift to a different paradigm where focus is more on preventive and early detection methodologies than just remedial action after the onset of the later stages.

On the other hand, recent developments in connectivity analysis for brain functionality through neuroimaging, shows increased potential for early detection of dementia both in clinical environment and in "home-lab" environments –as addition to an AAL platform- through the use of low-obtrusiveness sensors (such as Emotiv)

PATIENT MONITORING ENVIRONMENTS

Before examining the actual details and challenges the problem of early detection of dementia induces, we must initially lift our point of view one level and examine the setup of patient monitoring environments. We have already described how the current established paradigm focuses on monitoring patients after the onset of the disease. Unobtrusive monitoring methodologies are effective when subjects are already in an advanced stage of the disease, but monitoring of healthy -or even MCI subjects- is hindered by the psychological factor: Even though monitoring is unobtrusive, the subject knows that it is being monitored. So, in conjunction with the possible unfamiliar environment (i.e if tests are being performed in the premises of the clinic), we face the problem of changed behavior. The subject is moved away from the familiar comfort zone of the home and being subjected to various tests by clinical staff and strange-locking equipment (McKanna, Jimison, & Pavel, 2009). That of course raises stress levels and leads to perhaps exaggerated reactions to the monitoring protocol. The subject's perception of the monitoring environment directly affects the monitoring parameters (especially behavioral ones and even some physical) so to facilitate valid results we must induce the concept of *ecological validity* in our monitoring environment.

By "ecological validity" we mean that the methods, materials and setting of the experiment must approximate the real-world situation that is being examined (Brewer, 2014). This is particularly important in studies relating to fields such as cognitive psychology, neuropsychology and apply to aspects relating to decision making and judgment, factors of grave importance to the -early or not- detection of dementia and its results on the subjects' behavior.

Apart from ecological validity as a crucial factor in conducting research on the early detection of dementia, we should shortly digress on another important issue, that of the lack of existing data pool. Until the current paradigm shifts towards early detection of dementia, which means that more researchers and more institutions focus their efforts on this, current research lacks from available data on which algorithms, methodologies and detection pipelines can be applied. This combined with the wide timeframe needed (in the order of magnitude of years) to generate meaningful results, leads us to conclude that as much data can be available to as many researchers as possible. The scientific community has to simultaneously produce and share data as widely as possible to facilitate swift progress on the early detection of dementia. Thus, we come to the combined need for ecologically valid monitoring environments built on an open data scheme of dissemination for more accurate data combined with real-time dissemination capabilities.

THE OPEN DATA ECOLOGICALLY VALID LIVING LAB PARADIGM

There are quite a few ongoing research initiatives focused on the creation of integrated unobtrusive smart lab/home environments supporting the independent living of elderly people. The main goal of these smart environments is the ambient monitoring of the elderly through a set of monitoring devices (which comprises a common monitoring model in research efforts across the world). The subjects are continuously evaluated in ecologically valid living lab/home environments and monitoring parameters -behavior, gait, sentiment, activity, memory test results etc- are being recorded and stored -anonymized- for processing and pattern recognition methodologies to be applied on them . Subjects are being analyzed as unobtrusively as possible, just by performing routine tasks they would anyway perform at their homes, or on another level being prompted to perform some light physical exercises, in an overall wellness scheme, through the use of serious games promoting physical exercise or activity. Thus, we collect and can analyze a multitude of data, as little as possible unaffected by perception and stress related distortion.

Such an example of an ecologically valid living lab setup as in Figure 1 would consist of a living-room space, a bathroom-like space and a hall-kitchen space, all in the same room. In this scenario, a number of elderly volunteers visit this environment daily and perform a set of routine activities just as they would at home. An ICT infrastructure (for example, NoSQL databases, Kinect streaming services, etc.) supports the recording of the raw information of all the sources, comprising Kinect(RGB, skeleton and microphone array information), Smart Watch (acceleration), Wii Balance Board (center of gravity during ExerGames interaction, related to the balance ability of the elderly) and health measurements. The data generated by such a monitoring scheme would reach a mean throughput of 10GB per hour swiftly generating a big database of ready to be reproduced, shared and analyzed by the wide scientific community (playback) (Evdokimos I. Konstantinidis, Antoniou, Bamparopoulos, & Bamidis, 2014). On top of this, the paradigm exploits an RDF database contains semantic annotation of the datasets which can be provided by an external observer. In such a monitoring scheme, the infrastructure and ICT tools (streaming on demand, cloud storage and processing, etc.), are based on already developed services and frameworks (such as the cac-framework.com) (Evdokimos I. Konstantinidis et al., 2014) to make these data available on demand. As stated by Konstantinidis et al. (2014), the scientific community will be able to experiment and to test their algorithms on data stemmed from an ecologically valid environment in lab settings. This approach will enable developers and researchers of early detection algorithms that rely on information similar to the existing datasets, by enabling the design and developed algorithms and software tailored to the elder's daily living patterns. Most importantly a preliminary evaluation of the service adoption has already been conducted on the programmers/developers front with encouraging results.(E. Konstantinidis, Antoniou, et al., 2014; E. Konstantinidis, Billis, et al., 2014).Therefore, such an approach would facilitate the ulterior aim of speeding up innovation, collaboration as well as development and testing of more accurate services, which is achieved by an early involvement of users (playback already existing datasets of elderly in an ecologically valid living lab) as co-creators.

We have stressed the need to produce ecologically valid environment datasets in a real time format, which will support and accelerate the collaboration among

Figure 1. An ecologically valid living lab in laboratory settings resembling a real common living room and kitchen

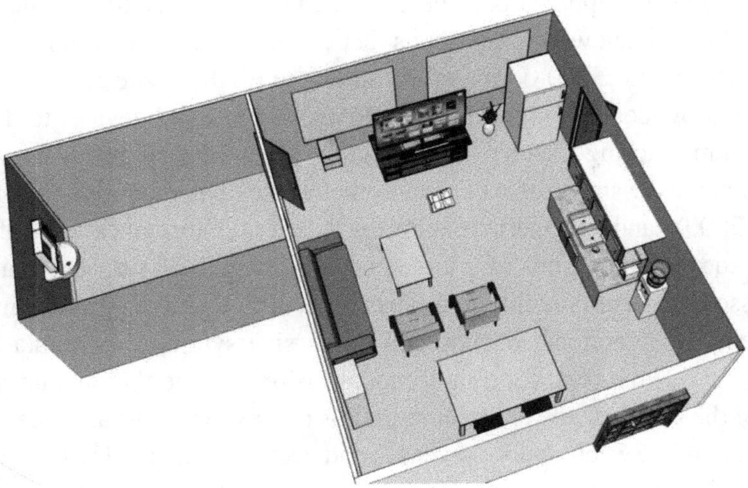

the scientific community, as well as in a datasets format for further exploitation of other entities, in a wide-open data scheme that will return back to the research community a wealth of information along with convenient tools for getting access to them.

ECOLOGICALLY VALID DATA COLLECTION

In the current monitoring paradigm, the assessment of a subject's cognitive and functional status is based on brief clinical visits, where various data is collected via short tests and compared with results from previous sessions. This is conventionally done by using a variety of validated clinical assessment tools and is heavily affected by the distorting lens of the subjects' and caregivers' recollection of events in the days preceding the tests as well as their capacity for self-assessment, which is -as already stated- affected by the "sterile" clinical environment. Moreover, infrequency and the actual short duration provide more confounding variables for the accuracy and efficacy of these tests.(Boise et al., 1999; Bradford et al., 2009)

So, the biggest challenge concerning not only the early detection of dementia, but also the more conventional monitoring of the progress of the disease itself, is the general lack of pervasive and unobtrusive environments that will exploit significant parameters, enhance adherence, provide constant monitoring by tracking activities and behaviors and thus a continuum of useful data, with underlying patterns that can be used to predict outcomes of mood, behavior, cognitive status and functionality, used as biomarkers for detecting trends towards dementia (Lyons et al., 2015). Moreover, although there is a plethora of ambient intelligence examples of home monitoring applications, these are mainly focused on life threatening acute events and less on slow varying trends that can indicate future conditions such as dementia (Mihailidis, 2008). Therefore, aiming to fill the above gap, we must focus on utilizing low-cost, off-the-self, unobtrusive sensors and devices to detect both short-term monitoring - such as the detection of emergency events as well as the detection and assessment of ADLs and other contextual situations (Storf, Becker, & Riedl, 2009)– and, long-term monitoring to detect abnormal patterns of health or behavior and continuous health assessment (Chiriac, Röll, Parada, & Rosales, 2012; Monekosso & Remagnino, 2010; Xefteris et al., 2011). Since cognitive impairment is coupled with functional decline and depressive symptoms, (Mehta, Yaffe, & Covinsky, 2002) the need for a multimodal fusion scheme that monitors multiple aspects of the subjects' life is apparent. In this context, we must also keep our mind on the tradeoff between unobtrusiveness and accuracy, coupled with the subjects' adherence. Unobtrusiveness seems to be a critical factor that enhances acceptance and compliance, while on the other hand obtrusive or even invasive methodologies provide more accurate data.

The transition from monitoring the disease to actually detecting it at the very early stages or even years before, calls for data acquisition and processing platforms, collecting and fusing data in a multimodal environment (sensors, exergames, questionnaires, etc.). The trending paradigm's objective is to integrate and extend state-of-the art technologies for:

- Fusing and interpreting the parameters uni-modally extracted from raw sensor data into a semantic representation of human behaviour and physiological status.
- Extracting correlations from sets of fused data (cognitive, emotional and physiological measurements). Utilisation of various soft computing, probabilistic and data mining techniques is crucial in order to operate on sensor data to provide least error prone analysis and decision support indicators.

The main parameters, based on Activities of Daily Living (ADLs) that can provide us with useful data, collected unobtrusively, for the possible early detection of dementia and help us make predictions are analysed in the following paragraphs.

Mobility

Since 1998 (Camicioli, Howieson, Oken, Sexton, & Kaye, 1998) has demonstrated that reduced mobility precedes cognitive impairment in the elderly. Researchers now, develop new algorithms for continuous in-home assessment of both variability in movement speeds and movement patterns, to discern underlying signs of risk. On one hand, researchers can employ a scheme of "passive" monitoring via sensors installed in various places inside a home and collecting data on speed, frequency of passage, total activity etc, or by "active" monitoring via the application of ExerGames that both aim to promote and sustain a healthy and active lifestyle and collect possible "anomalous" data in the performance of the various exercises.

Passive monitoring via dispersed sensors has many advantages but also some caveats. On one hand, passive, unobtrusive sensors solve the problem of compliance and adherence, because monitored people tend to either avoid or even forget to wear the common actigraphy devices used for mobility monitoring. Moreover, simple accelerometers do not provide location information - which is significant itself- coupled with the fact that since in-home movement is generally slow and non-linear, data interpretation is very difficult. Thus, in the case of older adults, the notion of ecologically valid unobtrusive monitoring comes back again as a very important factor. To that end, arrays of in-home sensors can be deployed supporting information collection of walking speed, location and frequency of passage. (Hagler, Austin, Hayes, Kaye, & Pavel, 2010; Hayes et al., 2008). The challenge remains though, to establish the individual activity patterns and manage to measure meaningful change that may have applications for predicting health parameters and functional status (Hagler et al., 2010) .

Exergames

The emergence of modern interaction interfaces (tablet, laptop with touch screen, smart tv) has been followed by the trend of transferring paper and pencil screening tests to computerized forms which are more acceptable from elders (Collerton et al., 2007). On top of this, and aligned with Plato's statement that "...you can discover more about a person in an hour of play than in a year of conversation..."(Robert et al., 2014), these computerized tests started turning into games with assessment aspects. Introduced with the term "Serious Games", these games are considered to provide more reliable assessment information compared to conventional methods (Bellotti, Kapralos, Lee, Moreno-Ger, & Berta, 2013; Robert et al., 2014). This can be attributed to the fact that users do not perceive serious games as a stressful testing procedure (Cassady & Johnson, 2002).

The assessment aspect of the cognitive serious games contribute to the early detection of neurological disease (Hagler, Jimison, & Pavel, 2014), while exergames, serious games promoting physical activity and exercise (S. Yang, 2010), are deemed as measuring physical health unobtrusively tools (E. Konstantinidis, Billis, et al., 2014; Staiano & Calvert, 2011). This has recently started to change and exergames have just introduced in the field of cognitive assessment(E. I. Konstantinidis, Bamidis, Billis, Kartsidis, & Papageorgiou, 2015). Only recent studies concerned correlations of physical activity features of SGs with cognitive assessment utilizing virtual environments and treadmills and correlating muscle strength and walking time with global cognitive measurements (Tarnanas et al., 2013). Touch screen serious games and a diversity of serious game have been lately employed towards cognitive Parkinson's Disease prediction(S. Liu, Shen, Mei, & Ji, 2013) and cognitive performance inference (Byun & Park, 2011) respectively. Konstantinidis et al. (2014) introduced the FitForAll exergaming platform towards physical exercise promotion. However, its potential role as contributor to the detection of early cognitive decline signs classifies it to a distinct position. The in-game metrics analysis exhibits classification accuracy greater than 72% when discriminating cognitively normal from mild cognitive impaired elderly. This study show also that FitForAll was more accurate than MMSE and comparable to the MOCA.

Sleep

Sleep patterns comprise a crucial indicator of various health problems, both stand-alone and as associated symptoms (i.e of pulmonary and cardio-vascular problems). In addition, sleep disruption have been identified as correlated with MCI and Alzheimer's disease. (Lyketsos et al., 2002; Tractenberg, Singer, & Kaye, 2005). Lately, sleep disruption has been linked with decreased performance on memory tests even on cognitively intact elderly (Seelye et al., 2015). In this context, it is obvious that in the framework of an unobtrusive monitoring platform that focuses on the early detection of increased risk factors for dementia, sleep patterns provide rich background information. Making use of off-the-shelf sensors like pressure mats and wrist-worn actigraphy monitors, we can employ a scenario of long term monitoring and assessment spanning months rather than a single day, providing a robust baseline that excludes outliers that skew our data and provide comparison backgrounds for between healthy and MCI subjects. In such a study (Hayes, Riley, Mattek, Pavel, & Kaye, 2014)it was found that amnestic MCI (aMCI) patients typically exhibit less sleep disruptions than non-amnestic MCI (naMCI) patients, who in their turn exhibited less than healthy (cognitively intact) individuals. Seelye et al.(2015) also showed that sustained periods of sleep disruptions have a clear impact on cognitive function in healthy adults. Duration of sleep was not related to the cognitive test performance. These findings suggest that continuous assessment of sleep patterns does provide significant information on factors that can contribute to variable or decreased cognitive function.

Social Engagement

Social engagement is an indirect sign of cognitive status. Moreover, higher levels of social activity have been shown to be a preventive measure for the avoidance of cognitive decline. (Akbaraly et al., 2009; Fratiglioni, Wang, Ericsson, Maytan, & Winblad, 2000; Scarmeas, Levy, Tang, Manly, & Stern, 2001)

As researchers now have a better grasp of the relationship between social engagement and cognitive decline, we can use this information in a twofold way:

1. Deployment of methodologies for the early identification of cognitive decline risks and
2. Development of intervention frameworks based on social engagement as a tool to improve cognitive function.

The greatest advantage of using social engagement metrics as cognitive decline risk for individuals is that most of its aspects can be easily measured in a passive way. These can include time spent out of home, frequency and duration of telephone use, frequency and duration of visitors as well as internet use (e-mail, chat etc).

Decision Support

In the previous paragraphs we examined the milieu of a patient monitoring paradigm that is established in an ecologically valid environment, with open access to monitoring data and input parameters spanning activities of daily living (ADL), behavioral aspects and physiological measurements with the express goal to detect adverse signs in order to enable the early detection of dementia. In this paragraph we go behind the monitoring front-end and try to provide a brief working example of a context-aware system that processes this data via pattern recognition and decision support methodologies to provide detection and prediction results on the subject's status. (Xefteris, Andronikou, Tserpes, & Varvarigou, 2010)

We will use the example of the USEFIL project (Artikis et al., 2012; Billis et al., 2015) which provides both short term monitoring for the detection of emergencies through context-aware detection and assessment of ADLs (Storf et al., 2009), and long-term monitoring for the detection of baseline divergent (abnormal) patterns of health, behavior and general health assessment (Chiriac, Röll, Parada, & Rosales, n.d.,2012).

USEFIL is an innovative data acquisition and processing platform that collects and fuses multimodal data (from sensors, exergames, questionnaires etc). Raw data collection is performed in-home and initial data are processed locally to provide user reminders and alerts, with group-level processing performed on a central database.

The DSS component of the USEFIL platform endeavors to recognize early deterioration signs for a multitude of medical problems as well as deviations from a behavioral baseline that indicate decline, alerting both formal and informal carers as soon as possible. The component performs these operations with the use of data mining and pattern recognition techniques in three steps:

1. Collect of the relevant data that is already filtered and pre-processed.
2. Project data segments into a time-series to enable pattern recognition.
3. Classify the occurring temporal fluctuations to diagnosis types.

The USEFIL DSS system is thus designed as a spatio-temporal model comprising A.I methods that process data related to user activity and physiological classification. The DSS utilizes soft computing, probabilistic and data mining techniques on the sensor acquired data to perform least error prone analysis and decision support.

Aiming to accomplish the aforementioned objectives, the USEFIL DSS system is designed to be a spatio–temporal model consisted of artificial intelligence methods manipulating data related with user activity and physiological classification. The progress beyond the current state-of-the art of the specific component is:

- Both short- and long-term monitoring.
- Hybrid decision support system, based on rule-based expert systems combined with fuzzy cognitive maps (FCM) -a type of fuzzy inference scheme.
- Involvement of medical experts in the design process of the DSS, in order to improve the targeting and acceptance of the system with professional carers (Papageorgiou, Billis, Frantzidis, Konstantinidis, & Bamidis, 2013).

The conceptual approach of the DSS component is shown in Figure 2.

The concept followed is that within the Data Fusion Tool the raw data are fused and activity states or transitions among them concerning behavioral and physiological states are stored as events. (Katzouris, Artikis, & Paliouras, 2014)

The Sensor Data Fusion tool outputs these events to the other DSS subcomponents that take care of detecting the various possible pathological states, extrapolate the possibility for future deterioration and identify possible pathological trends as well as suggest remedial approaches. These outputs are categorized in alarms/warnings/notifications or into prompts and suggestions, providing triggering flags to other USEFIL applications (such as an Alerting App) that interact with the subject or the carer. Long term analysis results may be also used as input to the other components (Billis, Papageorgiou, Frantzidis, Konstantinidis, & Bamidis, 2013).

The flowchart in Figure 3 provides a depiction of how the different DSS components are interconnected. (Panagiotis D. Bamidis, Tarnanas, Tsolaki, & Hadjileontiadis, 2015). The various outputs can be considered as standalone DSS results or be used by other DSS components for the production of further conclusions. As

Figure 2. USEFIL DSS conceptual architecture (I/Os and modules)

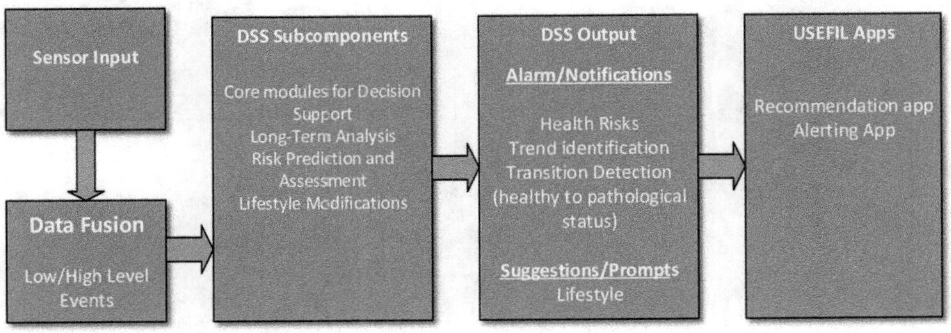

an example, the presence of severe symptoms can be used as a standalone result of the long-term analysis component or be combined with the DSS to classify a senior as suffering from a specific pathological condition.

These detected trends may be also used by the Risk Assessment Component, in order to provide estimation of potential future adverse situations. The DSS forms a "pool of evidence" comprising estimation of health trends, current health status and possible future outcomes, in order to procure the appropriate strategies for the alleviation of health problems and for helping the subject stay independent. The produced strategies are proposed via the "Lifestyle Modifications Suggestion". This transforms the DSS from a simple passive monitoring application to an active sug-

Figure 3. The interconnections between the USEFIL DSS components

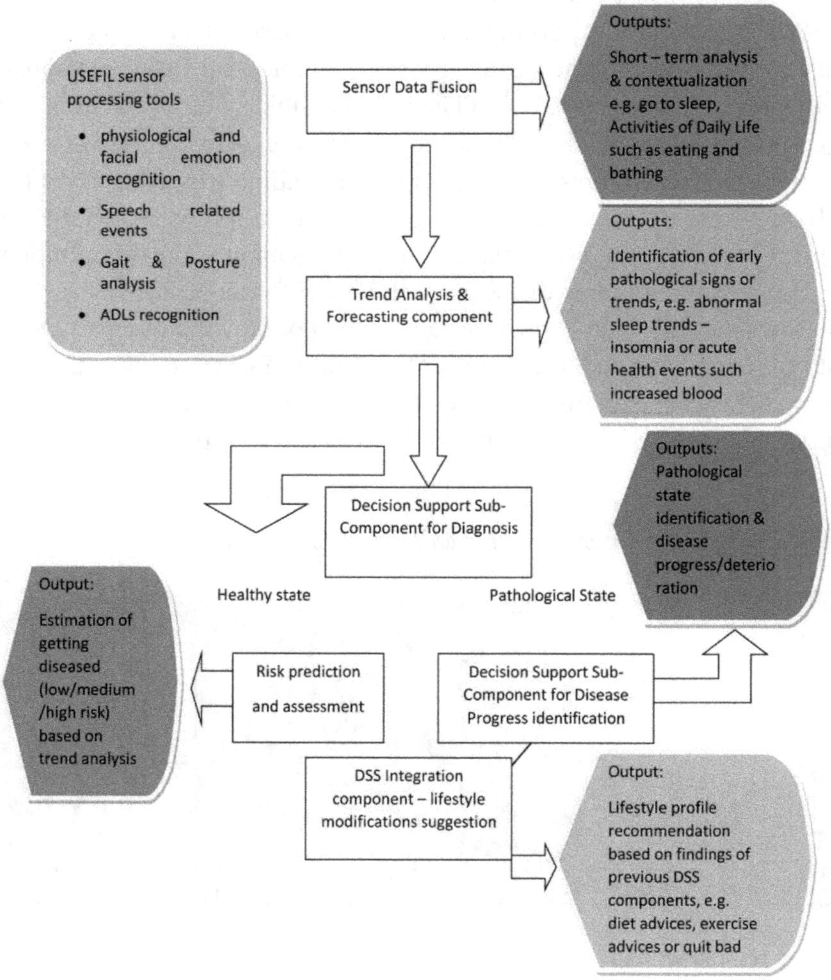

gestion system, not only detecting and predicting, but also being actively engaged in possible remedial actions.

The USEFIL DSS approach is encapsulating the essence of the early detection paradigm by actively engaging in long term monitoring for the identification of adverse trends, providing significant forecasting capabilities for the prognosis of potential future deterioration while at the same time providing possible solutions for delaying this deterioration by the application of certain life-style modifications.

In Vitro Detection with Neuroimaging

We have so far discussed the efficacy of unobtrusive methodologies as reliable markers for the detection of dementia. Nevertheless, reliable biomarkers for the early detection of dementia can be obtained from obtrusive methodologies as well, namely the most common techniques (see next section) usually employed in the field of neuroimaging. Indeed, recent research has shown promising results in the detection process by adding distinctive and reliable neuroimaging biomarkers to the diagnostic criteria of Alzheimer's disease (AD). For instance, (Dubois et al., 2007) demonstrated a significant potential for methodologies that aim to keep cognitive functions active or enhance their performance across the adult lifespan. Engaging seniors into computer based interventions of training schemes tailored to their specific capacities shows great promise in allowing for the longitudinal evaluation and monitor of their cognitive status (Bamidis et al., 2014; Busse, Gil, Santarém, & Filho, 2009; Colcombe & Kramer, 2003; Tardif & Simard, 2011). In parallel, our current understanding of neuroplasticity and the employment of neuroimaging biomarkers have the potential to offer additional solutions in the existing clinical routine for early detection and also for monitoring the disease's progression. The aim of this paragraph is to present recent neuroimaging findings on the dementia detection that can be employed to unravel the functional and structural reorganization of the aging brain.

Neuroimaging Modalities

The process of aging induces changes in the brain and directly in the activity of neurons and subsequently, the cognitive function. With recent advances and techniques, we are now able to study both brain structures and functions. Though obtrusive in nature, techniques such as EEG, MRI, fMRI, MEG, and DTI are non-invasive, painless and easy to apply, thus quite significant in the study of the aging brain in healthy as well as pathologic subjects. These methods enable us to reconstruct images of the structural (grey and white matter) and/or functional (electrophysiological, blood flow, metabolic) characteristics of the brain, in spatial scales ranging from a millimetre to several centimetre and temporal scales from a millisecond to hours. Each methodology has strengths and caveats in terms of resolution and thus, the decision on which to apply is dependent on the application.

Brain Plasticity

The process of aging is considered to be a progressive state of continuous decline. New research findings though provide us with quite a different milieu: It is apparent now that the brain retains its adaptability and flexibility across a person's lifespan and many cognitive abilities are preserved further than previously thought.

Plasticity refers to the ability of the brain to reorganize both structural and functional components. Plasticity is an ability that in healthy subjects remains active across the lifespan (Boyke, Driemeyer, Gaser, Buchel, & May, 2008).In contrast to an earlier notion that age-related neuroplastic changes were the result of cell death or dendritic deterioration, it is now well accepted that they are the result of lower synaptic densities in older adults (Hedden & Gabrieli, 2004). The aging process alters the biophysical properties of neurons and this affects the brain network dynamics resulting in poor signal to noise ration (SNR) (Burke & Barnes, 2006)and lower neuromodulatory system function in older brains (Mahncke et al., 2006). These changes mainly affect the prefrontal cortex and the medial temporal structures.

Therefore, intensive training of cognitive or motor processes, can stimulate brain plasticity, inducing changes in the underlying cortical structures (Mahncke et al., 2006). For instance, recent MEG findings indicate that two weeks of intensive multisensory training may induce neuroplastic changes in the functionality of frontotemporal cortical regions in adults (Paraskevopoulos, Kuchenbuch, Herholz, & Pantev, 2014). Inducing behavioral interventions enables the ability of the brain to reorganize itself, even in the case of the aging (Mahncke et al., 2006)

Since the cognitive deterioration of the brain may onset well before the aging process begins, and changes in plasticity at brain synapses combined with the loss of neurons are the key indicator for oncoming functional decline, it is apparent that detecting these changes at an early stage, can be instrumental in the early detection of dementia. These changes are precursors to dementia related impairments and precursors of AD, such as amyloid beta deposits, brain inflammation, tau tangles and ApoE4 proteins. They directly affect areas of the brain responsible for learning, memory and cognition by impairing synapses and contributing to cell death. Early neuron loss and changes in synapse function have been observed in the hippocampus and the neocortex, the regions involved in language, memory and higher cognitive functions, so using neuroimaging to detect such changes can alert clinicians to the future onset of dementia and provide a route to preventive actions, rather than the established remedial paradigm.

Structural Neuroimaging in Aging and Dementia

Age related structural changes in the brain have varying extents. The threshold between healthy and pathological aging is very thin as many of these brain changes extend in dementia and AD. The aging of the brain can range from a healthy (successful) state, where structure and volume is completely retained until almost the end of our lives, to a more typical or near pathological aging. Some typical dementia related structural changes can be also a part of a healthy aging curve in middle aged subjects as well as elderly subjects who are essentially cognitively intact. Some extent of brain atrophy can be present in healthy aging but when followed by cognitive decline it may induce an increased risk of neurodegenerative diseases. In this context, structural neuroimaging can be instrumental in detecting preclinical stages of age-related cognitive decline and be of great help in the early detection of the progression of dementia. In order to efficiently characterize age-related disorders such as dementia, we need to disentangle the mechanisms of the structural changes (i.e. atrophy) that take place in healthy aging.

MRI Detection of Dementia

In current clinical practice, structural MR imaging is widely available and reasonably inexpensive. The main challenge of MRI, concerning early detection of dementia or other neurodegenerative diseases is to discern MCI patients that will in the future fulfil the clinical criteria for dementia or AD. MRI can also be used to distinguish between non-AD and AD dementias -for instance, hippocampal atrophy is absent in dementia with Lewy bodies (McKeith et al., 2005)and vascular dementia (Barber et al., 1999). MRI is an efficient tool for the very early diagnosis of an individual suspected of dementia and its subtyping, through detection of hippocampal reductions. (Shi, Liu, Zhou, Yu, & Jiang, 2009). Moreover, MRI is employed for predicting the risk of AD progression in populations that are both cognitively healthy and MCI.

Though more research is needed to establish the clinical value of MRI in MCI, measuring these significant reductions due to AD can have a powerful impact on the early diagnosis of MCI and AD. In addition, MRI is employed for the prediction of the risk of dementia progression. (Risacher et al., 2009) established that the MRI biomarker measuring the degree of neurodegeneration of MTL structures was the best for imminent conversion and the biomarker of decreased hippocampal volume the most robust.

So, having established the as early as possible detection of the disease, MRI metrics such as brain volume fluctuations through time, can be used to evaluate and keep track of the disease (Fox & Freeborough, 1997).

DTI Detection of Dementia

Changes in grey and white matter are promising biomarkers of dementia. These markers are detected by microstructural abnormalities on DTI-based diffusivity indexes. These alterations enable the prediction of dementia progression independently of possible volume loss in prodromal situations (Canu et al., 2010; Fellgiebel et al., 2006; Oishi, Mielke, Albert, Lyketsos, & Mori, 2012) and are evident in both healthy brain aging as well as in MCI and dementia, but also in other neurodegenerative disorders (Kantarci et al., 2011; Oishi et al., 2012; Rogalski et al., 2012) .

In MCI patients, higher baseline diffusivity in the hippocampal head indexes a bigger risk of progression to AD. Thus, diffusion findings can be employed as complementary biomarkers to hippocampal atrophy in identifying progression. When taken in earlier stages of life, these findings can be indicators of the future appearance of symptoms.

Functional Neuroimaging and Resting State Analysis

To understand the effects of aging on neural plasticity, we have to initially examine the effect of age on the brain's functionality. Functional neuroimaging detects age-related increases and decreases of neural activity, in conjunction with cognitive decline. These approaches provide a link between the various implications of aging on our brains by measuring either resting state activity or neural activity while subjects perform cognitive tasks.

In this context, neuroimaging studies make use of resting state measurements for the definition of a baseline which is later compared with the results from the performed tasks. At rest, the cortex's functional characteristics show a high degree of reproducibility and stability and some brain regions show a consistent activity than during cognitive tasks (Greicius, Srivastava, Reiss, & Menon, 2004). The implicated brain regions include the posterior cingulate cortex (PCC), MTL structures, dorsal and ventromedical PFC and lateral (mainly inferior) parietal cortices (Mevel, Chételat, Eustache, & Desgranges, 2011). Due to its functional characteristics this is dubbed the Default Mode Network (DMN) (Raichle et al., 2001) . The DMN is characterised by a highly stable functionality which makes it a valuable tool for the evaluation of cognitive and neurological disorders such as amnsestic MCI (aMCI) (Garcés et al., 2014) and AD (Greicius et al., 2004).

Using fMRI for Resting State Analysis

fMRI is a highly promising biomarker for dementia, repeatable many times over the course of longitudinal studies. fMRI studies examining the effects of dementia in activation patterns and organization of DMN of dementia patients (Y. Liu et al., 2008) and age-matched healthy subjects revealed that dementia groups exhibit decreased resting state activity in almost all of the cortical regions involved in the DMN and most prominently in the hippocampus and the PCC, thus suggesting disrupted connectivity between these two regions in dementia(Greicius et al., 2004). In an earlier study (Shi et al., 2009)it was established that dementia patients exhibit diminished connectivity of the hippocampus to other regions, compared to healthy elderly individuals. In this study, a group of MCI patients had intermediate values, also significantly different from the dementia group. Lack of presence of this connectivity breakdown in the visual cortex suggests that the sensory systems may be affected only in later stages of the disease. Studies also revealed that the functional connectivity of the hippocampus with the medial PFC, ventral anterior cingulate cortec (ACC), right inferior temporal cortex, right cuneus (Cu) and precuneus (PCu), left Cu, right superior and middle temporal gurys and PCC was disrupted in dementia patients compared to healthy adults (L. Wang et al., 2006)

In Sheline et al.(2010) it is revealed that the functional connectivity breakdown of the DMN that dementia patients exhibit might predate the pathological effects of amyloid plaque toxicity.

Thus, detecting early connectivity breakdowns in the DMN via fMRI in resting state, could be of big help in a future early dementia detection paradigm.

Using MEG-EEG for Resting State Analysis

EEG has a high temporal resolution which makes it an ideal tool for studying the cortical connectivity of DMN. Several studies employed this approach searching for disrupted connectivity between cortical regions of the DMN, indicative of neurodegenerative diseases.

In a 2014 study, (Frantzidis et al., 2014) used EEG to reveal a significant reduction in the small-world brain architecture in both aMCI and mild demented patients relative to the group of healthy controls. These findings correlated significantly with the cognitive function as evaluated by MMSE. All of the above are in line with the notion that the AD may be grounded on a connectivity breakdown and may actually constitute a disconnection syndrome, as suggested by Delbeuck (Delbeuck, Collette, & Van der Linden, 2007).

Apart from structural and connectivity analyses, several studies have used another approach and ventured to identify the electrophysiological effects of dementia and MCI to the functionality of the DMN. These studies are focused on comparing the EEG activity measured across different frequency bands between dementia, MCI and healthy subjects. The results of such studies indicate that dementia patients in contrast to healthy subjects exhibit increases in the power of low frequency bands such as delta (-4Hz) and theta (4-7 Hz) in central and frontal electrode sites as well as a decrease in the power of posterior alpha (8-15Hz) and beta (16-30Hz) (Babiloni et al., 2004, 2013; Bennys, Rondouin, Vergnes, & Touchon, 2001). These findings are corroborated by MEG studies which exhibit increased power in the activity of parietal delta sources(Fernández et al., 2006) and more significantly, these abnormalities seem heavily correlated with global impairment of cognitive function via an MMSE evaluation (Jeong, 2004).

Comparing MCI patients with healthy controls, reveals the same pattern of findings (increase in power of low frequency bands in posterior sites and decrease of alpha and beta bands for MCI patients). Thus, we are led to pose the hypothesis that there can be a linear transition point between healthy and MCI and MCI and dementia, and that these EEG findings may provide stable screening biomarkers for the risk of onset of dementia and prediction regarding the progression from MCI to AD(Babiloni et al., 2013). Recently, an EEG study explored the effects of combined cognitive and physical training on resting state brain activity of MCI patients in comparison to the effects of solely cognitive or physical training as well as in comparison to active and passive control groups. The effect of the combined intervention was interpreted as beneficiary neuroplasticity changes (i.e. decrease delta and theta rhythms in the precuneus/posterior cingulate cortex) across MCI patients and these changes correlated with cognitive status improvement.(Styliadis, Kartsidis, Paraskevopoulos, Ioannides, & Bamidis, 2015).

FUTURE CHALLENGES

In 2013, over 35 million people around the world were estimated to have dementia. (Camicioli et al., 1998) The number of people worldwide with dementia is expected to increase to 65.7 million in 2030 and 115.4 million in 2050, which is approximately a doubling of sufferers every 20 years. ("WHO | Dementia: a public health priority," 2012). Dementia is a syndrome of progressive cognitive and functional deterioration which is incurable. There are diverse symptoms and various levels of impairment depended on affected brain regions and types of dementia. Contemporary medical technologies related to dementia have proven track record for detection and intervention but have also been distilled in more mild modalities to be implemented in the case of less severe needs. Recent technological advances that allow the in-vivo study of brain structures and functions in human subjects have greatly contributed to a better understanding of the brain changes that occur due to aging and are likely to impact the cognitive function and neuronal activity. The non-invasive nature of most of these techniques (i.e. Electroencephalography – EEG; Magnetoencephalography – MEG; Magnetic Resonance Imaging – MRI; functional MRI – fMRI;

Diffusion Tensor Imaging – DTI) makes them an invaluable tool in the study of the living brain in healthy as well as pathologic subjects (Styliadis, Kartsidis, & Paraskevopoulos, n.d.).

With diagnostic modalities providing significantly early detection of various dementia types the question becomes one of choice of interventions. Additionally, with studies outlining depressive symptoms, as a consistent factor which is negatively related to self-rated QoL of people with dementia living in long-term care facilities (Beerens, Zwakhalen, Verbeek, Ruwaard, & Hamers, 2013) as well as the self-evident costs related with long term care the Ambient Assisted Living (AAL) approach to the maintenance of quality of life and health care interventions provide greater flexibility and respectful interventions at the behavioral level with unobtrusive and transparent monitoring and interventions at familiar home environments.

Beyond the, now established, monitoring with unobtrusive sensors and devices that are natively ICT enabled an emergent field in elderly healthcare is the Internet of things (Ashton, 2009). Transparent and ubiquitous communication capacities by ad-hoc networking of various devices and actuators has begun finding application in elderly healthcare. This technology has been demonstrating, rather recently -e.g. (G. Yang et al., 2014), a significant number of enabling capacities in the field of elderly healthcare, especially for people with cognitive decline. Inkjet printed, flexible bio-patches that allow for portable and very unobtrusive ECG measurements; RFID enabled medication packaging that can sense how many medication slots have been opened, facilitating dramatic increase in medication adherence of elderly people; unique RFID tagged medical ids linked to detailed medical records for protection against false medical history. Such unobtrusive and transparent technologies provide critical quality of life improvement and subsequent lifestyle and healthcare maintenance.

With all these advances in ubiquitous networking and unobtrusive monitoring an area that appears to not have been heavily tapped into is the technologically enabled communication and collaboration between elderly that are suffering from one or another form of non-trivial age based cognitive decline. The effect of an existing, active and supporting social network in real life has been explored providing evidence that it is associated with the well-being of the elderly (X. Wang, 2014). What hasn't been explored so far in sufficient detail is the extent in which an electronic social network of dementia patients and their carers would impact in their quality of life. Although folksonomies (folk-generated taxonomies from custom subject tagging in social networks and forums (Adamic & Adar, 2005)) have led to emergent social networking the use of such provisions are still not sufficiently explored. In the context, however, of AAL environments and protected but ubiquitous networking there is significant potential for unobtrusive behavioral monitoring and intervention in the, now widely accepted, form of an electronic social network.

From the previous discussion, distilling content from this whole work three overall monitoring and intervention feedback loops emerge. In the purely biomedical level the aforementioned brain activity and anatomy monitoring and imaging capacities (e.g. EEG, PET, fMRI) provide immediate feedback to the medical doctor for medicinal or non-medicinal treatment of dementia's underlying pathogeny at the purely neurophysiological level. On a different level, ambient, unobtrusive sensor based monitoring and assessment in the home environment provides the necessary data that are usable for prescribing and suggesting personal behavioral modification that will improve or at least maintain quality of life (e.g. physical exercise programs, exergaming interventions). Furthermore, even though largely unexplored in the context of ICTs, real world support group interventions of elderly with varying degrees of dementia provide to the expert crucial data for intervening at the social level and creating a fertile social environment for the patients to maintain or even improve their way of life (Leung, Orrell, & Orgeta, 2015).

Medical diagnostic modalities, intervention protocols, unobtrusive ambient home monitoring and intervention as well as social support infrastructure have the capacity of creating an immense amount of data. From patient records and imaging to real time sensor data these are sources of information that can provide a wealth of additional meta-information using context, time evolution and aggregation techniques. In order to achieve "human activity recognition" (Rashidi & Mihailidis, 2013) a number of techniques must be applied in order to transform raw sensor data to human activity patterns. In that endeavor methods of either supervised learning through annotation, using annotated data and supervised machine learning algorithms can be utilized, or, even more abstractly, unsupervised data mining techniques can be incorporated (Rashidi & Mihailidis, 2013). These algorithms, in order to cope with the needs of interpreting activity in various contexts as well as discriminating outliers with significant anomalies in activities have widely adopted the use of modelling metadata and ontologies in order to codify both context and underlying semantic relationships.

Evolving from information theory, efforts are made to explain and exploit the cross-scale information processing that is apparent in natural dynamical systems. By viewing physical, biological, or social systems as networks of information exchange, statistical tools from information theory can be used to causally explain and quantify the effect that each participant of this network contributes to the overall behavior of the network (Quax, Apolloni, & Sloot, 2013). Through such toolbox, outcomes from contemporary physics, such as resonance phenomena and non-trivial propagation phenomena can be quantified and predicted (Czaplicka, Holyst, & Sloot, 2013). In that way specific structural changes in a network's characteristics can dramatically alter the dynamic evolution of various metrics of the system that is described by it. Such scientific paradigms can and have been used to explore the not only the fundamental processes on different and separate scales of dynamic systems, but also the cross-scale coupling of them and any possible resulting emergent properties that can be exploited for pattern recognition or efficient interventions (e.g.("dynanets.org," 2015)).

This kind of analysis tools have found use in a variety of disciplines and fields where implementing a specific hypothesis about a network, based on the characteristics of the participating nodes can lead to tangible conclusions about macroscopic and measurable characteristics of the whole system. For example information dissipation length (IDL) has been introduced as an index of global instability of the time series of USD and EUR interest rate swaps (IRS) presenting a specific pattern of gradual increase and subsequent decrease before and after the Lheman Brothers collapse, respectively (Quax, Kandhai, & Sloot, 2013). On another example by introducing the concept of transmission networks and proposing a filter reduction method in combined data from social networks and phylogenetic analysis, tangible results regarding correlation of cross-group sexual behavior and HIV transmission has been found (Zarrabi et al., 2013).

Bringing all these themes together, smart sensors and semantic technologies provide aggregated high level data about daily activities. Contemporary decision support and machine learning technologies can consume such high level data streams, in real time, providing intervention suggestions at both the physical and mental pathogeny level. Neuroscience advances provide assessment tools able to rapidly validate, and intervene with gamified and collaborative activities for mental health and overall wellbeing. What is at the moment missing is a formalization, both at a high level of abstraction, as well as at the prototype implementation level, of the role of these technologies and interventions, in the paradigm of maintaining wellness through structured interaction. Utilizing the aforementioned information theory background. Such a synergetic use of these technologies would provide both a conceptual paradigm and an implemented assessment and intervention prototype for more effective and impactful dementia monitoring and intervention. From this discussion of the previous sections on modalities and means, combining the previous discourse it becomes apparent that, apart from following through in researching specific aspects of dealing with the dementia patient, a significant future challenge will be the integration of the technologies and methods into something beyond an incoherent mashup of randomly interacting parts. Detailed data aggregation methods can provide detailed but also seamless exploration of various modalities' and interventions' impact. This methodology can explore, utilizing the previous theme of cross scale feedback propagation, the necessary exact prescriptions for all the components of this palette for achieving rigorous integration to protocols. In that effort the support from ecologically valid dementia oriented living labs in conjunction with the treatment space (hospital, personal physician) become an organic research testbed for this integration. Only through such a coordinated infrastructure of integrated research can, large scale trials explore the cross-scale and cross-modal impact of an emerging ecosystem of dementia prevention, treatment and care in order to provide an appropriate, immediate and personalized monitoring and intervention “prescription” that will ensure each individual patients length and quality of life.

REFERENCES

Adamic, L., & Adar, E. (2005). How to search a social network. *Social Networks*, *27*(3), 187–203. doi:10.1016/j.socnet.2005.01.007

Akbaraly, T. N., Portet, F., Fustinoni, S., Dartigues, J.-F., Artero, S., Rouaud, O., & Berr, C. et al. (2009). Leisure activities and the risk of dementia in the elderly: Results from the Three-City Study. *Neurology*, *73*(11), 854–861. doi:10.1212/WNL.0b013e3181b7849b PMID:19752452

Artikis, A., Bamidis, P. D., Billis, A., Bratsas, C., Frantzidis, C., Karkaletsis, V., … Spyropoulos, C. S. (2012). *Supporting tele-health and AI-based clinical decision making with sensor data fusion and semantic interpretation: The USEFIL case study*. Retrieved July 24, 2015, from http://airtlab.dii.univpm.it/netmed2012/sites/netmed2012.dii.univpm.it/files/papers/netmed2012.pdf#page=32

Ashton, K. (2009). That “Internet of Things” Thing. *RFiD Journal*, *4986*. Retrieved from http://www.itrco.jp/libraries/RFIDjournal-That Internet of Things Thing.pdf\npapers3://publication/uuid/8191C095-0D90-4A17-86B0-550F2F2A6745

Babiloni, C., Binetti, G., Cassetta, E., Cerboneschi, D., Dal Forno, G., Del Percio, C., & Rossini, P. M. et al. (2004). Mapping distributed sources of cortical rhythms in mild Alzheimer’s disease. A multicentric EEG study. *NeuroImage*, *22*(1), 57–67. doi:10.1016/j.neuroimage.2003.09.028 PMID:15109997

Babiloni, C., Carducci, F., Lizio, R., Vecchio, F., Baglieri, A., Bernardini, S., & Frisoni, G. B. et al. (2013). Resting state cortical electroencephalographic rhythms are related to gray matter volume in subjects with mild cognitive impairment and Alzheimer’s disease. *Human Brain Mapping*, *34*(6), 1427–1446. doi:10.1002/hbm.22005 PMID:22331654

Bamidis, P. D., Vivas, A. B., Styliadis, C., Frantzidis, C., Klados, M., Schlee, W., & Papageorgiou, S. G. et al. (2014). A review of physical and cognitive interventions in aging. *Neuroscience and Biobehavioral Reviews*, *44*, 206–220. doi:10.1016/j.neubiorev.2014.03.019 PMID:24705268

Barber, R., Gholkar, A., Scheltens, P., Ballard, C., McKeith, I. G., & O'Brien, J. T. (1999). Medial temporal lobe atrophy on MRI in dementia with Lewy bodies. *Neurology*, *52*(6), 1153–1153. doi:10.1212/WNL.52.6.1153 PMID:10214736

Beerens, H. C., Zwakhalen, S. M. G., Verbeek, H., Ruwaard, D., & Hamers, J. P. H. (2013). Factors associated with quality of life of people with dementia in long-term care facilities: A systematic review. *International Journal of Nursing Studies*, *50*(9), 1259–1270. doi:10.1016/j.ijnurstu.2013.02.005 PMID:23465959

Bellotti, F., Kapralos, B., Lee, K., Moreno-Ger, P., & Berta, R. (2013). Assessment in and of Serious Games: An Overview. *Advances in Human-Computer Interaction*, *2013*, 1–11. doi:10.1155/2013/136864

Bennys, K., Rondouin, G., Vergnes, C., & Touchon, J. (2001). Diagnostic value of quantitative EEG in Alzheimer's disease. *Neurophysiologie Clinique. Clinical Neurophysiology*, *31*(3), 153–160. doi:10.1016/S0987-7053(01)00254-4 PMID:11488226

Billis, A. S., Papageorgiou, E. I., Frantzidis, C., Konstantinidis, E. I., & Bamidis, P. D. (2013). Towards a hierarchically-structured decision support tool for improving seniors' independent living. In *Proceedings of the 6th International Conference on PErvasive Technologies Related to Assistive Environments - PETRA '13* (pp. 1–4). New York: ACM Press. http://doi.org/ doi:10.1145/2504335.2504362

Billis, A. S., Papageorgiou, E. I., Frantzidis, C. A., Tsatali, M. S., Tsolaki, A. C., & Bamidis, P. D. (2015). A Decision-Support Framework for Promoting Independent Living and Ageing Well. *IEEE Journal of Biomedical and Health Informatics*, *19*(1), 199–209. doi:10.1109/JBHI.2014.2336757 PMID:25073180

Boise, L., Morgan, D. L., Kaye, J., & Camicioli, R. (1999). Delays in the diagnosis of dementia: Perspectives of family caregivers. *American Journal of Alzheimer's Disease and Other Dementias*, *14*(1), 20–26. doi:10.1177/153331759901400101

Borson, S., Frank, L., Bayley, P. J., Boustani, M., Dean, M., Lin, P.-J., & Ashford, J. W. et al. (2013). Improving dementia care: The role of screening and detection of cognitive impairment. *Alzheimer's & Dementia : The Journal of the Alzheimer's Association*, *9*(2), 151–159. doi:10.1016/j.jalz.2012.08.008 PMID:23375564

Boyke, J., Driemeyer, J., Gaser, C., Buchel, C., & May, A. (2008). Training-Induced Brain Structure Changes in the Elderly. *The Journal of Neuroscience*, *28*(28), 7031–7035. doi:10.1523/JNEUROSCI.0742-08.2008 PMID:18614670

Bradford, A., Kunik, M. E., Schulz, P., Williams, S. P., & Singh, H. (2009). Missed and Delayed Diagnosis of Dementia in Primary Care. *Alzheimer Disease and Associated Disorders*, *23*(4), 306–314. doi:10.1097/WAD.0b013e3181a6bebc PMID:19568149

Brewer, M. (2014). Handbook of Research Methods in Social and Personality Psychology. Retrieved from http://books.google.com/books?id=NRWTAgAAQBAJ&pgis=1

Burke, S. N., & Barnes, C. A. (2006). Neural plasticity in the ageing brain. *Nature Reviews. Neuroscience*, *7*(1), 30–40. doi:10.1038/nrn1809 PMID:16371948

Busse, A. L., Gil, G., Santarém, J. M., & Filho, W. J. (2009). Physical activity and cognition in the elderly: A review. *Dementia Neuropsychologia, 3*(3), 204–208. Retrieved from http://search.ebscohost.com/login.aspx?direct=true&db=psyh&AN=2010-10986-005&site=ehost-live

Byun, S., & Park, C. (2011). *Serious Game for Cognitive Testing of Elderly HCI International 2011 – Posters' Extended Abstracts* (C. Stephanidis, Ed.). Berlin: Springer Berlin Heidelberg. doi:10.1007/978-3-642-22098-2

Camicioli, R., Howieson, D., Oken, B., Sexton, G., & Kaye, J. (1998). Motor slowing precedes cognitive impairment in the oldest old. *Neurology*, *50*(5), 1496–1498. doi:10.1212/WNL.50.5.1496 PMID:9596020

Canu, E., McLaren, D. G., Fitzgerald, M. E., Bendlin, B. B., Zoccatelli, G., Alessandrini, F., & Frisoni, G. B. et al. (2010). Microstructural diffusion changes are independent of macrostructural volume loss in moderate to severe Alzheimer's disease. *Journal of Alzheimer's Disease*, *19*(3), 963–976. doi:10.3233/JAD-2010-1295 PMID:20157252

Cassady, J. C., & Johnson, R. E. (2002). Cognitive Test Anxiety and Academic Performance. *Contemporary Educational Psychology*, *27*(2), 270–295. doi:10.1006/ceps.2001.1094

Chiriac, S., Röll, N., Parada, J., & Rosales, B. (2012). Towards combining validation concepts for short and long-term ambient health monitoring. *2012 6th International Conference on Pervasive Computing Technologies for Healthcare and Workshops, PervasiveHealth 2012*. http://doi.org/ doi:<ALIGNMENT.qj></ALIGNMENT>10.4108/icst.pervasivehealth.2012.248676

Colcombe, S., & Kramer, A. F. (2003). Fitness effects on the cognitive function of older adults: A Meta-Analytic study. *Psychological Science*, *14*(2), 125–130. doi:10.1111/1467-9280.t01-1-01430 PMID:12661673

Collerton, J., Collerton, D., Arai, Y., Barrass, K., Eccles, M., Jagger, C., & Kirkwood, T. et al. (2007). A comparison of computerized and pencil-and-paper tasks in assessing cognitive function in community-dwelling older people in the Newcastle 85+ Pilot Study. *Journal of the American Geriatrics Society*, *55*(10), 1630–1635. doi:10.1111/j.1532-5415.2007.01379.x PMID:17697099

Czaplicka, A., Holyst, J. A., & Sloot, P. M. A. (2013). Noise enhances information transfer in hierarchical networks. *Scientific Reports*, *3*, 1223. doi:10.1038/srep01223 PMID:23390574

Delbeuck, X., Collette, F., & Van der Linden, M. (2007). Is Alzheimer's disease a disconnection syndrome? Evidence from a crossmodal audio-visual illusory experiment. *Neuropsychologia*, *45*(14), 3315–3323. doi:10.1016/j.neuropsychologia.2007.05.001 PMID:17765932

Dubois, B., Feldman, H. H., Jacova, C., Dekosky, S. T., Barberger-Gateau, P., Cummings, J., & Scheltens, P. et al. (2007). Research criteria for the diagnosis of Alzheimer's disease: Revising the NINCDS-ADRDA criteria. *Lancet Neurology*, *6*(8), 734–746. doi:10.1016/S1474-4422(07)70178-3 PMID:17616482

dynanets.org. (2015). Retrieved July 25, 2015, from http://dynanets.org/

Fellgiebel, A., Dellani, P. R., Greverus, D., Scheurich, A., Stoeter, P., & Müller, M. J. (2006). Predicting conversion to dementia in mild cognitive impairment by volumetric and diffusivity measurements of the hippocampus. *Psychiatry Research: Neuroimaging*, *146*(3), 283–287. doi:10.1016/j.pscychresns.2006.01.006 PMID:16530394

Fernández, A., Turrero, A., Zuluaga, P., Gil, P., Maestú, F., Campo, P., & Ortiz, T. (2006). Magnetoencephalographic parietal delta dipole density in mild cognitive impairment: Preliminary results of a method to estimate the risk of developing Alzheimer disease. *Archives of Neurology*, *63*(3), 427–430. doi:10.1001/archneur.63.3.427 PMID:16533970

Flicker, L. (1999). Book: Dementia Reconsidered: the Person Comes First. *BMJ (Clinical Research Ed.)*, *318*(7187), 880–880. doi:10.1136/bmj.318.7187.880a PMID:10092286

Fox, N. C., & Freeborough, P. A. (1997). Brain atrophy progression measured from registered serial MRI: Validation and application to alzheimer's disease. *Journal of Magnetic Resonance Imaging*, *7*(6), 1069–1075. doi:10.1002/jmri.1880070620 PMID:9400851

Frantzidis, C. A., Vivas, A. B., Tsolaki, A., Klados, M. A., Tsolaki, M., & Bamidis, P. D. (2014). Functional disorganization of small-world brain networks in mild Alzheimer's Disease and amnestic Mild Cognitive Impairment: An EEG study using Relative Wavelet Entropy (RWE). *Frontiers in Aging Neuroscience*, *6*, 224. doi:10.3389/fnagi.2014.00224 PMID:25206333

Fratiglioni, L., Wang, H. X., Ericsson, K., Maytan, M., & Winblad, B. (2000). Influence of social network on occurrence of dementia: A community-based longitudinal study. *Lancet*, *355*(9212), 1315–1319. doi:10.1016/S0140-6736(00)02113-9 PMID:10776744

Garcés, P., Angel Pineda-Pardo, J., Canuet, L., Aurtenetxe, S., López, M. E., Marcos, A., & Maestú, F. et al. (2014). The Default Mode Network is functionally and structurally disrupted in amnestic mild cognitive impairment - a bimodal MEG-DTI study. *NeuroImage. Clinical*, *6*, 214–221. doi:10.1016/j.nicl.2014.09.004 PMID:25379433

Golle, P., & Partridge, K. (2009). Pervasive Computing (Vol. 5538). Berlin: Springer Berlin Heidelberg. http://doi.org/ doi:<ALIGNMENT.qj></ALIGNMENT>10.1007/978-3-642-01516-8_26

Greicius, M. D., Srivastava, G., Reiss, A. L., & Menon, V. (2004). Default-mode network activity distinguishes Alzheimer's disease from healthy aging: Evidence from functional MRI. *Proceedings of the National Academy of Sciences of the United States of America*, *101*(13), 4637–4642. doi:10.1073/pnas.0308627101 PMID:15070770

Hagler, S., Austin, D., Hayes, T. L., Kaye, J., & Pavel, M. (2010). Unobtrusive and ubiquitous in-home monitoring: A methodology for continuous assessment of gait velocity in elders. *IEEE Transactions on Bio-Medical Engineering*, *57*(4), 813–820. doi:10.1109/TBME.2009.2036732 PMID:19932989

Hagler, S., Jimison, H. B., & Pavel, M. (2014). Assessing executive function using a computer game: Computational modeling of cognitive processes. *IEEE Journal of Biomedical and Health Informatics*, *18*(4), 1442–1452. doi:10.1109/JBHI.2014.2299793 PMID:25014944

Hayes, T. L., Abendroth, F., Adami, A., Pavel, M., Zitzelberger, T. A., & Kaye, J. A. (2008). Unobtrusive assessment of activity patterns associated with mild cognitive impairment. *Alzheimer's & Dementia : The Journal of the Alzheimer's Association*, *4*(6), 395–405. doi:10.1016/j.jalz.2008.07.004 PMID:19012864

Hayes, T. L., Riley, T., Mattek, N., Pavel, M., & Kaye, J. A. (2014). Sleep habits in mild cognitive impairment. *Alzheimer Disease and Associated Disorders*, *28*(2), 145–150. doi:10.1097/WAD.0000000000000010 PMID:24145694

Hedden, T., & Gabrieli, J. D. E. (2004). Insights into the ageing mind: A view from cognitive neuroscience. *Nature Reviews. Neuroscience*, *5*(2), 87–96. doi:10.1038/nrn1323 PMID:14735112

Hughes, J. C., Robinson, L., & Volicer, L. (2005). Specialist palliative care in dementia. *BMJ (Clinical Research Ed.)*, *330*(7482), 57–58. doi:10.1136/bmj.330.7482.57 PMID:15637354

Jeong, J. (2004). EEG dynamics in patients with Alzheimer's disease. *Clinical Neurophysiology: Official Journal of the International Federation of Clinical Neurophysiology*, *115*(7), 1490–1505. doi:10.1016/j.clinph.2004.01.001 PMID:15203050

Kantarci, K., Senjem, M. L., Avula, R., Zhang, B., Samikoglu, A. R., Weigand, S. D., & Jack, C. R. et al. (2011). Diffusion tensor imaging and cognitive function in older adults with no dementia. *Neurology*, *77*(1), 26–34. doi:10.1212/WNL.0b013e31822313dc PMID:21593440

Katzouris, N., Artikis, A., & Paliouras, G. (2014). Event Recognition for Unobtrusive Assisted Living. In A. Likas, K. Blekas, & D. Kalles (Eds.), Lecture Notes in Computer Science: Vol. 8445. *Artificial Intelligence: Methods and Applications* (pp. 237–250). Cham: Springer International Publishing; doi:10.1007/978-3-319-07064-3

Konstantinidis, E., Antoniou, P., Billis, A., Bamparopoulos, G., Costas, P., & Bamidis, P. (2014). *Universal Access in Human-Computer Interaction. Aging and Assistive Environments* (C. Stephanidis & M. Antona, Eds.). Cham: Springer International Publishing. doi:10.1007/978-3-319-07446-7

Konstantinidis, E., Billis, A., Mouzakidis, C., Zilidou, V., Antoniou, P., & Bamidis, P. (2014). Design, implementation and wide pilot deployment of FitForAll: an easy to use exergaming platform improving physical fitness and life quality of senior citizens. *IEEE Journal of Biomedical and Health Informatics*, 1–1. http://doi.org/<ALIGNMENT.qj></ALIGNMENT>10.1109/JBHI.2014.2378814

Konstantinidis, E. I., Antoniou, P. E., Bamparopoulos, G., & Bamidis, P. D. (2014). A lightweight framework for transparent cross platform communication of controller data in ambient assisted living environments. *Information Sciences*, *300*, 124–139. doi:10.1016/j.ins.2014.10.070

Konstantinidis, E. I., Bamidis, P. D., Billis, A. S., Kartsidis, P., & Papageorgiou, S. G. (2015). Physical training in-game metrics for cognitive assessment: Evidence from extended trials with the FitForAll exergame platform. *PLoS ONE*.

Kotagal, V., Langa, K. M., Plassman, B. L., Fisher, G. G., Giordani, B. J., Wallace, R. B., & Foster, N. L. et al. (2015). Factors associated with cognitive evaluations in the United States. *Neurology*, *84*(1), 64–71. doi:10.1212/WNL.0000000000001096 PMID:25428689

Leung, P., Orrell, M., & Orgeta, V. (2015). Social support group interventions in people with dementia and mild cognitive impairment: A systematic review of the literature. *International Journal of Geriatric Psychiatry*, *30*(1), 1–9. doi:10.1002/gps.4166 PMID:24990344

Liu, S., Shen, Z., Mei, J., & Ji, J. (2013). Parkinson's Disease Predictive Analytics through a Pad Game Based on Personal Data. *Int. J. Inf. Technol, 19*(2).

Liu, Y., Wang, K., Yu, C., He, Y., Zhou, Y., Liang, M., & Jiang, T. et al. (2008). Regional homogeneity, functional connectivity and imaging markers of Alzheimer's disease: A review of resting-state fMRI studies. *Neuropsychologia*, *46*(6), 1648–1656. doi:10.1016/j.neuropsychologia.2008.01.027 PMID:18346763

Lyketsos, C. G., Lopez, O., Jones, B., Fitzpatrick, A. L., Breitner, J., & DeKosky, S. (2002). Prevalence of Neuropsychiatric Symptoms in Dementia and Mild Cognitive Impairment. *Journal of the American Medical Association*, *288*(12), 1475. doi:10.1001/jama.288.12.1475 PMID:12243634

Lyons, B. E., Austin, D., Seelye, A., Petersen, J., Yeargers, J., & Riley, T., … Kaye, J. a. (2015). Pervasive Computing Technologies to Continuously Assess Alzheimerâ€™s Disease Progression and Intervention Efficacy. *Frontiers in Aging Neuroscience*, *7*(June), 1–14. doi:10.3389/fnagi.2015.00102 PMID:25653617

Mahncke, H. W., Connor, B. B., Appelman, J., Ahsanuddin, O. N., Hardy, J. L., Wood, R. A., … Merzenich, M. M. (2006). Memory enhancement in healthy older adults using a brain plasticity-based training program: a randomized, controlled study. *Proceedings of the National Academy of Sciences of the United States of America*, *103*(33), 12523–8. http://doi.org/ doi:10.1073/pnas.0605194103

McCormick, W. C., Kukull, W. A., van Belle, G., Bowen, J. D., Teri, L., & Larson, E. B. (1994). Symptom Patterns and Comorbidity in the Early Stages of Alzheimer's Disease. *Journal of the American Geriatrics Society*, *42*(5), 517–521. doi:10.1111/j.1532-5415.1994.tb04974.x PMID:8176147

McKanna, J. A., Jimison, H., & Pavel, M. (2009). Divided attention in computer game play: analysis utilizing unobtrusive health monitoring. *Conference Proceedings: ... Annual International Conference of the IEEE Engineering in Medicine and Biology Society. IEEE Engineering in Medicine and Biology Society. Annual Conference, 2009*. http://doi.org/ doi:10.1109/IEMBS.2009.5334662

McKeith, I. G., Dickson, D. W., Lowe, J., Emre, M., O'Brien, J. T., Feldman, H., & Yamada, M. et al. (2005). Diagnosis and management of dementia with Lewy bodies: Third report of the DLB Consortium. *Neurology*, *65*(12), 1863–1872. doi:10.1212/01.wnl.0000187889.17253.b1 PMID:16237129

Mehta, K. M., Yaffe, K., & Covinsky, K. E. (2002). Cognitive Impairment, Depressive Symptoms, and Functional Decline in Older People. *Journal of the American Geriatrics Society*, *50*(6), 1045–1050. doi:10.1046/j.1532-5415.2002.50259.x PMID:12110064

Mevel, K., Chételat, G., Eustache, F., & Desgranges, B. (2011). The default mode network in healthy aging and Alzheimer's disease. *International Journal of Alzheimer's Disease*, *535816*. doi:10.4061/2011/535816 PMID:21760988

Mihailidis, A. (2008). *Technology and Aging: Selected Papers from the 2007 International Conference on Technology and Aging*. Retrieved from https://books.google.com/books?hl=el&lr=&id=OSCScvzDPrwC&pgis=1

Monekosso, D. N., & Remagnino, P. (2010). Behavior Analysis for Assisted Living. *IEEE Transactions on Automation Science and Engineering*, *7*(4), 879–886. doi:10.1109/TASE.2010.2049840

Oishi, K., Mielke, M. M., Albert, M., Lyketsos, C. G., & Mori, S. (2012). The fornix sign: A potential sign for Alzheimer's disease based on diffusion tensor imaging. *Journal of Neuroimaging : Official Journal of the American Society of Neuroimaging*, *22*(4), 365–374. doi:10.1111/j.1552-6569.2011.00633.x PMID:21848679

Panagiotis, D., Bamidis, Tarnanas, I., Tsolaki, M., & Hadjileontiadis, L. (2015). *Handbook of Research on Innovations in Database Technologies and Applications: Current and Future Trends*. Retrieved July 29, 2015, from http://www.igi-global.com/book/handbook-research-innovations-diagnosis-treatment/121164

Papageorgiou, E. I., Billis, A. S., Frantzidis, C., Konstantinidis, E. I., & Bamidis, P. D. (2013). A preliminary fuzzy cognitive map - based desicion support tool for geriatric depression assessment. In *2013 IEEE International Conference on Fuzzy Systems (FUZZ-IEEE)* (pp. 1–8). IEEE. http://doi.org/ doi:10.1109/FUZZ-IEEE.2013.6622485

Paraskevopoulos, E., Kuchenbuch, A., Herholz, S. C., & Pantev, C. (2014). Multisensory integration during short-term music reading training enhances both uni- and multisensory cortical processing. *Journal of Cognitive Neuroscience*, *26*(10), 2224–2238. doi:10.1162/jocn_a_00620 PMID:24669793

Quax, R., Apolloni, A., & Sloot, P. M. A. (2013). Towards understanding the behavior of physical systems using information theory. *The European Physical Journal. Special Topics*, *222*(6), 1389–1401. doi:10.1140/epjst/e2013-01933-9

Quax, R., Kandhai, D., & Sloot, P. M. A. (2013). Information dissipation as an early-warning signal for the Lehman Brothers collapse in financial time series. *Scientific Reports*, *3*, 1898. doi:10.1038/srep01898 PMID:23719567

Raichle, M. E., MacLeod, A. M., Snyder, A. Z., Powers, W. J., Gusnard, D. A., & Shulman, G. L. (2001). A default mode of brain function. *Proceedings of the National Academy of Sciences of the United States of America*, *98*(2), 676–682. doi:10.1073/pnas.98.2.676 PMID:11209064

Rashidi, P., & Mihailidis, A. (2013). A Survey on Ambient-Assisted Living Tools for Older Adults. *IEEE Journal of Biomedical and Health Informatics*, *17*(3), 579–590. doi:10.1109/JBHI.2012.2234129 PMID:24592460

Reiman, E. M., Quiroz, Y. T., Fleisher, A. S., Chen, K., Velez-Pardo, C., Jimenez-Del-Rio, M., & Lopera, F. et al. (2012). Brain imaging and fluid biomarker analysis in young adults at genetic risk for autosomal dominant Alzheimer's disease in the presenilin 1 E280A kindred: A case-control study. *Lancet Neurology*, *11*(12), 1048–1056. doi:10.1016/S1474-4422(12)70228-4 PMID:23137948

Risacher, S. L., Saykin, A. J., West, J. D., Shen, L., Firpi, H. A., & McDonald, B. C. (2009). Baseline MRI predictors of conversion from MCI to probable AD in the ADNI cohort. *Current Alzheimer Research*, *6*(4), 347–361. doi:10.2174/156720509788929273 PMID:19689234

Robert, P. H., König, A., Amieva, H., Andrieu, S., Bremond, F., Bullock, R., & Manera, V. et al. (2014). Recommendations for the use of Serious Games in people with Alzheimer's Disease, related disorders and frailty. *Frontiers in Aging Neuroscience*, *6*, 54. doi:10.3389/fnagi.2014.00054 PMID:24715864

Röcker, C., Hinske, S., & Magerkurth, C. (2007). Universal Access in Human-Computer Interaction. Ambient Interaction (Vol. 4555). Berlin: Springer Berlin Heidelberg. http://doi.org/ doi:<ALIGNMENT.qj></ALIGNMENT>10.1007/978-3-540-73281-5

Rogalski, E., Stebbins, G. T., Barnes, C. A., Murphy, C. M., Stoub, T. R., George, S., & deToledo-Morrell, L. et al. (2012). Age-related changes in parahippocampal white matter integrity: A diffusion tensor imaging study. *Neuropsychologia*, *50*(8), 1759–1765. doi:10.1016/j.neuropsychologia.2012.03.033 PMID:22561887

Scarmeas, N., Levy, G., Tang, M.-X., Manly, J., & Stern, Y. (2001). Influence of leisure activity on the incidence of Alzheimer's Disease. *Neurology*, *57*(12), 2236–2242. doi:10.1212/WNL.57.12.2236 PMID:11756603

Seelye, A., Mattek, N., Howieson, D., Riley, T., Wild, K., & Kaye, J. (2015). The Impact of Sleep on Neuropsychological Performance in Cognitively Intact Older Adults Using a Novel In-Home Sensor-Based Sleep Assessment Approach. *The Clinical Neuropsychologist*, *29*(1), 53–66. doi:10.1080/13854046.2015.1005139 PMID:25642948

Sheline, Y. I., Morris, J. C., Snyder, A. Z., Price, J. L., Yan, Z., D'Angelo, G., & Mintun, M. A. et al. (2010). APOE4 allele disrupts resting state fMRI connectivity in the absence of amyloid plaques or decreased CSF Aβ42. *The Journal of Neuroscience*, *30*(50), 17035–17040. doi:10.1523/JNEUROSCI.3987-10.2010 PMID:21159973

Shi, F., Liu, B., Zhou, Y., Yu, C., & Jiang, T. (2009). Hippocampal volume and asymmetry in mild cognitive impairment and Alzheimer's disease: Meta-analyses of MRI studies. *Hippocampus*, *19*(11), 1055–1064. doi:10.1002/hipo.20573 PMID:19309039

Staiano, A. E., & Calvert, S. L. (2011). The promise of exergames as tools to measure physical health. *Entertainment Computing*, *2*(1), 17–21. doi:10.1016/j.entcom.2011.03.008 PMID:23378860

Storf, H., Becker, M., & Riedl, M. (2009). Rule-based activity recognition framework: Challenges, technique and learning. In *Proceedings of the 3d International ICST Conference on Pervasive Computing Technologies for Healthcare* (pp. 1–7). ICST. http://doi.org/ doi:10.4108/ICST.PERVASIVEHEALTH2009.6108

Styliadis, C., Kartsidis, P., & Paraskevopoulos, E. (n.d.). *Neuroimaging Approaches for Elderly Studies*. IGI Global. Retrieved from http://www.igi-global.com/chapter/neuroimaging-approaches-for-elderly-studies/129268

Styliadis, C., Kartsidis, P., Paraskevopoulos, E., Ioannides, A. A., & Bamidis, P. D. (2015). Neuroplastic Effects of Combined Computerized Physical and Cognitive Training in Elderly Individuals at Risk for Dementia: An eLORETA Controlled Study on Resting States. *Neural Plasticity*, *12*(2). Retrieved from http://doi.org/ doi:10.1155/2015/172192 PMID:25945260

Tardif, S., & Simard, M. (2011). Cognitive stimulation programs in healthy elderly: A review. *International Journal of Alzheimer's Disease*, *378934*. doi:10.4061/2011/378934 PMID:21876829

Tarnanas, I., Schlee, W., Tsolaki, M., Müri, R., Mosimann, U., & Nef, T. (2013). Ecological validity of virtual reality daily living activities screening for early dementia: Longitudinal study. *JMIR Serious Games*, *1*(1), e1. doi:10.2196/games.2778 PMID:25658491

Tractenberg, R. E., Singer, C. M., & Kaye, J. (2005). Symptoms of sleep disturbance in persons with Alzheimer's disease and normal elderly. *Journal of Sleep Research*, *14*(2), 177–185. doi:10.1111/j.1365-2869.2005.00445.x PMID:15910515

Wang, L., Zang, Y., He, Y., Liang, M., Zhang, X., Tian, L., & Li, K. et al. (2006). Changes in hippocampal connectivity in the early stages of Alzheimer's disease: Evidence from resting state fMRI. *NeuroImage*, *31*(2), 496–504. doi:10.1016/j.neuroimage.2005.12.033 PMID:16473024

Wang, X. (2014). Subjective well-being associated with size of social network and social support of elderly. *Journal of Health Psychology*. http://doi.org/<ALIGNMENT.qj></ALIGNMENT>10.1177/1359105314544136

WHO. (2012). *Dementia: a public health priority*. Retrieved from http://www.who.int/mental_health/publications/dementia_report_2012/en/

Xefteris, S., Andronikou, V., Tserpes, K., & Varvarigou, T. (2010). Case-based approach using behavioural biometrics aimed at Assisted Living. *Journal of Ambient Intelligence and Humanized Computing*, *2*(2), 73–80. doi:10.1007/s12652-010-0029-8

Xefteris, S., Baboshin, A., Tserpes, K., Androulidakis, A., Glickman, Y., Varvarigou, T., … D'Andria, F. (2011). Enabling risk assessment and analysis by event detection in dementia patients using a reconfigurable rule set. In *Proceedings of the 4th International Conference on Pervasive Technologies Related to Assistive Environments - PETRA '11* (p. 1). New York: ACM Press. http://doi.org/doi:10.1145/2141622.2141678

Yang, G., Xie, L., Mantysalo, M., Zhou, X., Pang, Z., Xu, L., … Zheng, L.-R. (2014). A Health-IoT Platform Based on the Integration of Intelligent Packaging, Unobtrusive Bio-Sensor, and Intelligent Medicine Box. *IEEE Transactions on Industrial Informatics, 10*(4), 2180–2191. http://doi.org/<ALIGNMENT.qj></ALIGNMENT>10.1109/TII.2014.2307795

Yang, S. (2010). Defining Exergames & Exergaming. *Proceedings of Meaningful Play, 2010*, 1–17. Retrieved from http://meaningfulplay.msu.edu/proceedings2010/mp2010_paper_63.pdf

Zarrabi, N., Prosperi, M. C. F., Belleman, R. G., Di Giambenedetto, S., Fabbiani, M., De Luca, A., & Sloot, P. M. A. (2013). Combining social and genetic networks to study HIV transmission in mixing risk groups. *The European Physical Journal. Special Topics*, *222*(6), 1377–1387. doi:10.1140/epjst/e2013-01932-x

Chapter 5
Dementia and Language Bilingualism Helps Ward Off Alzheimer's Disease

Yiyang Yu
Northeast University, China

Yan Wu
Northeast Normal University, China

Sihan Lu
Northeast Normal University, China

Qiong Wu
Okayama University, Japan

Jinglong Wu
Okayama University, Japan

ABSTRACT

There has been extensive discussion with regard to whether bilingualism helps ward off dementia. However, there is still debate over bilingualism's effects. Researchers have determined that bilinguals have a greater advantage in delaying dementia than monolinguals. Researchers have used cognitive reserve to explain their views. However, recently, some researchers have arrived at a different conclusion, stating that bilinguals have no advantage compared with monolinguals in delaying dementia. In this review, we summarize a review of studies on bilingualism and dementia, supporting the viewpoint that bilinguals have an advantage in delaying dementia compared with monolinguals.

DOI: 10.4018/978-1-5225-0925-7.ch005

INTRODUCTION

As technology leads to advancements in medical treatment, life expectancy continues to increase, thus increasing the proportion of the elderly population. Adverse effects of brain diseases on the health of the elderly, particularly dementia, have become increasingly prominent. According to the report from the World Health Organization and the International Alzheimer's Association titled "Dementia: A public health priority" (World Health Organization, Alzheimer's Disease International, 2012), there were 35.6 million patients with dementia patient worldwide in 2012; this number is expected to increase to 65.7 million by 2030 and to 115.4 million by 2050. Moreover, $604 billion was spent on nursing care in 2012 alone. To benefit the health of mankind and save the resources of human society, it is imminent to find a way to resist dementia. Recently, resistance to dementia has received significant attention in society, and many efforts have been focused on this field, with some achievements. Many researchers focus on the study of dementia and language. Alzheimer's disease directly affects the patient's language skills. Researchers have found that different subtypes of dementia have different effects on the language ability of patients; for example, the language skills of patients with Alzheimer's disease will be reflected in the phoneme (Whitaker 1976, Balyes 1982), syntax, (Schwarts 1979, Obler 1983), semantics (Barker 1968, Bayles 1982, Nicholas 1985, Schwartz 1979, Bayles & Tomeda 1983, Gewirth 1984, Robinson 1996), discourse and pragmatic aspects (Nicholas 1985, Ripich 1988). Therefore, do language skills, particularly the number of language acquisitions, have effects on resisting dementia?

BACKGROUND

Classification of Dementia

The word 'Dementia' is derived from Latin, *de-men-tia*. *De* means away from, *men* means the mind, and *tia* is to the state. Dementia is a type of brain disease that results in memory and cognitive problems in patients; it is also characterized by degenerating functions of patient emotion, language and behavior. It can result in degeneration of the personal life, but the individual can still be physically maintained.

Sixty-five years old is used as the disease onset time boundary. If onset occurs before 65 years old, it is referred to as presenile dementia; if the onset occurs after 65 years old (including 65), it is referred to as senile dementia. Most patients have dementia in the senile stage. Smith (2013) believes that dementia is characterized by persistent changes in senile mental changes.

Current studies show that brain damage, aging and disease are the causes of dementia, which results in mental function degrading at a faster than typical rate at that age. Dementia is not one disease but rather a group of similar clinical manifestations of disease clusters.

Dementia can be divided into three types based on its cause: degenerative dementia, vascular dementia and post-traumatic dementia. Degenerative dementia includes Alzheimer's disease, front temporal dementia and Lewy body dementia. Vascular dementia is caused by cerebral vascular disease, and traumatic dementia is caused by a head trauma.

According to lesion location, dementia can be divided into cortical dementia and subcortical dementia. In cortical dementia (Corsellis, 1962), including Alzheimer's disease, the lesion is detected in the cerebral cortex. In subcortical dementia (Albert, 1974), the lesion area is detected in the cortex of the brain, such as in Parkinson's disease and Huntington's disease. In limbic dementia, the lesion area is detected in the limbic system (Gascon, 1973).

According to the possibility of cure, dementia can be divided into reversible and irreversible dementia. Some types of dementia can be cured, for example, when dementia is caused by a lack of vitamins or cancer. However, only approximately 5% of patients have reversible dementia. Most patients have irreversible dementia, which can only be prevented and relieved.

Diagnosis Tools of Dementia

Currently, people mainly use the CDR MMSE scale to diagnose dementia. In addition, brain science technology also plays an increasingly important role in the diagnosis of dementia.

Clinical Dementia Rating (CDR)

CDR is a clinical dementia rating scale that includes six dimensions: memory, orientation, judgment and problem-solving skills, work and social skills, family and personal preference and the ability to live independently. Each dimension has five levels corresponding to a different point value as follows: health (CDR = 0), suspected dementia (CDR = 0.5), mild dementia (CDR = 1), moderate dementia (CDR = 2) and severe dementia (CDR = 3). Doctors obtain assessment scores through communication with patients and their relatives.

When the patient receives a CDR score of 0 and does not display obvious symptoms, the patient is in a healthy state. A CDR score of 0.5 indicates that the patient is essentially normal, with only minor damage. A CDR score of 1 indicates that the patient has more obvious symptoms and cannot complete complex tasks. A CDR score of 2 indicates that the patient's cognitive ability is greatly affected and that they can complete only simple tasks; the patient must be taken care of. A CDR score of 3 indicates that the patient's cognitive ability is severely damaged and that the patient cannot perform independent activities.

Mini Mental Status Examination (MMSE)

The MMSE is a simple psychological scale, also known as the Folstein Test (Folstein, 1975); this test was originally designed for intellectual impairment evaluation and was only later used to diagnose dementia. It is currently used to diagnose Alzheimer's disease in clinical situations. The diagnosis includes time and place orientation, language, mental arithmetic, short-term memory, graphics imitation and other projects. A correct answer receives one point, and the test has scores ranging from 0-30. A score above 24 represents a normal score. A score of 18-24 indicates mild dementia, a score of 16-17 indicates moderate dementia, and a score of 15 or less indicates severe dementia.

Other Diagnostic Tools

The DRS scale was designed by Mattis (1976). It contains five dimensions: attention, boot protection, concept formation, structure and memory. Compared with the MMSE scale, the DRS scale has more content. However, according to the Stuss (1996) survey, the DRS does not have a significant advantage compared with the MMSE scale in the diagnosis of dementia. The ADAS, CERAD, ADL and other tools are also used in the diagnosis of dementia.

Structural brain imaging includes MRI and CT. Brain imaging technology can identify degradations of the patient's brain. Additionally, we can explore the relationship between the degrees of brain atrophy in patients with individual differences. MRI is better than CT for the technical analysis of dementia.

Functional brain imaging includes positron emission tomography (PET) and single photon emission computed tomography (SPECT). The PET technique is more sensitive than SPECT technology in the diagnosis of early stage Alzheimer's. In recent years, functional magnetic resonance imaging (FMRI) has increasingly been used in the diagnosis of dementia. FMRI and PET diagnostic results are similar. However, the advantage of FMRI is that it can conduct brain function tests while the patient is performing cognitive tests.

Electroencephalography (EEG) has low costs, and it can be frequently repeated. The test results of the elderly differ significantly from those of normal young people.

According to Berger (1937), the brain waves of elderly people are similar those of young people with brain disease. However, as Alzheimer's disease progresses, EGG changes will become more apparent.

It is possible to diagnose Alzheimer's disease by neuropsychological indicators (Wu 2012), in addition to using a variety of scales to diagnose Alzheimer's disease. Researchers have made successful diagnosis through visual, auditory, tactile and multisensory integration. (Wu 2012) In clinical diagnosis, neuropsychological testing has the following advantages:

First, wide range of applications. Scale diagnostic requests subjects have knowledge and language background. Neuropsychological indicators diagnosis according to visual auditory and tactile, which has good adaptability for subjects.

Second, cost saving. Current neuroimaging method for diagnosing Alzheimer's costs more. Therefore, taking neuropsychological screening in advance is necessary, and then do further examination to the patients who have a high risk on Alzheimer's disease.

Third, high accuracy. Neuropsychological index can test the subject's visual, auditory and tactile cognitive abilities, rather than indirectly inferred through questionnaires.

However, this experimental method also has disadvantages, such as survey conditions are difficult to unify and the operation is too complex. To solve this problem, researchers invented a tactile testing equipment which can improve the efficiency and accuracy of neuropsychological examination, and reduce the difficulty of surveying at the same time (Yang, 2012, 2015). This equipment diagnoses MCI by subject's ability that can distinguish different tactile stimuli.

DEMENTIA LANGUAGE PERFORMANCE

Language Performance with Alzheimer's Disease

The cause of Alzheimer's disease is brain degeneration, which occurs at a much faster rate than the normal rate of aging. Although the pathology of Alzheimer's disease is different from that of aphasia, the symptoms of Alzheimer's disease in different stages are similar to the different types of aphasia; thus, we can learn from the research experience of aphasia. Currently, the disease cannot be cured (Selkoe, 2012), but it can be intervened through drugs. Researchers have discovered factors that influence the age of onset and have identified a series of cognitive training methods: a non-drug treatment for this disease prevention intervention, in which foreign language training is one of the most important cognitive training methods.

Alzheimer's disease is not equivalent to dementia; however, it is the most common type of dementia. Currently, many researchers are focusing on Alzheimer's disease because the proportion of patients with Alzheimer's disease accounts for approximately 70% of the total patients with dementia. Moreover, Alzheimer's disease is caused by brain degeneration, and this type of dynamic process of change has more research value.

Alzheimer's disease seriously affects the patient's language skills in the late stages of illness. Outsiders do not easily perceive the patient's condition in early illness, but patients themselves have a feeling and will use certain strategies to avoid the loss of verbal communication function (Bayles 1982). As the disease progresses, the patient will have more obvious language problems, such as naming obstacles. The main impaired language ability problem of patients with mid-term Alzheimer's is expressing one's intended meaning. Fluency, pronunciation, and grammar are not problems, but the ability of description is damaged. Late in the illness, the patient's language is completely meaningless.

Language Performance in Patients with Other Sub-Types

Pick's disease is another multiple sub-type of presenile dementia. Researchers have found that the language performance of patients with Pick's disease is different from that of patients with Alzheimer's disease. Language skills are greatly impacted in early illness (Holland, 1985). In late illness, patients with Alzheimer's disease will have the same performance as patients in the early stage of Pick's disease. The effect of sub-cortical dementia on language ability, such as in Parkinson's disease, does not have as much of an effect as that of cortical dementia (Bayles, 1982; Luo 2001).

COGNITIVE DIFFERENCES OF BILINGUALS AND MONOLINGUALS

A bilingual person is someone who can communicate in two languages. According to the mastery of the language, they can be divided into balanced and unbalanced bilinguals. Balanced bilinguals can maintain and master two languages at a similar level. Unbalanced bilinguals can master two languages, but one of the languages is more dominant. Prior studies have shown that bilinguals differ from monolinguals in cognitive ability. Researchers compared bilinguals and monolinguals and found that both bilinguals and monolinguals have advantages and disadvantages in cognitive ability.

Language Cognitive Differences

Some researchers believe that bilinguals have disadvantages in language ability. Since the 1960s, many studies have supported this view (Hakuta, 1986; Gollan, Montoya 2002; Lvanova 2008). For example, bilinguals cannot keep up with monolinguals on the following aspects: speed and fluency in picture naming, language fluency, word recall, and other aspects of the development of child language ability.

Li (2012) stated that compared with monolinguals, bilinguals have the following disadvantages: first, second language learners have a slower learning speed. Researchers found that this condition exists only in early child bilinguals and that the situation will be improved after attending school; however, they are still at a disadvantage in language examinations. Second, in terms of vocabulary, bilinguals are limited compared with monolinguals. (Páez Tabors & López 2007; Colier 1995, French & Llorente 2008). In both adults and children, bilinguals' vocabulary is smaller than that of monolinguals (Bialystck, E. Barac, R. Blaye, A. & Poulin-Dubois, D., 2010).

Conversely, some researchers believe that second language learners have no disadvantages in language ability. Petitto (2009) believes that bilingual children do not differ from monolingual children regarding language learning speed. Moreover, some researchers believe that adults' disadvantages in the vocabulary of their second language will gradually disappear (Hamers & Blanc, 2000).

However, some research shows that bilinguals have advantages in language ability. The studies of Blumenfeld (2011), Bosch (2001), Costa (2004), and Kaushanskaya (2009) have validated this view. These researchers found that bilinguals received better results in the following tasks: bilingual discrimination, language switching, and new word learning. In addition, bilinguals were more dominant in meta-language capability (Bialystok, 2003; Baker, 2001).

Both bilinguals and monolinguals display different performances in cognitive ability. For tasks involving only one language, monolinguals have an advantage over bilinguals. If the task involves cross-language, language learning, or meta-language capability, bilinguals are more dominant.

Central Executive Functions of Bilinguals

Central executive function is responsible for the processing mechanisms that occur when humans process various types of information. It is responsible for attention and the inhibition of the conversion of control (Baddeley, 2010). Bilinguals have more obvious advantages in nonverbal cognitive tasks, particularly in terms of attention selection and cognitive control (He, 2011).

Specifically speaking, there are three aspects to the advantages of bilinguals (Li, 2011). First, it is easier for bilinguals to concentrate and inhibit other irrelevant interferences. This advantage is shown in both verbal tasks and non-verbal tasks (Bialystok 2010; Morereno, Bialystok, Wodniecka, & Alain, 2010). Second, bilinguals have advantages in attention allocation, such as in task switching (Prior & Mac Whinnry, 2010). Third, bilinguals' short-term memory capacity is greater than that of monolinguals (Michael & Gollan, 2009).

A study has indicated that Broca's area, which exists in the prefrontal cortex, has executive control function regarding language function (Bialystok, 2005). Moreover, there are interactions between these two functions. In addition, Bialystok found that in conflict control tasks, bilinguals are dominant and activate more brain regions. Diamond believes that when using one language, bilinguals must inhibit the activation of the other language, which indicates that bilinguals are engaged in control suppression training throughout their lives (Jared, 2010). Under brain training, bilinguals will have better central executive function. As bilinguals continue to use both languages, the cognitive ability and processing modes of the brain will become exercised and improved.

THE EFFECT OF BILINGUAL EXPERIENCE ON DEMENTIA

In a study that strictly controlled occupation, gender, immigrant experience, language level and other factors, the average onset age of dementia in bilinguals was postponed by four years; in addition, the onset age in Alzheimer's patients was postponed for five years (Bialystok, 2007, 2010). A researcher from India (Suvarna, 2013) classified different sub-types of dementia and then observed the effects of bilingual experience on dementia. He found that Alzheimer's disease, vascular dementia and frontotemporal dementia are delayed in onset as a result of bilingual experience. Even illiterate patients benefited from their bilingual experience with postponed onset. The question becomes: how can the bilingual experience resist dementia?

Researchers found that cognitive abilities are not affected in approximately 25% of the elderly (Esiri, 2001) in whom brain physiological degeneration has reached the clinical criteria for Alzheimer's disease. This indicates that some people have stronger resistance to brain degradation. Stern proposed a hypothesis called cognitive reserve (Stern, 2002). If dementia patients receive more training before onset, this training will slow down the speed of the onset.

We can assume that when using language, bilinguals' brains receive more training than monolinguals; thus, their central control is enhanced. More training results in more reserves in the brain. Consequently, bilinguals who have better control and more brain reserves have an advantage over monolinguals.

However, recently, researchers have doubted the bilingual effect against dementia. Researchers found that the bilingual experience of Spanish users cannot combat dementia (Zahodne, 2014).

FUTURE RESEARCH DIRECTIONS

Research on bilingualism and dementia has continued in recent years, but controversy remains in the following areas.

At present, researchers believe that the bilingual experience does not play a significant role in defense against dementia. If we can obtain a more detailed distinction of the language level of bilinguals, we will have more accurate answers. Gollan found that the higher language levels of bilinguals resulted in lower possibilities of suffering from dementia (Gollan, 2011). Previous studies have shown that balanced bilinguals have more obvious advantages than unbalanced bilinguals in cognitive ability. Thus, in terms of resistance to dementia, do balanced bilinguals still have advantages? Additionally, which level must unbalanced bilinguals reach to effectively resist Alzheimer's disease?

Because it is possible that bilingual experience can resist dementia, is it possible to reduce the risk of suffering dementia by learning a foreign language? Research has shown that cognitive training can resist dementia. As a type of cognitive training, foreign language learning can be effective for the prevention of dementia. However, further study is necessary to determine whether the time-period, the type of language, and the language level are factors that will affect resistance to dementia. Questions remain regarding which aspects of second language ability play a significant role in resisting dementia. Indian researchers found that some respondents who are illiterate still have the ability to resist dementia, similar to bilinguals who are literate.

Is there a possibility that the more languages people can master, the greater the ability of people to resist dementia? This issue remains a controversy. Chertkow's (2010) study shows that each additional language can delay the onset of Alzheimer's. However, Suvarna (2013) found that in terms of resisting dementia, multilinguals do not have a significant advantage compared with bilinguals. This issue is meaningful because in non-English speaking countries, students currently spend a significant amount of time learning English; thus, they can be considered unbalanced bilinguals. If people who can master two or more foreign languages have a greater ability to resist dementia, learning a new foreign language is significant because those people can more effectively resist dementia. If there is no evidence to support this view, then there is no need to learn a new foreign language to reduce the risk of dementia.

CONCLUSION

Currently, language studies on dementia are still being conducted. Researchers in every field are working on this subject. Researchers have found that bilinguals and monolinguals display differences in many cognitive aspects throughout life. There is an even greater need for bilingual word-guessing activities that cause speculation in the case of incomplete information; however, this can lead to the degeneration of the brain and missing information, and this lack of knowledge will result in incomplete information. There are many strengths and weaknesses in the different cognitive abilities of bilinguals and monolinguals. The brains of bilinguals and monolinguals function differently. The cognitive ability and brain differences appear to be caused by learning language. Language learning is a type of cognitive training. A number of studies have shown that cognitive training can reduce the risk of Alzheimer's; therefore, people who learn a second language should have this ability. However, some researchers have questioned whether bilingualism can reduce the risk of dementia; thus, a more detailed study is necessary.

ACKNOWLEDGMENT

My deepest gratitude goes to Professor Jinglong Wu, for his constant encouragement and guidance. He has walked me through the stages of this work. Without his consistent, I could not finish the paper. Second, I would like to express my collaborators, they give me a lot of advice to idealize the paper. I am also indebted my partner in the lab, who improve the paper in English.

REFERENCES

Albert, M. L., Feldman, R. G., & Willis, A. L. (1974). The 'subcortical dementia' of progressive supranuclear palsy. *Journal of Neurology, Neurosurgery, and Psychiatry*, *37*(2), 121–130. doi:10.1136/jnnp.37.2.121 PMID:4819905

Baddeley, A. (2010). Exploring the central executive. *Quarterly Journal of Experimental Psychology A, 1*(1), 5-28.

Barker, M. G., & Lawson, J. S. (1968). Nominal aphasia in dementia. *The British Journal of Psychiatry*, *114*(516), 1351–1356. doi:10.1192/bjp.114.516.1351 PMID:5702274

Bayles, K. A. (1982). Language function in senile dementia. *Brain and Language*, *16*(2), 265–280. doi:10.1016/0093-934X(82)90086-4 PMID:7116128

Bayles, K. A., & Tomoeda, C. K. (1983). Confrontation naming impairment in dementia. *Brain and Language*, *19*(1), 98–114. doi:10.1016/0093-934X(83)90057-3 PMID:6222782

Bialystok, E. (2007). Cognitive effects of bilingualism: How linguistic experience leads to cognitive change. *International Journal of Bilingual Education and Bilingualism*, *10*(3), 210–223. doi:10.2167/beb441.0

Bialystok, E. (2010). Global-local and trail-making tasks by monolingual and bilingual children: Beyond inhibition. *Developmental Psychology*, *46*(1), 93–105. doi:10.1037/a0015466 PMID:20053009

Bialystok, E., Barac, R., Blaye, A., & Poulin-Dubois, D. (2010). Word mapping and executive functioning in young monolingual and bilingual children. *Journal of Cognition and Development*, *11*(4), 485–508. doi:10.1080/15248372.2010.516420 PMID:21197133

Bialystok, E., Craik, F. I. M., Cheryl, G., Wilkin, C., Ryouhei, I., & Atsuko, G. et al.. (2005). Effect of bilingualism on cognitive control in the simon task: Evidence from meg. *NeuroImage*, *24*(1), 40–49. doi:10.1016/j.neuroimage.2004.09.044 PMID:15588595

Bialystok, E., Majumder, S., & Martin, M. M. (2003). Developing phonological awareness: Is there a bilingual advantage. *Applied Psycholinguistics*, *24*(1), 27–44. doi:10.1017/S014271640300002X

Blumenfeld, H. K., & Marian, V. (2011). Bilingualism influences inhibitory control in auditory comprehension. *Cognition*, *118*(2), 245–257. doi:10.1016/j.cognition.2010.10.012 PMID:21159332

Bosch, L., & Sebastián-Gallés, N. (2000). Evidence of early language discrimination abilities in infants from bilingual environments. *Infancy*, *2*(1), 29–49. doi:10.1207/S15327078IN0201_3

Chertkow, H., Whitehead, V., Phillips, N., Wolfson, C., Atherton, J., & Bergman, H. (2010). Multilingualism (but not always bilingualism) delays the onset of Alzheimer disease: Evidence from a bilingual community. *Alzheimer Disease and Associated Disorders*, *24*(2), 118–125. doi:10.1097/WAD.0b013e3181ca1221 PMID:20505429

Collier, V. P. (1995). Acquiring a second language for school. *Directions in Language & Education*, *1*, 14.

Corsellis, J. A. N. (1963). Encephalitides. *British Journal of Psychiatry the Journal of Mental Science,* (459), 324.

Costa, A., Hernández, M., & Sebastián-Gallés, N. (2008). Bilingualism aids conflict resolution: Evidence from the ant task. *Cognition, 106*(1), 59–86. doi:10.1016/j.cognition.2006.12.013 PMID:17275801

Costa, A., & Santesteban, M. (2004). Lexical access in bilingual speech production: Evidence from language switching in highly proficient bilinguals and l2 learners. *Journal of Memory and Language, 50*(4), 491–511. doi:10.1016/j.jml.2004.02.002

Esiri, M., Matthews, F., Brayne, C., Ince, P., Matthews, F., & Xuereb, J. (2001). Pathological correlates of late-onset dementia in a multicenter, community-based population in England and Wales. *Lancet, 357*(9251), 169–175. doi:10.1016/S0140-6736(00)03589-3 PMID:11213093

Folstein, M. F., Folstein, S. E., & Mchugh, P. R. (1975). "Mini-mental state". A practical method for grading the cognitive state of patients for the clinician. *Journal of Psychiatric Research, 12*(1), 189–198. doi:10.1016/0022-3956(75)90026-6 PMID:1202204

French, C., & Llorente, A. M. (2008). *Language: Development, Bilingualism, and Abnormal States. Principles of Neuropsychological Assessment with Hispanics.* Springer New York.

Gascon, G. G., & Gilles, F. (1973). Limbic dementia. *Journal of Neurology, Neurosurgery, and Psychiatry, 36*(3), 421–430. doi:10.1136/jnnp.36.3.421 PMID:4714104

Gewirth, L. R., Shindler, A. G., & Hier, D. B. (1984). Altered patterns of word associations in dementia and aphasia. *Brain and Language, 21*(21), 307–317. doi:10.1016/0093-934X(84)90054-3 PMID:6704703

Gollan, T. H., Montoya, R. I., & Werner, G. A. (2002). Semantic and letter fluency in Spanish-English bilinguals. *Neuropsychology, 16*(4), 562–576. doi:10.1037/0894-4105.16.4.562 PMID:12382994

Gollan, T. H., Salmon, D. P., Montoya, R. I., & Galasko, D. R. (2011). Degree of bilingualism predicts age of diagnosis of Alzheimer's disease in low-education but not in highly educated Hispanics. *Neuropsychologia, 49*(14), 3826–3830. doi:10.1016/j.neuropsychologia.2011.09.041 PMID:22001315

Hakuta, K. (1986). Cognitive development of bilingual children. *Acculturation, 44*(1), 36–54.

Hamers, J. F., & Blanc, M. (2000). *Bilinguality and Bilingualism*. Cambridge University Press. doi:10.1017/CBO9780511605796

Holland, A. L., Mcburney, D. H., Moossy, J., & Reinmuth, O. M. (1985). The dissolution of language in pick's disease with neurofibrillary tangles: A case study. *Brain and Language*, *24*(1), 36–58. doi:10.1016/0093-934X(85)90096-3 PMID:3971135

Jared, D. (2010). Social science. The benefits of multilingualism. *Science*, *330*(6002), 332–333. doi:10.1126/science.1195067 PMID:20947754

Kaushanskaya, M., & Marian, V. (2009). The bilingual advantage in novel word learning. *Psychonomic Bulletin & Review*, *16*(4), 705–710. doi:10.3758/PBR.16.4.705 PMID:19648456

Li, Wu, & Liu. (2012). the effect of bilingual experiences on cognition abilities. *Advances in Psychological Science, 20*(7), 995-1002.

Luo & Peng. (2001). Perspective on Dementia. *Contemporary Linguistics,* (2), 109-118.

Mattis, S., & Mattis, S. (1976). *Mental status examination for organic mental syndrome in the elderly patient*. Grune & Stratton Inc.

Michael, E. B., & Gollan, T. H. (2009). Being and becoming bilingual. Handbook of bilingualism, 389.

Moreno, S., Bialystok, E., Wodniecka, Z., & Alain, C. (2010). Conflict resolution in sentence processing by bilinguals. *Journal of Neurolinguistics*, *23*(6), 564–579. doi:10.1016/j.jneuroling.2010.05.002 PMID:21057658

Nicholas, M., Obler, L., Albert, M., & Goodglass, H. (1985). Lexical retrieval in healthy aging. *Cortex*, *21*(4), 595–606. doi:10.1016/S0010-9452(58)80007-6 PMID:4092486

Obler, L. K. (1983). *Language and brain dysfunction in dementia - language functions and brain organization*. Language Functions & Brain Organization. doi:10.1016/B978-0-12-635640-3.50020-5

Páez, M. M., Tabors, P. O., & López, L. M. (2007). Dual language and literacy development of Spanish-speaking preschool children. *Journal of Applied Developmental Psychology*, *28*(2), 85–102. doi:10.1016/j.appdev.2006.12.007 PMID:20396646

Petitto, L. A. (2009). New discoveries from the bilingual brain and mind across the life span: Implications for education. *Mind Brain & Education*, *3*(4), 185–197. doi:10.1111/j.1751-228X.2009.01069.x

Portocarrero, J. S., Burright, R. G., & Donovick, P. J. (2007). Vocabulary and verbal fluency of bilingual and monolingual college students. *Archives of Clinical Neuropsychology the Official Journal of the National Academy of Neuropsychologists*, *22*(3), 415–422. doi:10.1016/j.acn.2007.01.015 PMID:17336036

Prior, A., & Macwhinney, B. (2010). A bilingual advantage in task switching. *Bilingualism: Language and Cognition*, *13*(2), 253–262. doi:10.1017/S1366728909990526

Ripich, D. N., & Terrell, B. Y. (1988). Patterns of discourse cohesion and coherence in Alzheimer's disease. *The Journal of Speech and Hearing Disorders*, *53*(1), 8–15. doi:10.1044/jshd.5301.08 PMID:3339870

Robinson, K. M., Grossman, M., White-Devine, T., & D' Esposito, M. (1996). Category-specific difficulty naming with verbs in Alzheimer's disease. *Neurology*, *47*(1), 178–182. doi:10.1212/WNL.47.1.178 PMID:8710073

Schwartz, M. F., Marin, O. S., & Saffran, E. M. (1979). Dissociations of language function in dementia: A case study. *Brain and Language*, *7*(3), 277–306. doi:10.1016/0093-934X(79)90024-5 PMID:455049

Smith, G. E., & Bondi, M. W. (2013). *Mild cognitive impairment and dementia: definitions, diagnosis, and treatment*. Oxford University Press.

Stern, Y. (2002). Stern y. what is cognitive reserve? Theory and research application of the reserve concept. *Journal of the International Neuropsychological Society*, *8*(3), 448–460. doi:10.1017/S1355617702813248 PMID:11939702

Stuss, D. T., & Levine, B. (1996). The dementias: Nosological and clinical factors related to diagnosis. *Brain and Cognition*, *31*(2), 99–113. doi:10.1006/brcg.1996.0036 PMID:8811985

Suvarna, A., Bak, T. H., Vasanta, D., Bapiraju, S., Mekala, S., & Anuj Kumar, S. et al.. (2013). Bilingualism delays age at onset of dementia, independent of education and immigration status. *Neurology*, *81*(22). PMID:24198291

Whitaker, H. (1976). 1–a case of the isolation of the language function. *Studies in Neurolinguistics,* 1-58.

World Health Organization & Alzheimer's Disease International. (2012). *Dementia: a public health priority.* Author.

Wu, J. (2012). Delayed audiovisual integration of patients with mild cognitive impairment and Alzheimer's disease compared with normal aged controls. *Journal of Alzheimer's Disease*, *32*(2), 317–328. PMID:22810093

Wu, J., Yu, Y., & Yang, J. (2012). Neuropsychological Parameters as Potential Biomarkers for Alzheimer's Disease. *Current Translational Geriatrics and Experimental Gerontology Reports, 1*(2), 68–75. doi:10.1007/s13670-012-0007-4

Yang, J. (n.d.). Decline of human tactile angle discrimination in patients with mild cognitive impairment and Alzheimer's disease. *Journal of Alzheimer's Disease, 22*(1), 225-234.

Yang, J., Usairy Syafiq, M., Yu, Y., Takahashi, S., Zhang, Z., & Wu, J. (2015). Development and Evaluation of a Tactile Cognitive Function Test Device for Alzheimer's Disease Early Detection. *Neuroscience and Biomedical Engineering, 3*(2), 58–65. doi:10.2174/2213385203666150804001349

Zahodne, L. B., Schofield, P. W., Farrell, M. T., Stern, Y., & Manly, J. J. (2014). Bilingualism does not alter cognitive decline or dementia risk among Spanish-speaking immigrants. *Neuropsychology, 28*(2), 238–246. doi:10.1037/neu0000014 PMID:24188113

KEY TERMS AND DEFINITIONS

Alzheimer's Disease: An onset of dementia that results in memory, thinking and behavioral problems. Alzheimer's disease develops slowly and becomes worse as time goes on, becoming severe enough to interfere with daily life. Alzheimer's is the most common form of dementia, accounting for 60 to 80 percent of dementia cases. Although the most important risk factor for Alzheimer's is age and most people who suffer from Alzheimer's disease are 65 years old or older, this disease is an abnormal result of aging. However, old age is not the only factor that results in Alzheimer's disease. Approximately 5 percent of people with this disease have early-onset Alzheimer's disease (presenile dementia), which often occurs by age 40 or 50. Alzheimer's disease is a progressive disease that causes deterioration over several years. In the early stages of Alzheimer's disease, memory loss is mild, but in the last stage of Alzheimer's disease, individuals lose their ability to respond to the environment. Alzheimer's disease is the sixth leading cause death in the US. When a patient has had Alzheimer's disease for eight years, their symptoms become obvious to others, but the patient can survive for 4 to 20 years with the disease. There is no cure for Alzheimer's disease, but we can continue to research the symptoms to alleviate the worsening of dementia symptoms and improve the quality of life for those with Alzheimer's disease. However, there is an ongoing effort to find a better way to treat Alzheimer's disease (Wiki.org *Alzheimer's disease* https://en.wikipedia.org/wiki/Alzheimer%27s_disease).

Bilingual / Multilingual: The use of two or more languages, by an individual speaker or a speaker community. Bilingualism / multilingualism is the ability of a bilingual / multilingual. There are more multi-language speakers than monolingual speakers in the world. Multilingualism is becoming increasingly common because of the development of the Internet, which promotes the ease of access to spread information. The frequency of people who use more than one language has increased, thus promoting the necessity to master other languages (by Wiki.org *Multilingualism*https://en.wikipedia.org/wiki/Multilingualism).

Cognitive Reserve: Describes the ability to resist damage to the brain using the mind. There are two models that can be used to explore the concept of "reserve": brain reserve and cognitive reserve; these terms are often used interchangeably in the literature. Using a computer analogy, brain reserve and cognitive reserve can be thought of as hardware and software respectively. At present, all of these factors are thought to contribute to global reserves. Cognitive reserve is usually used to refer to the brain and cognitive reserve in the literature. (Wiki.org *Cognitive reserve*https://en.wikipedia.org/wiki/Cognitive_reserve).

Dementia: A cluster of diseases that interfere with daily life because a person's mental abilities decline. Dementia is not a specific disease; it is a general term that describes a wide range of use in thinking skills severe enough to interfere with a person's ability. Dementia symptoms can vary widely, but at least two of the following core mental functions must be significantly impaired to be diagnosed with dementia: Memory, Communication and language, Ability to focus and pay attention, Reasoning and judgment, and Visual perception. There are many areas of the brain that are responsible for different functions. When a particular area is destroyed, the function of that area cannot be implemented properly. The cause of dementia is brain cell damage. This damage can affect how brain cells communicate. When brain cells cannot communicate properly, mind, behavior and emotion are all affected (Alz.org *what is dementia*http://www.alz.org/what-is-dementia.asp).

Chapter 6

Stimulation Devices for Human Haptic Perception and Their Applications in Cranial Nerve Diseases

Jian Zhang
Beijing Institute of Technology, China

Liancun Zhang
Beijing Institute of Technology, China

Jinglong Wu
Beijing Institute of Technology, China

ABSTRACT

Tactile perception is a class of complicated sensations that can be divided into categories including concrete pressure, shape, and temperature perception. In different parts of the human body, the distribution of tactile sensitivity clearly differs. Various stimulatory devices are becoming increasingly widely used in studies of human haptic perception. New methods and devices that can be used to explore tactile stimulation are also being developed and have yielded many important results. This paper introduces such tactile stimulation devices, which can be divided into many categories according to qualities, including their geometric properties, temperature, force, and vibration. This article also introduces some devices that can be used to guide clinical diagnosis and treatment. These devices can be used to examine a patient's haptic perception to help the patient's doctors diagnose their illness.

DOI: 10.4018/978-1-5225-0925-7.ch006

INTRODUCTION

This chapter focuses on human haptic perception. It is intended to introduce the rapidly evolving field of stimulation devices.

In the first part, we describe the basics of human haptic perception and provide a simple introduction to the essentials of tactile stimulation devices.

In the second part, we begins with a review of the different types of stimulation devices. Because a variety of tactile displays and body parts exist, different academic research projects have different requirements for tactile stimulation devices, and this has led to the development of a wide variety of methods and devices that can be used for tactile stimulation.

Finally, the applications of devices used to stimulate human haptic perception have been extended into medical fields. Many studies have indicated that there is a correlation between tactile perception and some diseases. Because of the advantages of their simple structure, low cost, and non-intrusive nature, these devices will be useful for a wide variety of prospective applications in the medical field. In recent years, research into the development of equipment that can monitor Alzheimer's disease and be used in therapeutic approaches for treating and diagnosing it have been at the forefront of such medical studies.

BACKGROUND

In everyday life, we attach great value to vision and hearing because of the roles they play in making us aware of our surroundings. Touch is also important to cognition (James, Kim & Fisher, 2007). The blind rely heavily on the sense of touch in their normal activities, and even deaf-blind individuals come to know much about the world around them and to function well within it (Gazzaniga, Ivry & Mangun, 2013). Touch is a method that is used to identify objects according to tactile sensation, which is a class of complicated sensations that can be divided into categories including concrete pressure, shape, and temperature perception.

Different parts of the human body are associated with clearly different distributions of brain activity (as shown in Figure 1) (Penfield & Rasmussen, 1950). Moreover, because of the inhomogeneity in the skin tissue structures that lie beneath different sites of measurement, the distribution of tactile sensitivity is also clearly different. For the purpose of studies into human haptic perception, various stimulation devices are becoming increasingly widely used. New methods and devices used to explore tactile stimulation are also being developed and have yielded many important results, especially in the medical field.

Figure 1. Brain areas involved in haptic perception

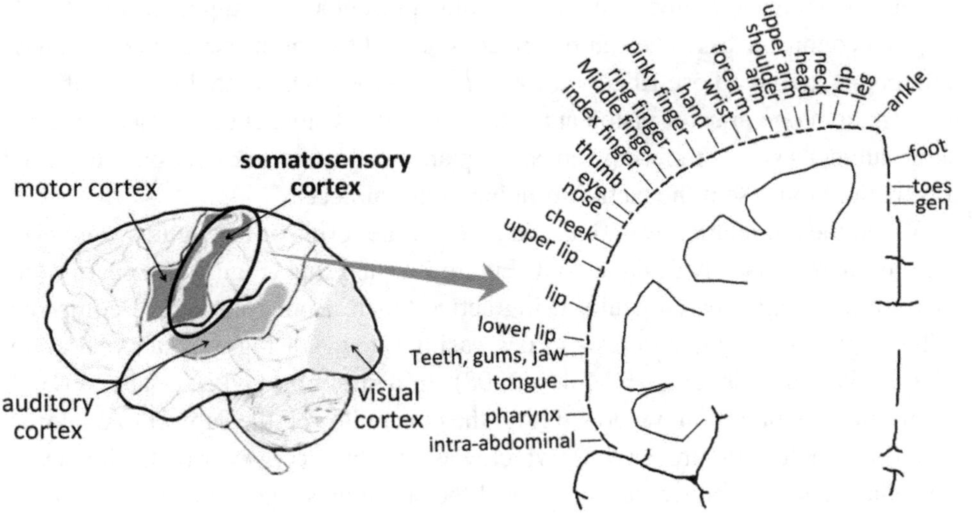

STIMULATION DEVICES OF HUMAN HAPTIC PERCEPTION

In numerous experiments, many types of devices have been used, each of which provides different types of stimulation, depending on a number of factors. Because they are used in different environments, the construction and properties of these instruments show a large amount of divergence. Functional Magnetic Resonance Imaging (fMRI) has been widely applied in the field of brain cognition research. To use fMRI, the automatic functions and magnetic fields of stimulatory devices must be strictly controlled.

Stimulation devices can be divided into many categories according to the type of stimuli they produce, which can include geometric properties, temperature, force, or vibration. This paper summarizes the typical stimulation devices that are used to study human haptic perception.

Geometric Stimulation

Geometric properties describe the structure of a sample object. Geometric properties have been extensively studied in the field of tactile perception. Geometric properties generally comprise shape and size. Size can be measured using a number of metrics, including the total area, volume, and perimeter. However, shape is determined based on the integration of size information, so it is particularly hard to measure. Therefore, several types of stimulation equipment have been developed to test geometric properties.

To decrease the effect of extra finger motion as much as possible, Yang, Liu and Zhang (2010) made a type of tactile stimulus presentation equipment for a tactile length recognition task. The equipment consisted of two of the same injectors, with both connected to a hose filled with water. Therefore, when moving a quantity of water held in one injector piston at the experimenter's side, another injector piston at the subject's side is moved by an equal quantity in a reverse direction. They used this method to present the tactile stimulus to the subjects.

When the stimulation was figure in a plane, the forms of the figures were even more numerous. Newly designed dot (Figure 2A) and ring (Figure 2B) charts were used to test tactile spatial acuity using active touch. Both charts were composed of four symbols arranged in rows of decreasing size in 0.1 log-unit steps (Gordon, Cindee, Vaughn, Cheong, & Miller, 2008). In a study by Dykes et al (2007), A 9-cm square exploration window within the cover allowed the subject to explore a specific stimulus (Figure 3A&B), which was sent by a conveyor belt. The device was composed of a conveyor that moved the stimulus shapes, a belt platform, an air-driven piston and an electronic control module. Yang, Wu and He (2010) developed a novel tactile presentation system for assessing and training cognitive functions using tactile senses while under MRI. The primary components of the system include a finger movement control unit, a disk for multiple tactile pattern delivery, and a force-sensing unit. It is worth mentioning that the system could supply two experimental conditions including active and passive touch.

Savini et al (2010) used different types of shapes (square, circle, triangle, and ellipse) for passive tactile recognition of 2D geometrical shapes. To standardize the force applied to the hand, the pieces were mounted on flexible bars using a graduated scale (Figure 3C). Moreover, a device allowed the investigator to manually present the shapes using the same force (4 N) across all subjects and trials. In other studies, the same device was used to study the working memory of somatosensory stimuli (Savini, Brunetti, Babilonib, & Ferretti, 2012).

In the above studies, the stimulations used plane figures, but other researchers have studied three dimensional (3-D) haptic shape perception. In 2009, to investigate the saliency of 3-D shape features, Plaisier, Tiest and Kappers (2009) developed a task to approximate 3-D haptic shape perception. In the task, the stimuli consisted of brass shapes that were suspended from flexible wires. The shapes were spheres, cubes, ellipsoids, cylinders, and tetrahedrons. Bodegard, Geyer, Grefkes, Zilles, and Roland (2001) and Mirela, Tiest, and Kappers (2011) have extensively researched this question using similar stimulations.

Figure 2. A) Illustration of the dot chart (top). B) Illustration of the ring chart (bottom). Both charts are composed of four symbols arranged in rows of decreasing size in 0.1 log-unit steps (26% change in size).

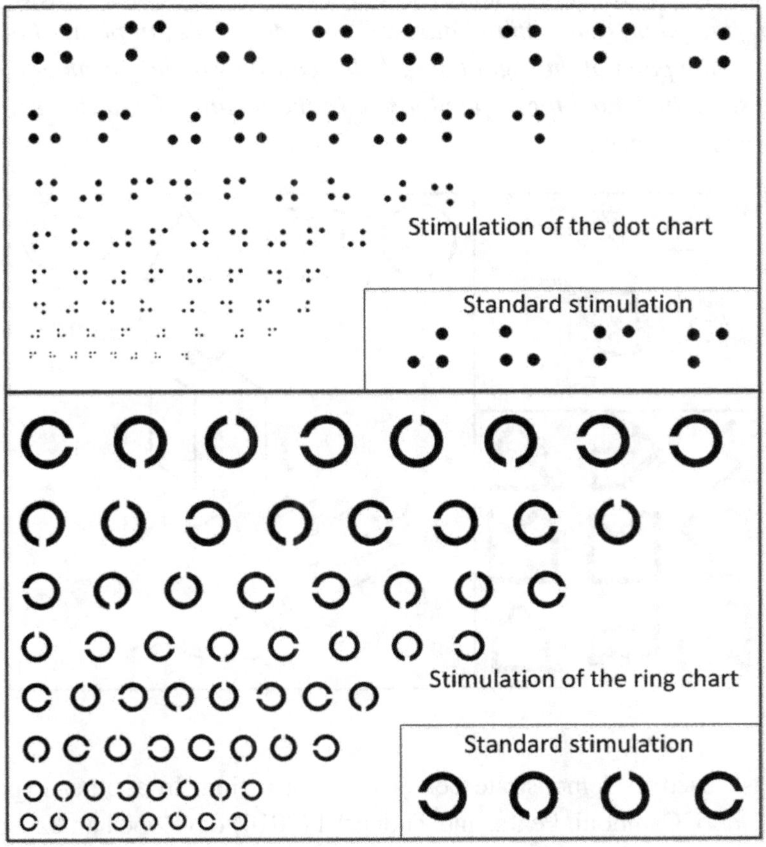

Thermal Stimulation

Thermal properties describe the apparent warmth or coolness of a contacted surface, and this sense is mediated by thermal receptors. These receptors respond within a temperature range of 5°C–45°C (Lederman, 1981). Temperature perception is different at different locations on the body. With age, this ability tends to decrease, as does the capacity to process perceived information in real-time. When studying temperature perception, participants are stimulated via contact with surfaces on objects with different temperatures.

Silva, Restivo, & Gzbriel (2013) completed a study that addressed temperature perception in elderly males. In this experiment, they used a temperature-controlled element (a Peltier element) on which the subjects placed one hand and then performed

Figure 3. Illustration showing the plane figure stimulations. A) The dimensions of a typical stimulus showing the aspects that were constant for all shapes: a 1.5 mm thick base, a 2 mm elevation and a 3 mm thickness. All shapes are formed within an area of 4.5 cm×4.5 cm at the center of the 9.5 cm square base. B) These Illustrations show the plane figure stimulations. C) Wooden pieces in plane shapes were pressed into the palm of the right hand. A device with wooden flexible bars and a reference scale indicated the applied force. In the picture, the device bearing the square shape is shown.

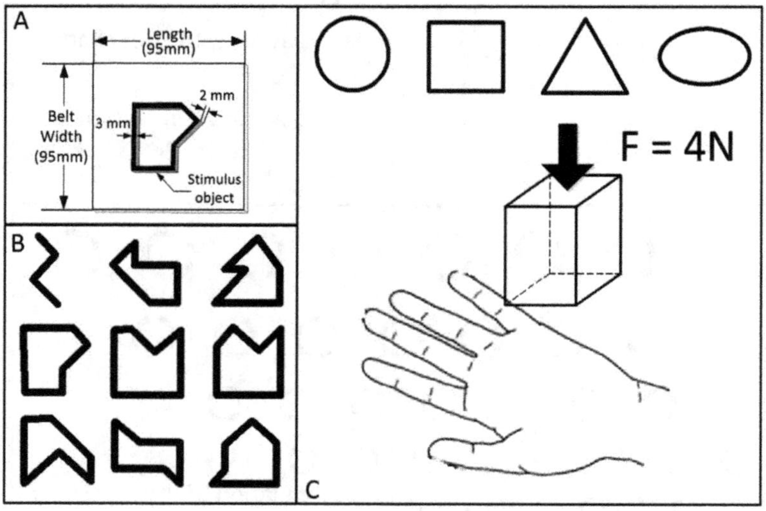

a basic task used to demonstrate perceived information. In another experiment, Klocker, Oddo, Camboni, Penta, and Thonnard (2014) developed an experimental apparatus that consisted of three thermal stimulation modules. Each module allowed the temperature of an aluminum plate to be regulated between 10 °C and 50 °C using two high-performance Peltier elements, two heat sinks, and two exhaust fans that helped to remove excess heat from the Peltier elements. Two Negative Temperature Coefficient thermistors were embedded in the aluminum plates, and two linear proportional-integral temperature controllers allowed the stimulus temperature to be measured and provided thermal feedback. A custom mounting system allowed the aluminum plate on top of the thermal stimulation modules to be rapidly replaced.

Furthermore, because temperature perception is different for different body location, Frank and Greenlee (2014) studied temperature perception in the vestibular cortex using fMRI. In this experiment, they used hot (47–49 °C), cold (5–7.5 °C), and warm to establish a baseline (30–32.5 °C). The following equipment was used to build the system: three plastic barrels, two temperature sensors, two mini-pumps, eight plastic tubes, a switching device to stimulate the left and right ears using water at different temperatures, two rigid glass pods (each connected to a water influx and efflux tube) that were integrated into the left and right side of the MRI ear protection device, and a plastic relay plate with a belt that was worn by the participant (as shown in Figure 4). In the experiment, temperature-controlled water was pumped into one or both of the ear canals via a closed-loop tube system. Water temperature was transmitted to the surface of the ear canal via a small glass pod.

Some companies currently provide specialized products for studying temperature perception. For example, the Medoc company specializes in producing PATHWAY, which can be used for temperature stimulation between -10 °C and 54 °C and can alter temperature at a speed of 7 °C/s. The equipment has been used in the research studies performed on related topics by Chen, Dillenburger, Wang and Tang (2012).

Figure 4. Scheme and functions of the thermal stimulation device. Two barrels containing hot and cold water were located in the scanner control room. Every barrel contained a mini-pump that pumped temperature-controlled water to the switching device via two tubes. Four tubes (solid lines), one containing hot water and one containing cold water for each side of the head, passed from the switching panel through the waveguide to the scanner room to transport the water to the participant. The participant wore a relay plate and a belt to which the tubes were attached. The two tubes containing hot and cold water on either side of the subject's head were conjoined to a single tube at the relay plate. This tube terminated in a small glass pod that was contained in the MRI ear protection device. Two more tubes (dotted lines) were attached to the pods to return the used water to a collecting barrel in the scanner control room. Arrows indicate the direction of water flow.

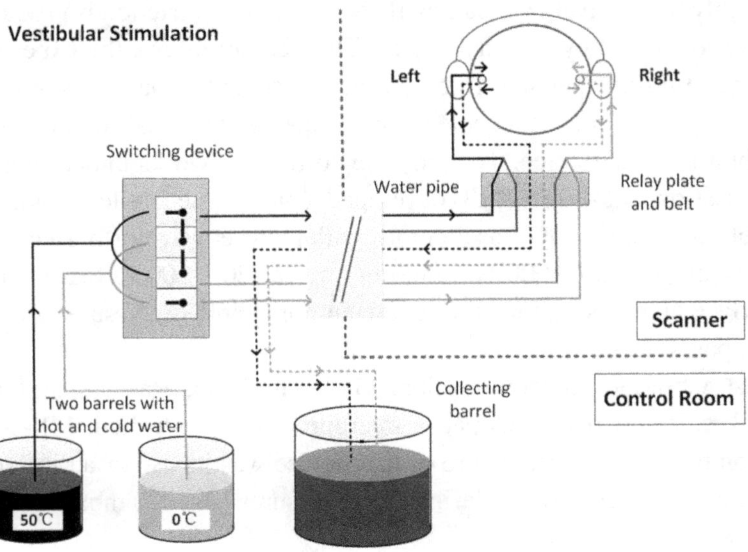

Vibration Stimulation

Touch perception depends on obtaining both spatial and temporal information from tactile stimuli. There is strong evidence showing that slowly and rapidly adapting neural afferents are the main mediators of the spatial and temporal aspects of tactile information (Hegner, Grodd & Braun, 2010). The present fMRI study was designed to obtain a better understanding of the brain regions that are involved in vibrotactile to tactile events and to ascertain to what extent their activation was correlated. The devices provided vibration stimulation using different methods to implement the stimulation. The most popular application is the pneumatic driving system. However, when designing the program, we also considered factors including the choice of the objects, the stimulation duration, and the stimulation intensity.

In one study, a device was designed by Chakravarty, Broadbenta, Rosa-Neto, Lambert and Collins (2009) to perform the experiments related to vibrotactile sensations. The device stimulated the right hand of the subject while fMRI was performed. In the design of the device, the authors exploited the physical characteristics of and object being rotated about a simple single axis of rotation. For smooth rotation to occur about an axis, both static and dynamic balance must be achieved. In the design, they exploited these characteristics to build a turbine that converted the kinetic energy of flowing compressed air into rotary mechanical power. Vibration was achieved by including an off-center mass. The stimulator delivered stimulation to the participant in the 40–50 Hz range.

In other study by Golaszewski et al (2006), vibrotactile stimulation with a frequency of 50 Hz and a displacement of 1 mm was applied to the sole of the right foot during fMRI using an MRI-compatible moving magnet actuator. This actuator type is highly back-drivable, meaning that practically no friction is produced when the magnet is moved by external forces. This feature allows the experimenter to generate position-independent forces, which is advantageous for keeping the indentor in contact with the foot sole of the subject and at small foot displacements while vibration was applied. To study the cortical networks underlying foot sole somatosensation, Hao et al (2013) developed a pneumatic tactile stimulator that as capable of producing 1-DOF oscillations with a preset waveform, frequency (≤10 Hz), force magnitude (5-500 N), and duty cycle (20%-100%) that contacted the target surface area. Using this device, the authors applied pressure to the soles of the participants' feet.

To test vibration somatosensation, Gallasch, Fend, Rafolt, Nardone, Kunz and Kronbichler (2010) developed a microprocessor-controlled, MR-compatible stimulation device. A main feature of this device was its use of an inflatable cuff that allowed the application of defined test pressures (0–1000 mbar) to the surface of the skin. The cuff was pressurized by a piezoelectric proportional valve with an embedded closed-loop controller. The distortion of the pressure pulses, which were introduced by the tube between the valve and the cuff (using tube lengths of 2 and 6 m), was then evaluated. Two types of stimulation patterns were implemented using the microprocessor: constant frequency stimulation (selectable between 1 and 20 Hz) and stimulation in which the frequencies were changed in a stepwise manner according to a pseudorandom sequence.

Force Stimulation

Forces can be classified as pressure (normal force) or friction (tangential force). In experiments to explore touch sensation, a force transducer is the key device used in force testing equipment. In experiments performed by Klocker, Oddo, Camboni, Penta and Thonnard (2014), a task was performed using an apparatus with a force transducer during passive fingertip stimulation. The contribution of force to tactile perception was investigated while in contact with the surface of an object, with a particular focus on the topography of model surfaces.

Srinivasan and Lamotte (1995) investigated the ability of humans to tactually discriminate the softness of elastic objects with deformable and rigid surfaces. For objects with deformable surfaces, the authors cast transparent rubber specimens with variable compliances. For objects with rigid surfaces (spring cells), the authors fabricated telescoping hollow cylinders in which the inner cylinder was supported by several springs. He performed psychophysical experiments using active touch and passive touch conditions.

Pressure on the skin is generally unavoidable, but little is understood about the pressure sensitivity of some regions of the body. Xiong, Goonetilleke and Jiang (2011) measured pressure discomfort thresholds and pressure pain thresholds to determine the pressure sensitivity map of the foot. An indentation apparatus that allowed the precise control of indentation speed and the ability to measure pressure thresholds and the mechanical properties of foot tissues *in vivo* was developed and used to measure pressure perception. The system consisted of a replaceable indentation probe, a stepper motor, a load cell and potentiometer, and a personal computer with the Labview program. The stepper motor controlled the speed of indentation. The load cell and the potentiometer recorded reactive force and tissue deformation, respectively.

The skin compresses and undergoes tensile mechanical deformation when it comes in contact with the surface of an object. Furthermore, force can also cause the deformation of muscle, tendons, and joints. Some studies have examined wrist force, finger-bending force (Allievi, Mellendez-Calderon, Arichi, Edwards, & Burdet, 2012), and resistive force in the hand (Khanicheh et al, 2006) using special devices.

Surface Texture Stimulation

The fine structural details of surfaces give rise to a perceptual property that is generally called texture (Klatzky, & Lederman, 2010). While any definition of texture will designate it as a surface property, as opposed to the geometry of the object as a whole, beyond that point of consensus there is little agreement as to what constitutes texture. Roughness is an important perceptual dimension of tactile surface textures. It describes the gaps between the elements that constitute the surface, and it can also describe the microstructures of the surface geometry. The perceived roughness of a tactually explored surface is a subjective sensation that depends on the physical characteristics of the surface. Some brain imaging experiments have investigated the existence and localization of roughness perception using the following devices and others similar to them (Ciesielska-Wrobe, Langenhove, & Grabowska, 2014; Lederman, 1981).

In a study by Simoes-Franklin, Whitaker and Newell (2011), the participants either actively explored a surface (active touch) or the surface was moved under the participant's stationary finger (passive touch). The stimuli consisted of three different grades of aluminum oxide sandpaper, which the participants were required to categorize as either coarse, medium, or fine. The baseline was one flat smooth surface (paper). The apparatus comprised a plain wooden disc to which a wooden dowel was attached through the center. This dowel allowed the researchers to rotate and provide stability to the device. Each stimulus surface was cut to fit one quarter of the wooden disc and subsequently glued onto the surface of the disc.

Unlike the above-described study, another study (Meftah, Belingard, & Chapman, 2000) investigated the ability of humans to estimate roughness. In this study, three series of eight surfaces were prepared on flexible letterpress plates. The surfaces consisted of cylindrical raised dots (0.6 mm diameter) that were arranged in a rectangular array. The tactile stimulator consisted of a cylindrical drum with a 400 mm circumference that was mounted on a drive shaft and rotated using a DC motor by a 100:1 reduction gear.

All of the above stimulation devices provide only one type of stimulation. However, these stimulations act together to stimulate the skin during daily life. Therefore, Klocker et al (2014) designed an experiment in which tactile exploration using the fingertips provided information regarding the physical properties of surfaces and their relative pleasantness. In these experiments, an apparatus was constructed that consisted of three stimulation modules: force, temperature, and surface texture.

The design of the device was relatively complicated to satisfy the requirements of the experiment.

Array Tactile Stimulation

Probe-type stimulation is a special kind of stimulation equipment that can be incorporated into a variety of stimulation devices. It is mainly used to study the localization of skin perception via the stimulation of different skin parts. Two classical methods for performing these types of experiments are known as the two-point touch threshold and the point-localization threshold method (Lederman S & Klatzky, 2009). The results of these studies indicate that point localization thresholds are usually lower than the corresponding two-point values but that these measurements are highly correlated, as shown in Table 1. It is to be expected that test equipment will require additional refinements to enhance the precision with which results are detected.

Dresel et al (2008) developed a novel computer-controlled MR-compatible stimulation device for mapping somatosensory-evoked brain activity using fMRI. The device employed von Frey-filaments, which are commonly used for quantitative sensory testing, to deliver punctate tactile stimuli to the face and other body surfaces with a high degree of spatiotemporal accuracy. The stimulation device was a modular assembly of six main components, as shown in Figure 5, that consisted of a control unit, a signal converter, a driving unit, and multiple mediators, positioning units and applicators. In this study, von Frey-filaments were used as applicators. It was used to apply punctate tactile stimuli with a maximum frequency of 10 Hz at full extension of the piston. Higher frequencies could be achieved using shorter bowden lengths and smaller stroke amplitudes.

The above-mentioned equipment is a single channel stimulation device. Son et al (2015) presented a new flexible multimodal tactile stimulation system that delivered stimulation information simultaneously using a single actuator. The average vibration amplitude of 30 μm was measured over a wide dynamic range (25–650 Hz). He developed the implemented 4x1 multimodal tactile display array. However, a 3x3 array tactile display was designed by Sofia, Jones and Member (2013). This array was composed of pancake motors. The array for stimulation could be taped to the skin on the palm or to other body surfaces. Phung et al (2015) also developed a similar device with a tactile display, and another array was designed with 100 contactor pins that were arranged on a 1 mm × 1 mm square matrix over an area of 1 cm^2 by Summers, Chanter, Southall and Brady. It was designed to simulate sensations on the fingertip by artificially generating the appropriate patterns of tactile stimulation.

Devices such as those described in this review could be applied to body surfaces to explore somatosensory mapping. Stringer, Chen, Friedman, Gatenby, & Gore

Table 1. Two-point touch and point localization thresholds of various body sites (mm). Data are presented only for women. The corresponding data for males showed that there general patterns were closely paralleled. The data represent mean threshold values for the left and right sides of the body because with few exceptions, there was no effect of laterality. Although the point localization thresholds were usually lower than the corresponding two-point values, the measurements were highly correlated. The results indicated that the more distal parts of the body sense spacial information more accurately.

body sites	forehead	cheek	nose	upper lip	breast	shoulder	upper arm	forearm	palm	thumb	index finger	middle finger	ring finger	pinky finger	back	belly	thigh	calf	sole	hallux
2-point threshold	17	8	9	6	38	47	44	41	11	3	3	3	3	3.5	42	32	44	45	22	13
Point localization	3	2	2.5	1.5	11	9	10	9	8	2	1	1.5	2	2	10	9	11	9	9	3.5

Figure 5. Schematic illustration of the tactile stimulation device. 5-V TTL pulses from the PC-based control unit were converted by the signal converter into 24-V actuation signals for the magnetic valves in the driving unit. The magnetic valves released the pressure from the pressurized air supply to the appropriate side of the double-action pneumatic cylinders, which drove eight separate von Frey-filaments (applicators) via nonmagnetic bowden wires (mediators). Each von Frey-filament could be individually oriented using a positioning unit. The stimulus application was synchronized with the MR image acquisition by the MRI trigger signal.

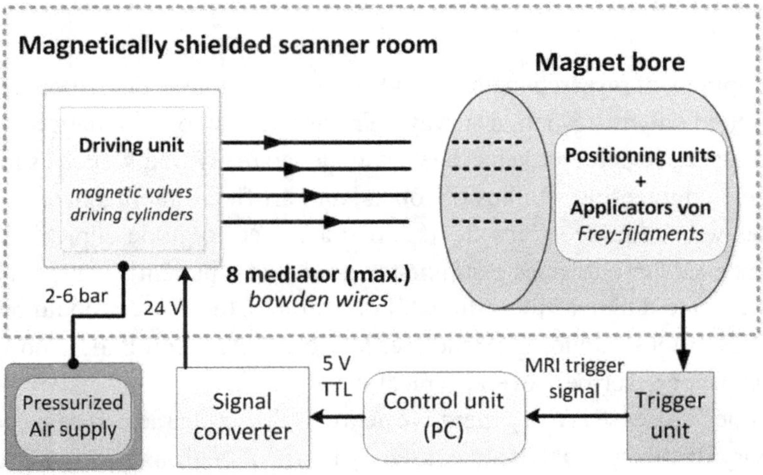

(2011) performed an experiment in which a hand and finger cast was connected to an air pressure generator by plastic tubing. Stretchable fabric was fitted across each opening in the cast to allow restricted skin displacement in response to an air puff. Air puffs were delivered to the glabrous skin of selected distal finger pads. This equipment was used to evaluate the ability of bold signals at a high MRI field to map fine-scale, single-digit activity in subdivisions of the human primary somatosensory cortex.

Besle, Sánchez-Panchuelo, Bowtell, Francis and Schluppeck (2013, 2014) used another experimental design to study the activation of the human primary somatosensory cortex following stimulation of different fingertips. The fingertips of each subject's left hand were stimulated using five independently controlled, piezoelectric devices to deliver suprathreshold vibrotactile stimuli (50 Hz) to 1 mm2 of the skin. Another team (Overduin & Servos, 2004, 2008) used a custom Plexiglas frame to deliver pulses of air via an array of shallow 0.5-cm wide depressions that were designed to conduct reflected air away from the hand surface. Flexible tubes that led to a series of air valves were connected to 16 of these depressions. The tubing length and aperture was consistent across channels. The air valves were computer-controlled and received air from a compressor at a steady-state pressure of 240–275 kPa.

The above devices were used for somatosensory mapping experiments. Stimulation was applied to body surfaces during fMRI. The improved properties of these devices required their precise positioning on the skin. In particular, the safety and compatibility of the devices when using MRI is crucial but also difficult to achieve.

APPLICATION

The development of research methods and applications for the described equipment are not applied only in academic surveys. The application of stimulation devices to study human haptic perception has been extended to many fields, such as medicine, biomedicine engineering, studies of robots, and artificial intelligence. Forthcoming articles will introduce some devices that are used to guide clinical diagnoses and treatments. These devices examine the ability of a patient's haptic perception to help doctors to diagnose their illness. For example, the devices could be used to diagnose conditions including Alzheimer's disease (AD) and Parkinson's disease (PD). This paper describes several typical devices.

Alzheimer's disease is a degenerative neurosis that is characterized by cognitive and memory dysfunctions that are caused by a loss of neurons and synapses in the cerebral cortex and certain subcortical regions. Based on the characteristics of the disease, some researchers (e.g., Yang, Ogasa, Ohta, Abe, & Wu, 2010; Wu, Yang, & Ogasa, 2010) have developed a tactile angle discrimination system to examine whether the ability to discriminate tactile angles differs between patients with AD and individuals in the NC group. One reference angle and eight comparison angles were used. During each trial, one pair of angles that consisted of the reference angle and a comparison angle was presented to the subject. Figure. 6A is an illustration of the angles. During the experiment, all of the subjects were asked to place their right index finger on a plate, as shown in Figure 6B.

The results showed that there were significant differences in the angle discrimination thresholds between AD patients and individuals in the NC group, which has important implications for medicine and basic science. Recently, the team presented another new generation device (Figure 6C). A number of hospitals have also started to conduct clinical research involving these products. Because of their advantages, including a simple structure, low cost, and non-intrusive nature, these devices will be useful for a wide variety of applications in the medical field.

Konczak, Sciutti, Avanzino, Squeri, Gori, Masia et al (2012) studied how Parkinson's disease alters haptic perception in addition to studying the underlying

Figure 6. Tactile angle discrimination device. A) An illustration of the reference angle (60°) and one of eight comparison angles (110°) that were used in these experiments. B) A zoom-in of the angle movement apparatus and the subject's finger position. C) A new generation device.

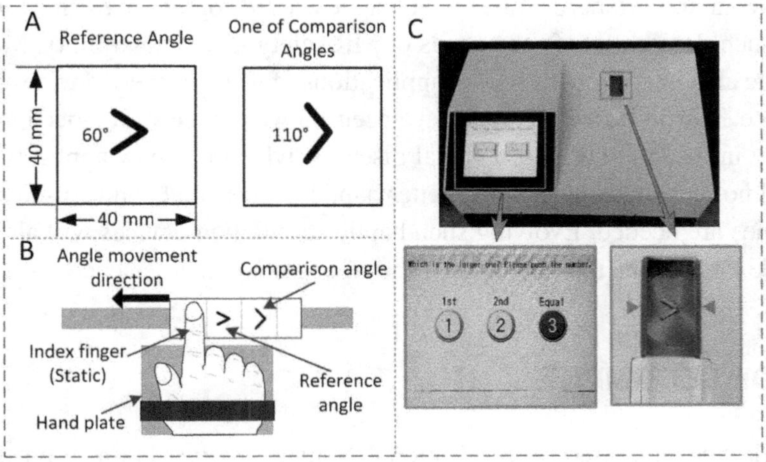

mechanisms involved in somatosensory and sensorimotor integration. Changes in haptic sensitivity and acuity. The ability to detect and discriminate between haptic stimuli resulting from Parkinson's disease was systematically quantified and contrasted to performance. In these experiments, virtual contours of various curvatures were presented using a robotic force device. The robotic manipulandum was a two-degrees-of-freedom planar manipulandum with a large elliptical workspace (80x40 cm). Please see the online supplementary material for a detailed technical description of the robot.

Cao, Xu, Zhao, Long and Zhang (2011) also used two different tiny wooded wheels as the stimuli in an experiment studying PD. The study illustrated that early PD was associated not only with altered brain activation but also with altered functional connectivity related to tactile perception. Fiorio, Marotta, Ottaviani, Pozzer and Tinazzi (2014) designed an experiment to investigate whether Aristotle's illusion is reduced in the affected hand of patients with PD. Other studies have also indicated that there is a correlation between tactile perception and PD (Juri, Rodriguez-Oroz, & Obeso, 2010; Gierthmuhlen et al, 2010; Conte et al, 2010).

The above review describes the main characteristics of haptic devices that are used in medical applications. Stimulation devices used to study human haptic perception are also used to study other diseases, such as diabetes, headache, and skin grafts.

CONCLUSION

This article reviews stimulation devices used to study human haptic perception and expounds on the developmental status of various types of such devices. Because fMRI plays an important role in clinical diagnoses and cognitive research, it is critical that such devices satisfy the needs of MR safety and compatibility. Moreover, this article also introduces the novel applications of some of these devices in medical science. The proposed methods have been shown to be useful tools for doctors, especially in the study of neurological diseases, which is a new application field. With technological advancements, better haptic devices that can be used in scientific studies are needed. Evolving such haptic stimulation devices will allow them to provide larger contributions to the field of cognitive neuroscience.

ACKNOWLEDGMENT

This work was supported by the National Natural Science Foundation of China (Grants 61473043).

REFERENCES

Allievi, A. G., Mellendez-Calderon, A., Arichi, T., Edwards, A. D., & Burdet, E. (2012). An fMRI compatible wrist robotic interface to study brain development in neonates. *Annals of Biomedical Engineering*, *41*(6), 1181–1192. doi:10.1007/s10439-013-0782-x PMID:23475437

Besle, J., Sánchez-Panchuelo, R., Bowtell, R., Francis, S., & Schluppeck, D. (2013). Single-subject fMRI mapping at 7 T of the representation of fingertips in S1: A comparison of event-related and phase-encoding designs. *Neurophysiol*, *109*(9), 2293–2305. doi:10.1152/jn.00499.2012 PMID:23427300

Besle, J., Sánchez-Panchuelo, R., Bowtell, R., Francis, S., & Schluppeck, D. (2014). Event-related fMRI at 7T reveals overlapping cortical representations for adjacent fingertips in S1 of individual subjects. *Human Brain Mapping*, *35*(5), 2027–2043. doi:10.1002/hbm.22310 PMID:24014446

Bodega, A., Geyer, S., Grefkes, C., Zilles, K., & Roland, P. E. (2001). Hierarchical processing of tactile shape in the human brain. *Neuron*, *31*(2), 317–328. doi:10.1016/S0896-6273(01)00362-2 PMID:11502261

Cao, H., Xu, X., Zhao, Y., Long, D., & Zhang, M. (2011). Altered brain activation and connectivity in early parkinson disease tactile perception. *AJNR. American Journal of Neuroradiology*, *32*(10), 1969–1974. doi:10.3174/ajnr.A2672 PMID:21998100

Chakravartya, M. M., Broadbenta, S., Rosa-Neto, P., Lambert, C. M., & Collins, L. (2009). Design, construction, and validation of an MRI-compatible vibrotactile stimulator intended for clinical use. *Journal of Neuroscience Methods*, *184*(1), 129–135. doi:10.1016/j.jneumeth.2009.07.018 PMID:19631690

Chen, L. M., Dillenburger, B. C., Wang, F., & Tang, C. H. (2012). Differential fMRI activation to noxious heat and tactile stimuli in parasylvian areas of new world monkeys. *Pain*, *153*(1), 158–169. doi:10.1016/j.pain.2011.10.006 PMID:22115923

Ciesielska-Wrobel, I. L., Langenhove, L. V., & Grabowska, K. (2014). Fingertip skin models for analysis of the haptic perception of textiles. *Journal of Biomedical Science and Engineering*, *7*(01), 1–6. doi:10.4236/jbise.2014.71001

Conte, A., Modugno, N., Lena, F., Dispenza, S., Gandolfi, B., Iezzi, E., & Berardelli, A. et al. (2010). Subthalamic nucleus stimulation and somatosensory temporal discrimination in Parkinson's disease. *Brain*, *133*(9), 2656–2663. doi:10.1093/brain/awq191 PMID:20802206

Dresel, C., Parzinger, A., Rimpau, C., Zimmer, C., Ceballos-Baumann, A. O., & Haslinger, B. (2008). A new device for tactile stimulation during fMRI. *NeuroImage*, *39*(3), 1094–1103. doi:10.1016/j.neuroimage.2007.09.033 PMID:17997331

Dykes, R. W., Miquee, A., Xerri, C., Zennou-Azogui, Y., Rainville, C., Dumoulin, A., & Marineau, D. (2007). A delivery device for presentation of tactile stimuli during functional magnetic resonance imaging. *Journal of Neuroscience Methods*, *159*(2), 308–317. doi:10.1016/j.jneumeth.2006.07.020 PMID:16945420

Fiorio, M., Marotta, A., Ottaviani, S., Pozzer, L., & Tinazzi, M. (2014). Aristotle's illusion in parkinson's disease: Evidence for normal interdigit tactile perception. *PLoS ONE*, *9*(2), e88686. doi:10.1371/journal.pone.0088686 PMID:24523929

Frank, S. M., & Greenlee, M. W. (2014). An MRI-compatible caloric stimulation device for the investigation of human vestibular cortex. *Journal of Neuroscience Methods*, *235*, 208–218. doi:10.1016/j.jneumeth.2014.07.008 PMID:25064191

Gallasch, E., Fend, M., Rafolt, D., Nardone, R., Kunz, A. B., Kronbichler, M., & Golaszewski, S. et al. (2010). Cuff-type pneumatic stimulator for studying somatosensory evoked responses with fMRI. *NeuroImage*, *50*(3), 1067–1073. doi:10.1016/j.neuroimage.2010.01.014 PMID:20079447

Gazzaniga, M. S., Ivry, R. B., & Mangun, G. R. (Eds.). (2013). *Cognitive neuroscience: the biology of the mind* (4th ed.). W. W. Norton & Company.

Gierthmuhlen, J., Schumacher, S., Deuschl, G., Fritzer, E., Llein, C., & Baron, R. (2010). Somatosensory function in asymptomatic Parkin-mutation carriers. *European Journal of Neurology*, *17*(3), 513–517. doi:10.1111/j.1468-1331.2009.02797.x PMID:19863651

Golaszewsk, S. M., Siedentopf, C. M., Koppelstaetter, F., Fend, M., Ischebeck, E., & Gonzalez-Felipe, V. et al.. (2006). Human brain structures related to plantar vibrotactile stimulation: A functional magnetic resonance imaging study. *NeuroImage*, *29*(3), 923–929. doi:10.1016/j.neuroimage.2005.08.052 PMID:16253525

Gordon, E. L., Cindee, M., Vaughn, B. N., Cheong, A. M. Y., & Miller, J. C. (2008). Retention of high tactile acuity throughout the life span in blindness. *Perception & Psychophysics*, *70*(8), 1471–1488. doi:10.3758/PP.70.8.1471 PMID:19064491

Hao, Y., Manor, B., Liu, J., Zhang, K., Chai, Y., Lipsitz, L., & Fang, J. et al. (2013). A novel MRI-compatible tactile stimulator for cortical mapping of foot sole pressure stimuli with fMRI. *Magnetic Resonance in Medicine*, *69*(4), 1194–1199. doi:10.1002/mrm.24330 PMID:22678849

Hegner, Y. L., Lee, Y., Grodd, W., & Braun, C. (2010). Comparing Tactile Pattern and Vibrotactile Frequency Discrimination: A Human fMRI Study. *Journal of Neurophysiology*, *103*(6), 3115–3122. doi:10.1152/jn.00940.2009 PMID:20457848

James, T. W., Kim, S., & Fisher, J. S. (2007). The neural basis of haptic object processing. *Canadian Journal of Experimental Psychology*, *61*(3), 219–229. doi:10.1037/cjep2007023 PMID:17974316

Juri, C., Rodriguez-Oroz, M., & Obeso, J. A. (2010). The pathophysiological basis of sensory disturbances in Parkinson's disease. *Neurological Sciences*, *289*(1-2), 60–65. doi:10.1016/j.jns.2009.08.018 PMID:19758602

Khanicheh, A., & Muto, A., Triantafyllou, C., Weinberg, B., Astrakas, L., Mavroidis, C., et al. (2006). fMRI-compatible rehabilitation hand device. *Journal of Neuroengineering and Rehabilitation*, *3*(24), 1–11. PMID:17022828

Klatzky, R. L., & Lederman, S. J. (2010). Multisensory texture perception. In Multisensory Object Perception in the Primate Brain (pp. 211-230). Springer-Verlag. doi:10.1007/978-1-4419-5615-6_12

Klocker, A., Oddo, C. M., Camboni, D., Penta, M., & Thonnard, J. (2014). Physical factors influencing pleasant touch during passive fingertip stimulation. *PLoS ONE*, *9*(7), e101361. doi:10.1371/journal.pone.0101361 PMID:25000561

Konczak, J., Sciutti, A., Avanzino, L., Squeri, V., Gori, M., Masia, L., & Sandini, G. et al. (2012). Parkinson's disease accelerates age-related decline in haptic perception by altering somatosensory integration. *Brain*, *135*(11), 3371–3379. doi:10.1093/brain/aws265 PMID:23169922

Lederman, S. J. (1981). The perception of surface roughness by active and passive touch. *Bulletin of the Psychonomic Society*, *18*(5), 253–255. doi:10.3758/BF03333619

Lederman, S. J., & Klatzky, R. L. (2009). Tutorial review haptic perception: A tutorial. *Attention, Perception & Psychophysics*, *71*(7), 1439–1459. doi:10.3758/APP.71.7.1439 PMID:19801605

Meftah, E. M., Belingard, L., & Chapman, C. E. (2000). Relative effects of the spatial and temporal characteristics of scanned surfaces on human perception of tactile roughness using passive touch. *Experimental Brain Research*, *132*(3), 351–361. doi:10.1007/s002210000348 PMID:10883383

Mirela, K., Tiest, W. M. B., & Kappers, A. M. L. (2011). Discrimination thresholds for haptic perception of volume, surface area, and weight. *Attention, Perception & Psychophysics*, *73*(8), 2649–2656. doi:10.3758/s13414-011-0202-y PMID:21870206

Overduin, S. A., & Servos, P. (2004). Distributed digit somatotopy in primary somatosensory cortex. *NeuroImage*, *23*(2), 462–472. doi:10.1016/j.neuroimage.2004.06.024 PMID:15488396

Overduin, S. A. & Servos, P. (2008). Symmetric Sensorimotor Somatotopy. *PLoS One, 3*(1), e1505.

Penfield, W., & Rasmussen, T. (Eds.). (1950). *The cerebral cortex of man*. New York: Macmillan.

Phung, H., Nguyen, C. T., Nguyen, T. D., Lee, C., Kim, U., Lee, D., & Choi, H. R. et al. (2015). Tactile display with rigid coupling based on soft actuator. *Meccanica*, *50*(11), 2825–2837. doi:10.1007/s11012-015-0270-5

Plisier, M. A., Tiest, W. M. B., & Kappers, A. M. L. (2009). Salient features in 3-D haptic shape perception. *Attention, Perception & Psychophysics*, *71*(2), 421–430. doi:10.3758/APP.71.2.421 PMID:19304631

Savini, N., Babilonib, C., Brunetti, M., Caulo, M., Gratta, C. D., & Ferretti, A. et al.. (2010). Passive tactile recognition of geometrical shape in humans: An fMRI study. *Brain Research Bulletin*, *83*(5), 223–231. doi:10.1016/j.brainresbull.2010.08.001 PMID:20696217

Savini, N., Brunetti, M., Babilonib, C., & Ferretti, A. (2012). Working memory of somatosensory stimuli: An fMRI study. *International Journal of Psychophysiology*, *86*(3), 220–228. doi:10.1016/j.ijpsycho.2012.09.007 PMID:23044088

Silva, A., Restivo, M. T., & Gzbriel, J. (2013). Haptic device demo using temperature feedback.*International Conference IEEE, 2*, 172-173.

Simoes-Franklin, C., Whitaker, T. A., & Newell, F. N. (2011). Active and passive touch differentially activate somatosensory cortex in texture perception. *Human Brain Mapping*, *32*(7), 1067–1080. doi:10.1002/hbm.21091 PMID:20669167

Sofia, K. O., Jones, L. A., & Member, S. (2013). Mechanical and psychophysical studies of surface wave propagation during vibrotactile stimulation. *IEEE Transactions On Haptics*, *6*(3), 320–329. doi:10.1109/TOH.2013.1 PMID:24808328

Son, C., Ko, K., Lee, H. J., Na, K., Han, J., & Yun, K. S. et al.. (2015). A flexible multimodal tactile display array for virtual shape and texture. *Microsystem Technologies*, 1–8.

Srinivasan, M. A., & Lamotte, R. H. (1995). Tactual discrimination of softness. *Journal of Neurophysiology*, *73*, 88–105. PMID:7714593

Stringer, E. A., Chen, L. M., Friedman, B. M., Gatenby, C., & Gore, J. C. (2011). Differentiation of somatosensory cortices by high-resolution fMRI at 7T. *NeuroImage*, *54*(2), 1012–1020. doi:10.1016/j.neuroimage.2010.09.058 PMID:20887793

Summers, I. R., Chanter, C. M., Southall, A. L., & Brady, A. C. (2011). Results from a tactile array on the fingertip. *Eurohaptics*, 26-28.

Wu, J. L., Yang, J. J., & Ogasa, T. (2010). Raised-angle discrimination under passive finger movement. *Perception*, *39*(7), 903–1006. doi:10.1068/p6264 PMID:20842975

Xiong, S., Goonetilleke, R. S., & Jiang, Z. H. (2011). Pressure thresholds of the human foot: Measurement reliability and effects of stimulus characteristics. *Ergonomics*, *54*(4), 292–293. doi:10.1080/00140139.2011.571831 PMID:21390958

Yang, J. J., Ogasa, T., Ohta, Y., Abe, K., & Wu, J. L. (2010). Decline of human tactile angle discrimination in patients with mild cognitive impairment and alzheimer's disease. *Journal of Alzheimer's Disease*, *22*, 225–234. PMID:20847416

Yang, J. J., Wu, J. L., & He, J. P. (2011). Programmable tactile pattern presentations operational under MRI to investigate neural mechanisms of tactile shape discrimination. *Journal of Neuroscience Methods*, *201*(1), 17–26. doi:10.1016/j.jneumeth.2011.06.030 PMID:21763724

Yang, W. H., Liu, J. H., & Zhang, W. L. (2010). The study about human information processing in tactile recognition.*International Conference on Mechatronics and Automation* (pp. 905-997). Xi'an. doi:10.1109/ICMA.2010.5589960

ADDITIONAL READING

Adams, M. J., Briscoe, B. J., & Johnson, S. A. (2007). Friction and lubrication of human skin. *Tribology Letters*, *26*(3), 239–253. doi:10.1007/s11249-007-9206-0

Anderson, N. H. (1974). Algebraic models in perception. In E. Carterette & M. Friedman (Eds.), *Handbook of perception II* (pp. 215–298). New York: Academic Press.

Asamura, N., Yokoyama, N., & Shinoda, H. (1998). Selectively stimulating skin receptors for tactile display. *IEEE Computer Graphics and Applications*, *18*(6), 32–37. doi:10.1109/38.734977

Backman, L., & Small, B. J. (2007). Cognitive deficits in preclinical Alzheimer's disease and vascular dementia: Patterns of findings from the Kungsholmen Project. *Physiology & Behavior*, *92*(1-2), 8086. doi:10.1016/j.physbeh.2007.05.014 PMID:17573076

Becerra, L. R., Breiter, H. C., Stojanovic, M., Fishman, S., Edwards, A., Comite, A. R., & Borsook, D. et al. (1999). Human brain activation under controlled thermal stimulation and habituation to noxious heat: An fMRI study. *Magnetic Resonance in Medicine*, *41*(5), 1044–1057. doi:10.1002/(SICI)1522-2594(199905)41:5<1044::AID-MRM25>3.0.CO;2-M PMID:10332889

Boecker, H., Ceballos-Baumann, A., Bartenstein, P., Weindl, A., Siebner, H. R., & Fassbender, T. et al.. (1999). Sensory processing in Parkinson's and Huntington's disease. *Brain*, *122*(9), 1651–1665. doi:10.1093/brain/122.9.1651 PMID:10468505

Briggs, R. W., Dy-Liacco, I., Malcolm, M. P., Lee, H., Peck, K. K., Gopinath, K. S., & Tran-Son-Tay, R. et al. (2004). A pneumatic vibrotactile stimulation device for fMRI. *Magnetic Resonance in Medicine*, *51*(3), 640–643. doi:10.1002/mrm.10732 PMID:15004811

Garcia-Hernandez, N., Sarakoglou, I., Tsagarakis, N., & Caldwell, D. (2012). Exploration of virtual surface features with a high performance tactile and force feedback interface. *IEEE international conference on systems, man, and cybernetics,* 2998-3003.

Graham, S. J., Staines, W. R., Nelson, A., Plewes, D. B., & McIlroy, W. E. (2001). New devices to deliver somatosensory stimuli during functional MRI. *Magnetic Resonance in Medicine*, *46*(3), 436–442. doi:10.1002/mrm.1211 PMID:11550233

Harrington, G. S., Wright, C. T., & Downs, J. H. (2000). A new vibrotactile stimulator for functional MRI. *Human Brain Mapping*, *3*(3), 140–145. doi:10.1002/1097-0193(200007)10:3<140::AID-HBM50>3.0.CO;2-0 PMID:10912593

Hatwell, Y., Streri, A., & Gentz, E. (Eds.). (2003). *Touching for knowing*. Amsterdam: Benjamins. doi:10.1075/aicr.53

Hayward, V., Astley, O. R., Cruz-Hernandez, M., Grant, D., & Robles-DeLa-Torre, G. (2004). Haptic interfaces and devices. *Sens Rev*, *24*(1), 16–29. doi:10.1108/02602280410515770

Hollins, M., Bensmaia, S. J., & Washburn, S. (2001). Vibrotactile adaptation impairs discrimination of fine, but not coarse, textures. *Somatosensory & Motor Research*, *18*, 253–262. doi:10.1080/01421590120089640 PMID:11794728

Johansson, R. S., & Vallbo, A. B. (1979). Tactile sensibility in the human hand: Relative and absolute densities of four types of mechanoreceptive units in glabrous skin. *The Journal of Physiology*, *286*(1), 283–300. doi:10.1113/jphysiol.1979.sp012619 PMID:439026

Kalman, K., Magloczky, E., & Janka, Z. (1995). Disturbed visuospatial orientation in the early stage of Alzheimer's dementia. *Archives of Gerontology and Geriatrics*, *21*(1), 2734. doi:10.1016/0167-4943(95)00639-3 PMID:15374221

Kampe, K. K., Jones, R. A., & Auer, D. P. (2000). Frequency dependence of the functional MRI response after electrical median nerve stimulation. *Human Brain Mapping*, *9*(2), 106–114. doi:10.1002/(SICI)1097-0193(200002)9:2<106::AID-HBM5>3.0.CO;2-Y PMID:10680767

McGlone, F., & Reilly, D. (2010). The cutaneous sensory system. *Neuroscience and Biobehavioral Reviews*, *34*(2), 148–159. doi:10.1016/j.neubiorev.2009.08.004 PMID:19712693

Oddo, C. M., Controzzi, M., Beccai, L., Cipriani, C., & Carrozza, M. C. (2011). Roughness Encoding for Discrimination of Surfaces in Artificial Active-Touch. *IEEE Transactions on Robotics*, *27*(3), 522–533. doi:10.1109/TRO.2011.2116930

Peltier, S., Stilla, R., Mariola, E., LaConte, S., Hu, X., & Sathian, K. (2007). Activity and effective connectivity of parietal and occipital cortical regions during haptic shape perception. *Neuropsychologia*, *45*(3), 476–483. doi:10.1016/j.neuropsychologia.2006.03.003 PMID:16616940

Petersen, R. C. (2004). Mild cognitive impairment as a diagnostic entity. *Journal of General Internal Medicine*, *256*, 183194. PMID:15324362

Poletto, & Christopher, J. (Eds.) (2006). Tactile Stimulation. *John Wiley & Sons.*

Saito, D. N., Okada, T., Morita, Y., Yonekura, Y., & Sadato, N. (2003). Tactile-visual cross-modal shape matching: A functional MRI study. *Brain Research. Cognitive Brain Research*, *17*(1), 14–25. doi:10.1016/S0926-6410(03)00076-4 PMID:12763188

Skedung, L., Danerlov, K., Olofsson, U., Johannesson, C. M., Aikala, M., & Kettle, J. et al.. (2011). Tactile perception: Finger friction, surface roughness and perceived coarseness. *Tribology International*, *44*(5), 505–512. doi:10.1016/j.triboint.2010.04.010

Talbi, A., Ducloux, O., Tiercelin, N., Deblock, Y., Pernod, P., & Preobrazhensky, V. (2006). Vibrotactile using micromachined electromagnetic actuators array. *Journal of Physics: Conference Series*, *34*, 637–642. doi:10.1088/1742-6596/34/1/105

Van-Kuilenburg, J., Masen, M. A., & Heide, E. (2015). A review of fingerpad contact mechanics and friction and how this affects tactile perception. *Proceedings of the Institution of Mechanical Engineers. Part J, Journal of Engineering Tribology*, *299*(3), 243–258. doi:10.1177/1350650113504908

Vega-Bermudez, F., Johnson, K. O., & Hsiao, S. S. (1991). Human tactile pattern recognition: Active versus passive touch, velocity effects, and patterns of confusion. *Journal of Neurophysiology*, *65*, 531–546. PMID:2051193

Yamamoto, A., Nagasawa, S., Yamamoto, H., & Higuchi, T. (2006). Electrostatic tactile display with thin film slider and its application to tactile telepresentation systems. *IEEE Transactions on Visualization and Computer Graphics*, *12*(2), 168–177. doi:10.1109/TVCG.2006.28 PMID:16509376

KEY TERMS AND DEFINITIONS

Array Tactile Stimulation: Tactile stimulation is provided in the form of an array distribution.

Cognition Impairment: A measurable change in cognitive function that affects processes including the ability to think, concentrate, formulate ideas, or remember.

Force Stimulation: Tactile stimulation used to indicate pressure and friction information.

Geometric Stimulation: Tactile stimulation used to indicate the structure of a sample object.

Haptic Perception: The way that a person gains information about his or her environment using touch.

Surface Texture Stimulation: Tactile stimulation used to indicate the structural details of a surface.

Tactile Stimulation: Stimulation using tactile information.

Thermal Stimulation: Tactile stimulation used to indicate the warmth or coolness of a surface.

Vibration Stimulation: Tactile stimulation used to indicate fast or slow in combination with spatial and temporal information.

Chapter 7
Transfer of Training between Working Memory Task and Attentional Task

Ting Guo
Northeast Normal University, China

Hong Chen
Northeast Normal University, China

Yanna Ren
Okayama University, Japan

Satoshi Takahashi
Okayama University, Japan

Xiaotong Zhu
Northeast Normal University, China

Jinglong Wu
Okayama University, Japan

ABSTRACT

The present studies indicate that training effects in a certain domain may result in the acquired skills being transferred to other domains that require similar abilities. Cognitive training involves structured exercises that are prescribed and undertaken with the purpose of enhancing cognitive abilities, such as attention, memory, and problem solving. In contrast to symptomatic pharmacotherapy, non-pharmacological approaches may further improve patients' situations. Our aim was to summarize the empirical evidence for the rehabilitation of individuals with cognitive disorders by using training tasks to enhance specific cognitive functions to combat against cognitive degradation and transfer the benefits to other widely used domains.

DOI: 10.4018/978-1-5225-0925-7.ch007

INTRODUCTION

1. Working Memory

Working memory (WM) is the ability to store and manipulate information for short periods of time. It is an important predictor of scholastic aptitude and a critical bottleneck underlying higher-order cognitive processes, including controlled attention and reasoning (Au et al., 2015).

Working memory (WM) refers to the temporary storage of information for managing daily functioning and the learning of skills (Baddeley & Hitch, 1974; Bo, Borza, & Seidler, 2009). According to Baddeley (1992), WM is composed of the central executive, the visuospatial sketchpad, and the phonological loop (see other conceptions of Engle, 2002). The central executive performs executive functions, such as updating, manipulating, and coordinating information from the visuospatial sketchpad and the phonological loop (Baddeley, 1996). The phonological loop is responsible for processing speech-related information, whereas the visuospatial sketchpad is used to store and manipulate visuospatial information. The functions of the visuospatial sketchpad and the phonological loop are domain-specific, whereas the executive functions are domain-general (Baddeley, 1992, 1996). The WM in high-level cognitive processes is important; many experiences have demonstrated the importance in reading comprehension, and the acquisition of motor skills (Daneman & Carpenter, 1980; Kane et al., 2004; McNay & Willingham, 1998).

Recently, there have been many interesting studies regarding the prospects of WM training for improving cognition function. The conclusion of these studies is that improvements in WM performance as a function of training may be transferable to other similar mental activities related to WM capacity (Klingberg, 2010; Morrison and Chein, 2011; Buschkuehl et al., 2012).

2. Attention Network

Attention is the ability to attend to some objectives and ignore others. There are three basic concepts in the attention system. First, the attention system is anatomically separate from the processing systems, which handle incoming stimuli, make decisions, and produce outputs. Second, attention utilizes a network of anatomical areas. Third, these anatomical areas perform different functions that can be specified in cognitive terms (Petersen & Posner, 2012).

Some researchers had previously described attention networks in 1990, and they thought that attention networks included three networks. The first is an alerting network that focuses on brain stem arousal systems along with right hemisphere systems related to sustained vigilance; the second is an orienting network that focuses on the parietal cortex; and the last is an executive network that includes the midline frontal/anterior cingulate cortex (Petersen & Posner, 2012).

An important function of attention is the ability to prepare and sustain alertness to process high priority signals, which is defined as alerting. Some studies about letter and word matching have demonstrated a relationship between the alert state and other aspects of information processing (Posner, 1978). The orienting network is focused on the ability to prioritize sensory input by selecting a modality or location. Anatomically, the base of the orienting effect is part the network involved in the parietal, subcortical, and frontal areas (Petersen & Posner, 2012). The third major system was presented under the heading of target detection because the moment of target detection captures awareness in a very specific way. The moment of target detection produces interference across the system, slowing the detection of another target, although it continues monitoring for targets in many processing streams without too much difficulty (Duncan, 1980). This set of processes is related to the limited capacity of the attention system and has often been called focal attention.

3. The Interaction of Working Memory and the Attention Network

Traditionally, attention and working memory have always been viewed as distinct cognitive domains. However, a growing number of psychological and neuroscientific studies have revealed that these two function constructs may overlap substantially in certain areas (Table 1) (Hubacher et al., 2015).

The common involvement of the frontoparietal networks during the retention of verbal and visual information in working memory (WM) tasks has been highlighted. These common networks have been observed both for overall activation levels during verbal and visual WM tasks (Steve Majerus et al., 2010; Nystrom et al., 2000; Rämä, Sala, Gillen, Pekar, & Courtney, 2001) and for WM load effects. WM load effects, specifically comparing high-load with low-load retention conditions, have been considered to reflect a key index of WM storage capacity (Ravizza, Delgado, Chein, Becker, & Fiez, 2004; Todd, Fougnie, & Marois, 2005). Studies exploring load effects in WM have shown the involvement of the posterior parietal cortex and the intraparietal sulcus (IPS) in the WM load for both verbal and visual WM tasks, whereas the amount of activation within sensory cortices does not appear to be sensitive to the WM load (Ravizza et al., 2004; Todd et al., 2005; Todd & Marois, 2004). This has led to the proposal that common, attention-based principles support the retention of information in the verbal and visual WM. In many current theoretical accounts of WM, attentional mechanisms such as atten-

Table 1. Interaction of working memory and attention network

Working Memory		Attention Network	
Function	**Structures**	**Function**	**Structures**
Encoding	Prefrontal cortex	Orient	Superior parietal cortex
	Right inferior frontal junction		Temporal parietal junction
	Middle frontal gyrus		Frontal eye fields
	Intraparietal sulcus		Superior colliculus
Maintenance	Left inferior frontal gyrus	Alert	Locus coeruleus
	Right posterior parietal cortex		Right frontal cortex
	Cerebellum		Parietal cortex
Retrieval	Anterior insulation	Executive control	Anterior cingulate cortex
	Cerebellum		Lateral ventral cortex
			Prefrontal cortex
			Basal ganglia

(Beatty et al., 2015; Gazzaley & Nobre, 2012; Hubacher et al., 2015)

tional focalization and selection are considered to be central for efficient WM performance because they allow temporary representations of the WM content to remain active and in the focus of attention (e.g., Cowan 1995; Fuster 1999; Lavie 2005; Gazzaley and Nobre 2012). Cowan (1995) argued that limitations in the scope of attention define the WM capacity: the scope of attention is defined by the amount of information that can be consciously attended at one time (S. Majerus et al., 2014).

4. Training

Certain cultural factors and parenting factors interact with genes and influence people's behavior; consequently, we should be able to develop specific training methods that can be used to influence the underlying brain networks. Some training methods have been used in the literature. Several studies, such as those on attention and working memory training, have shown improved executive attention function and have produced changes in task-related brain areas (Rueda, Rothbart, McCandliss, Saccomanno, & Posner, 2005). The practice of a form of meditation has been used to change the brain state in a way that improves attention, reduces stress, and improves functional connectivity between the anterior cingulate gyrus and the striatum (Petersen & Posner, 2012; Tang et al., 2009; Tang et al., 2007).

Cognitive training involves structured exercises that are prescribed and undertaken with the intention of enhancing cognitive abilities, such as attention, memory, and problem solving (Lawlor-Savage & Goghari, 2014). The aim of cognitive training in older people is to create far transfer from the training to broadly enhance cognitive functioning. Transfer often occurs readily when the training and target tasks are very similar (Thorndike & Woodworth, 1901); however, transfer to target task abilities that share few perceptual and cognitive elements with training has been harder to interpret. Nevertheless, as a result of working memory training, several investigators have recently shown far transfer in young people, resulting in fluid ability; this was assessed by the Raven's Progressive Matrices (Jaeggi et al., 2008, 2010, 2011; Klingberg et al., 2002, 2005). Thus, training can considerably enhance academic, professional, and personal success abilities (Gottfredson, 1997). However, in healthy elderly individuals, studies that trained reasoning, speed, or memory did not obtain far transfer (Ball et al., 2002; Edwards et al., 2002; Neely and Backman, 1995), whereas studies that trained complex strategy use, task-switching, and problem solving did obtain far transfer (Basak et al., 2008; Karbach & Kray, 2009; Stine-Morrow et al., 2008). It should be noted that the literature is not balanced; by contrast, working memory training is the predominant type studied in young people, whereas complex task training is the predominant type studied in older people (Strenziok et al., 2014).

NEURAL PLASTICITY

Electrical activity plays significant roles in the structural and functional refinement of neural circuits throughout an organism's lifetime (Buonomano & Merzenich, 1998; Gilbert, 1998; Karmarkar & Dan 2006; Katz & Shatz, 1996) (Caporale & Dan, 2008). Manipulations of sensory experiences that disrupt normal activity patterns can lead to largescale network remodeling and marked changes in neural response properties. Learning and memory are also likely to be mediated by activity-dependent circuit modifications. Understanding the cellular mechanisms underlying such functional plasticity has been a longstanding challenge in neuroscience (Martin et al. 2000).

In his influential postulate on the cellular basis for learning, Hebb stated that "when an axon of cell A is near enough to excite cell B and repeatedly or persistently takes part in firing it, some growth process or metabolic change takes place in one or both cells such that A's efficiency, as one of the cells firing B, is increased" (Hebb, 1949). The finding of long-term potentiation (LTP) of synaptic transmission supported this postulate. LTP was initially discovered in the hippocampus (Bliss & Gardner-Medwin, 1973; Bliss & Lømo, 1973) and was subsequently reported in a large number of neural circuits, including the amygdala (Chapman, Kairiss, Keenan, & Brown, 1990; Clugnet & LeDoux, 1990), neocortical areas (Artola & Singer, 1987), and the midbrain reward circuit (Liu et al. 2005, Pu et al. 2006). Traditionally, LTP is induced by pairing low-frequency stimulation (LFS) with large postsynaptic depolarization (> 30 mV) or by high-frequency stimulation (HFS) of the presynaptic afferent neurons. In contrast, long-term depression (LTD) is induced by LFS, either alone or paired with a small postsynaptic depolarization (Artola et al. 1990, Dudek & Bear 1993, Kirkwood & Bear 1994, Linden & Connor 1995, Mulkey & Malenka 1992, Stanton & Sejnowski 1989). Together, LTD and LTP allow the activity-dependent bidirectional modification of synaptic strength, thus serving as promising candidates for the synaptic basis of memory and learning (Bliss & Collingridge, 1993; Caporale & Dan, 2008; Ito, 2005; Siegelbaum & Kandel, 1991).

In the last decade, there has been growing interest in the benefits of learning influences produced by training programs, with the aim of improving cognitive abilities and brain plasticity. Cognitive training consists of voluntarily engaging in the practice of training, which has been designed to increase experience in a specific ability (Jolles & Crone, 2012). The nature of training exercises may produce either a specific effect on the efficiency of the targeted brain network or a more general influence affecting the dynamic state of the brain (Tang & Posner, 2009).

TRAINING BASED ON NEURONAL PLASTICITY

Several studies that used training interventions have shown efficacy gains in the attention network (Rueda et al., 2005), cognitive control (Anguera et al., 2013), working memory (Gazzaley & Nobre, 2012), general fluid intelligence (Jaeggi, Buschkuehl, Jonides, & Perrig, 2008), task switching (Karbach & Kray, 2009), and inhibitory control processes (Thorell, Lindqvist, Bergman Nutley, Bohlin, & Klingberg, 2009) following training. To understand how post-training improvements are related to training-induced brain plasticity, several training studies have been conducted in combination with neuroimaging techniques. Reported findings show that cognitive training influences brain plasticity at different levels. Using EEG, Rueda and colleagues (2005) studied training-induced changes in the efficiency of the executive attention networks in a sample of preschool-aged children. Their results revealed that attention training produces a reduction in latency and a shift of topography of the N2 component, suggesting a more mature pattern of activation after training. However, increased activation of the pre-frontal (middle frontal gyrus) and parietal (intra-parietal and inferior parietal) regions was reported after working memory training (Olesen, Westerberg, & Klingberg, 2004). Additionally, Jolles and colleagues (2013) have shown that fifteen sessions of training with a working memory program resulted in increased functional connectivity at rest within the frontoparietal network (Jolles, van Buchem, Crone, & Rombouts, 2013). Moreover, it has been reported that training induces changes in the binding potential of dopamine D1 receptors in the parietal and prefrontal cortices (McNab et al., 2009). Thus, interventions designed to increase experience with specific cognitive processes produce changes in multifarious neural mechanisms, which very likely underlie the effects in competency observed in the behavioral and cognitive functions.

Cognitive training studies have been important to assess and understand to what extent we can affect the efficiency of brain networks with theoretically grounded interventions. Data have been reported that show the potential of modifying brain systems to improve self-regulatory processes. Although more studies are required to replicate and validate these findings, current evidence has shed light on the beneficial effects of training interventions in different processes that promote mental capital (Rosario Rueda, P. Pozuelos, & M. Cómbita, 2015).

1. Memory Training

There are plenty of tasks for memory training, such as finger sequence learning, dMTS (delayed Matching-to-Sample Task), n-back, digit span, running memory tasks, arithmetic tasks, etc. An influential working memory task is the n-back task; it has plentiful variants, such as the dual n-back task (Figure 1) (Jaeggi et al., 2008) and the spatial n-back task (Chan, Wu, Liang, & Yan, 2015); this task can demonstrate different patterns. However, researchers believe that suitable training tasks may transfer to other cognitive abilities, such as working memory capacity, attentional network, fluid intelligence, and problem solving; furthermore, we believe that the training effect will improve daily function.

As shown in Figure 1, the dual n-back training task in previous studies required participants to simultaneously maintain and manipulate auditory and visual stimuli at increasing levels of difficulty (Lawlor-Savage & Goghari, 2014). Specifically, the participants had to remember the position of an image on a quadrate and an auditory stimulus such as a letter, word, or number. The participants then responded when the visual or auditory stimulus matched the presented stimulus. A previous study that used the n-back training task in children with attention-deficit/hyperactivity disorder (ADHD) demonstrated that the working memory training could enhance attentional function and treatment in children with ADHD (Green et al., 2012).

2. Attentional Training

Moruzzi & Magoun (1949) created the concept of arousal when they first attempted to research the role of the brain stem reticular system in maintaining alertness. As

Figure 1. A training task that used the n-back paradigm, with dual 2-back conditions
Source: Jaeggi et al., 2008; Lawlor-Savage & Goghari, 2014; Morales, Padilla, Gomez-Ariza, & Bajo, 2015

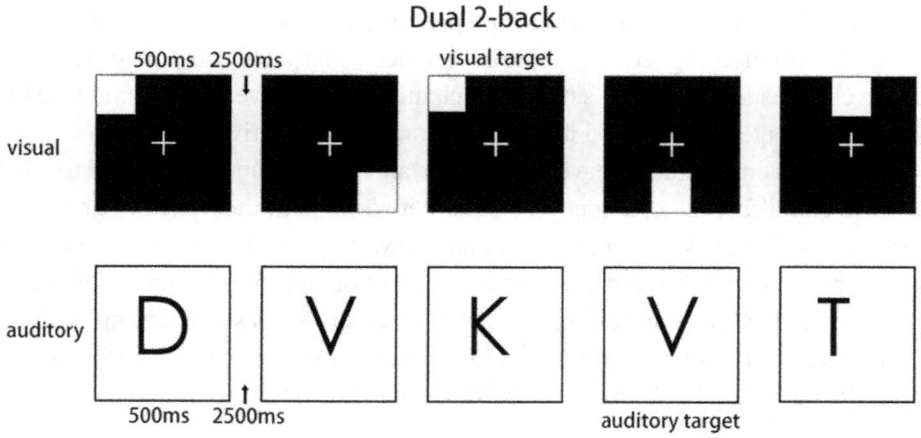

more became known regarding the neuromodulatory systems of the brain stem and thalamus, it was necessary to qualify the general concept of arousal into more differentiated components. Within cognitive psychology, a major emphasis has been placed on producing and maintaining optimal vigilance and performance during tasks; this is the sense of alertness that Petersen & Posner (1990) discussed in their article.

The influence of attention travels via bottom-up signals that arrive in sensory-specific areas: for vision, this occurs in the primary visual cortex and extra striate areas moving forward toward the temporal lobe. That this remote influence involves synchronization between activity in the more dorsal attention areas and activity in the more ventral visual areas is an influential idea (Womelsdorf et al., 2007). The synchronization apparently leads to greater sensitivity in the visual system, allowing faster responses to visual targets and thus improving the priority for processing targets.

One may think of focal attention as the entry to the conscious state, which may involve widespread connections from the midline cortex and the anterior cingulate cortex (ACC) to produce the global work space frequently associated with consciousness (Dehaene & Changeux 2011). Recent research suggests that the ACC is involved in conflict detection and monitoring, whereas the lateral frontal areas are in charge of solving the conflict (Botvinick, Barch, Carter, & Cohen, 2001). This brain region has been highly studied by imaging experiments partly because of its frequent activation (Rosario Rueda et al., 2015).

Training for attentional function has always used conflict tasks, such as the Stroop, Simon, and flanker tasks (Figure 2). A recent study with the flanker task was used to test long-term training effects; the participants were presented with a black fixation cross for a random short period of time; then, they were presented with a row of five arrows pointing either left or right, and the target was the central arrow. The target presentation could be presented by a warning tone and/or a visual cue (a black asterisk). The distance between the central target arrow and the flankers could be either centered or significantly displaced to the left or right. The cue has four conditions, with four different targets that combine to create a conflict situation and force the participants to solve the conflict (Morales et al., 2015). In other studies, researchers also found that the conflict training task could change the encephalic region of memory (Gazzaley & Nobre, 2012).

Previously, studies have combined the theory of working memory and cognitive control. Researchers have used working memory tasks or the conflict paradigm for training and have used the conflict task to assess the training effect (Bogg & Lasecki, 2014; Lawlor-Savage & Goghari, 2014). However, there are also other opinions indicating that the experimental paradigm of cognitive control that contains the conflict task is closely associated with problem solving, self-control, attention maintenance and other cognitive abilities. Thus, training that involves solving the

Figure 2. One of the conflict tasks
Source: Morales et al., 2015

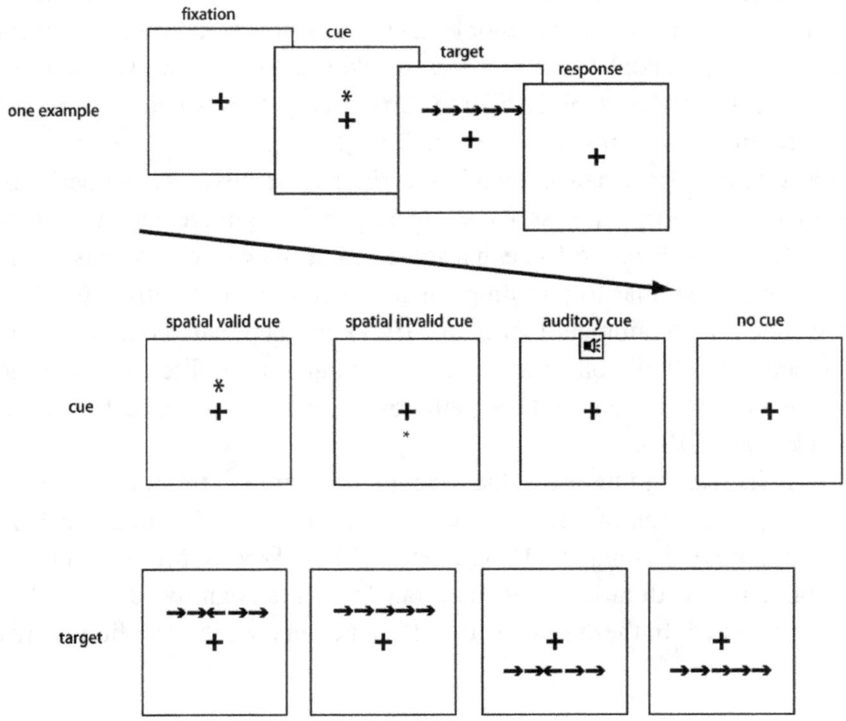

conflict task should transfer to other correlating domains and should improve cognitive functions as a whole.

APPLICATION IN ALZHEIMER'S DISEASE

The World Alzheimer's Report and World Health Organization (WHO) have highlighted dementia care as a public health priority (Organization, 2012). Despite the increased understanding of the retrogression of the brain and the putative pathological mechanisms of cognitive impairment, the treatment options remain limited for dementia. Previous studies have demonstrated that factors that influence the integrity and function of neuronal networks may help to combat the emergence of disabling clinical symptoms. Interventions that improve the neuroplasticity response through stimulation may affect cognitive impairments and possibly attenuate the trajectories of decline (Cheng et al., 2015).

Cognitive impairment is the core syndrome of dementia. It also determines the loss of independent functioning. There has been long-standing interest as to whether cognitive training and programs with structured training of specific cognitive domains would help to improve cognition and function in people suffering from dementia (Herrera, Chambon, Michel, Paban, & Alescio-Lautier, 2012; Lee, Yip, Yu, & Man, 2013). A recent study demonstrated that in people with cognitive impairment, the improvement in cognitive functions or behavior measures associated with cognitive training were limited (Bahar-Fuchs, Clare, & Woods, 2013). However, other recent studies suggested the possibility of transferring cognitive benefits with working memory training paradigms (Cheng et al., 2015).

Cognitive training can help individuals' in the early stages of Alzheimer's disease by addressing their forgetfulness and enhancing their cognitive competence. In recent years, there has been evidence that some actions may protect against cognitive decline progress. Similar to multilingualism (Chertkow et al., 2010; Craik et al., 2010), educational attainment (Yu et al., 1989) and habitual "cognitive activity" (Wilson et al., 2003) all confer some protection against late-life cognitive decline and even against Alzheimer's-related pathology (Landau et al., 2012; Li et al.,2013) (Strenziok et al., 2014).

There is increasing interest in the function of cognitive training in potentially slowing the progression of AD (Jean, Bergeron, Thivierge, & Simard, 2010). The effects of cognitive training in AD are modest (Clare, Woods, Moniz Cook, Orrell, & Spector, 2003), with little evidence of transferring to cognitive domains beyond those being trained. In these studies, the efficiency in cognitive abilities may have been limited by training schedules. Some modest changes have been reported with training programs, including improvements in working memory, processing speed, and learning ability (Clare et al., 2003); improvements in recall and recognition related to practiced material (Cahn-Weiner, Malloy, Rebok, & Ott, 2003); recall and verbal attention (Davis, Massman, & Doody, 2001); and recall and face-name association tests (Belleville et al., 2006; Kanaan et al., 2014).

In clinical therapy, plentiful treatment programs have been integrated by various cognitive tasks to remediate the individuals with cognitive impairments. For example, constraint-induced therapy (CIT) is a successful model to regain upper extremity function after stroke. Kanaan, McDowd et al. (2014) used a variant of the CIT model in individuals with Alzheimer's disease (AD); their tasks are presented in Table 2.

The individuals' performances were better after training than at baseline for some of the statistical tests, specifically MMSE scores, letter fluency, and 3 of the trail making tasks: visual scanning, number sequencing, and letter sequencing (Kanaan et al., 2014). This study demonstrated that in the early stages of Alzheimer's disease, training with a variety of combined tasks can be a very important and effective method in the treatment and intervention of the disease. We must continue to explore these results through laboratory studies to identify which training tasks are suitable and easy to measure.

Table 2. Training task schedule

Region	Task	Measure of Performance
Working Memory	Forward digit span	Longest digit span / Number of correct trials
	Backward digit span	Longest digit span / Number of correct trials
	Running memory task	Percentage of correct responses / Median response time
Memory& Attention	Arithmetic task	Percentage of correct responses / Median response time
Attention	Sustained attention	Percentage of correct responses / Number of incorrect responses / Number of responses missed
Attention	Divided attention	Dual task cost of proportion of correct responses / Dual task cost of median response time
Attention	Alternating switching	Alternating switch cost of proportion of correct responses / Alternating switch cost of median response time
Memory& Attention	Cued switching	Cued cost of proportion of correct responses / Cued cost of median response time
Memory& Movement	Paper-and-Pencil Training Tasks	Data from paper and pencil tasks are not recorded for statistical analysis

DISCUSSION

The previous study demonstrates that several weeks of working memory training enhances performance on measures of general fluid intelligence and other cognitive abilities. We expect that future studies will outdistance our attempt to answer the question of whether transfer occurs and instead seek to explore the nature and degree of how these improved test scores may reflect "true" improvements in cognitive function, which can translate into practical, real-world settings. Theoretically, the observed improvements are plausible because general fluid intelligence, working memory and attention network performance draw upon overlapping cognitive and neural processes, including shared demands on working memory and conflict resolution (Burgess et al., 2011; Buschkuehl, Hernandez-Garcia, Jaeggi, Bernard, & Jonides,2014; von Bastian & Oberauer, 2013). Because working memory and the attention network are essential cognitive skills that underlie a wide range of life functions, even modest improvements may have significant changes in societal ramifications; therefore, it is becoming very clear that training involving working memory and conflict tasks with the goal of attempting to increase holistic cognitive skills holds much promise.

Plenty of reviews and meta-analyses have reported positive effects of general forms of cognitive remediation on patients who suffer from cognitive deficits; however, little is known about how more specific forms, such as working memory training, may be beneficial. A more targeted and easily accessible form of computerized cognitive training, such as adaptive n-back working memory training, has demonstrated positive behavioral and neural effects in healthy populations. Such findings are beginning to emerge for individuals with cognitive deficits, with potential benefits not only for aspects of cognition (e.g., problem solving, attention network, working memory, processing speed) but also for more generalized functioning, such as social and occupational performance. However, regarding the details of training, several questions remain regarding (e.g., intension, duration, type) how training exerts an impact (e.g., improved attention, improved working memory), the long term benefits of training, and how training must be adapted for the special needs of an individual with cognitive deficits (e.g., effects of medication, symptoms, illness duration, and other individual differences).

There is sufficient room for well-controlled, methodologically rigorous investigations and attempts to identify moderators or mediators of training related benefits. Such work is necessary to extend working memory training to a population and individuals experiencing severe and cognitive deficits. Previous results have suggested that high-intensity, short duration cognitive training is feasible in individuals in the earliest stages of AD and results in clear training-related improvements in practiced tasks. Moreover, modest cognitive benefits were present in unpracticed tasks, suggesting some carryover to more generalizable cognitive domains, with some evidence of durability of these benefits at a few months follow-up. These findings support further development and testing for the effectiveness of cognitive training in those with cognitive impairment.

CONCLUSION

The present studies have indicated that the attention network and working memory have some overlapping regions on a neurological level. Training that involves basic cognitive functioning and that activates and stimulates specific brain regions may produce benefits in a wider range of cognitive functions. It will be important to identify a form of cognitive training that is accessible, sustainable, and practical for both individuals and service providers within public or private health systems.

ACKNOWLEDGMENT

This study was supported in part by Japan Society for the Promotion Of Science (JSPS) kakenhi, grant numbers: 25249026 and 25303013 and a Grant-in-Aid for Strategic Research Promotion from Okayama University; National Natural Science Foundation of China (NSFC61473043).

REFERENCES

Anguera, J. A., Boccanfuso, J., Rintoul, J. L., Al-Hashimi, O., Faraji, F., Janowich, J., & Gazzaley, A. et al. (2013). Video game training enhances cognitive control in older adults. *Nature*, *501*(7465), 97–101. doi:10.1038/nature12486 PMID:24005416

Artola, A., & Singer, W. (1987). Long-term potentiation and NMDA receptors in rat visual cortex. *Nature*, *330*(6149), 649–652. doi:10.1038/330649a0 PMID:2446147

Au, J., Sheehan, E., Tsai, N., Duncan, G. J., Buschkuehl, M., & Jaeggi, S. M. (2015). Improving fluid intelligence with training on working memory: A meta-analysis. *Psychonomic Bulletin & Review*, *22*(2), 366–377. doi:10.3758/s13423-014-0699-x PMID:25102926

Bahar-Fuchs, A., Clare, L., & Woods, B. (2013). Cognitive training and cognitive rehabilitation for mild to moderate Alzheimer's disease and vascular dementia. *Cochrane Database of Systematic Reviews*, 6. PMID:23740535

Beatty, E. L., Jobidon, M. E., Bouak, F., Nakashima, A., Smith, I., Lam, Q., & Vartanian, O. et al. (2015). Transfer of training from one working memory task to another: Behavioural and neural evidence. *Frontiers in Systems Neuroscience*, *9*, 86. doi:10.3389/fnsys.2015.00086 PMID:26082694

Belleville, S., Gilbert, B., Fontaine, F., Gagnon, L., Ménard, É., & Gauthier, S. (2006). Improvement of episodic memory in persons with mild cognitive impairment and healthy older adults: Evidence from a cognitive intervention program. *Dementia and Geriatric Cognitive Disorders*, *22*(5-6), 486–499. doi:10.1159/000096316 PMID:17050952

Bliss, T., & Collingridge, G. L. (1993). A synaptic model of memory: long-term potentiation in the hippocampus. *Nature, 361*(6407), 31-39.

Bliss, T., & Gardner-Medwin, A. R. (1973). Long-lasting potentiation of synaptic transmission in the dentate area of the unanaesthetized rabbit following stimulation of the perforant path. *The Journal of Physiology, 232*(2), 357-374.

Bliss, T., & Lømo, T. (1973). Long-lasting potentiation of synaptic transmission in the dentate area of the anaesthetized rabbit following stimulation of the perforant path. *The Journal of Physiology, 232*(2), 331-356.

Bogg, T., & Lasecki, L. (2014). Reliable gains? Evidence for substantially underpowered designs in studies of working memory training transfer to fluid intelligence. *Frontiers in Psychology*, *5*, 1589. doi:10.3389/fpsyg.2014.01589 PMID:25657629

Botvinick, M. M., & Barch, T. S. (2001). Conflict Monitoring and Cognitive Control. *Psychological Review*, *108*(3), 624–652. doi:10.1037/0033-295X.108.3.624 PMID:11488380

Cahn-Weiner, D. A., Malloy, P. F., Rebok, G. W., & Ott, B. R. (2003). Results of a randomized placebo-controlled study of memory training for mildly impaired Alzheimer's disease patients. *Applied Neuropsychology*, *10*(4), 215–223. doi:10.1207/s15324826an1004_3 PMID:14690802

Caporale, N., & Dan, Y. (2008). Spike timing-dependent plasticity: A Hebbian learning rule. *Annual Review of Neuroscience*, *31*(1), 25–46. doi:10.1146/annurev.neuro.31.060407.125639 PMID:18275283

Chan, J. S., Wu, Q., Liang, D., & Yan, J. H. (2015). Visuospatial working memory training facilitates visually-aided explicit sequence learning. *Acta Psychologica*, *161*, 145–153. doi:10.1016/j.actpsy.2015.09.008 PMID:26398484

Chapman, P. F., Kairiss, E. W., Keenan, C. L., & Brown, T. H. (1990). Long-Term synaptic potentiation in the amygdala. *Synapse (New York, N.Y.)*, *6*(3), 271–278. doi:10.1002/syn.890060306 PMID:2237784

Cheng, C. P., Chan, S. S., Mak, A. D., Chan, W. C., Cheng, S. T., Shi, L., & Lam, L. C. et al. (2015). Would transcranial direct current stimulation (tDCS) enhance the effects of working memory training in older adults with mild neurocognitive disorder due to Alzheimer's disease: Study protocol for a randomized controlled trial. *Trials*, *16*(1), 479. doi:10.1186/s13063-015-0999-0 PMID:26499250

Clugnet, M.-C., & LeDoux, J. E. (1990). Synaptic plasticity in fear conditioning circuits: Induction of LTP in the lateral nucleus of the amygdala by stimulation of the medial geniculate body. *The Journal of Neuroscience*, *10*(8), 2818–2824. PMID:2388089

Davis, R. N., Massman, P. J., & Doody, R. S. (2001). Cognitive intervention in Alzheimer disease: A randomized placebo-controlled study. *Alzheimer Disease and Associated Disorders*, *15*(1), 1–9. doi:10.1097/00002093-200101000-00001 PMID:11236819

Gazzaley, A., & Nobre, A. C. (2012). Top-down modulation: Bridging selective attention and working memory. *Trends in Cognitive Sciences*, *16*(2), 129–135. doi:10.1016/j.tics.2011.11.014 PMID:22209601

Green, C. T., Long, D. L., Green, D., Iosif, A.-M., Dixon, J. F., Miller, M. R., & Schweitzer, J. B. et al. (2012). Will working memory training generalize to improve off-task behavior in children with attention-deficit/hyperactivity disorder? *Neurotherapeutics: The Journal of the American Society for Experimental NeuroTherapeutics*, *9*(3), 639–648. doi:10.1007/s13311-012-0124-y PMID:22752960

Hebb, D. (1949). *The Organization of Behaviour: A Neuropsychological Theory*. Academic Press.

Herrera, C., Chambon, C., Michel, B. F., Paban, V., & Alescio-Lautier, B. (2012). Positive effects of computer-based cognitive training in adults with mild cognitive impairment. *Neuropsychologia*, *50*(8), 1871–1881. doi:10.1016/j.neuropsychologia.2012.04.012 PMID:22525705

Hubacher, M., Kappos, L., Weier, K., Stocklin, M., Opwis, K., & Penner, I. K. (2015). Case-Based fMRI Analysis after Cognitive Rehabilitation in MS: A Novel Approach. *Front Neurol*, *6*, 78. doi:10.3389/fneur.2015.00078 PMID:25904893

Ito, M. (2005). Bases and implications of learning in the cerebellum—adaptive control and internal model mechanism. *Progress in Brain Research, 148*, 95–109. doi:10.1016/S0079-6123(04)48009-1 PMID:15661184

Jaeggi, S. M., Buschkuehl, M., Jonides, J., & Perrig, W. J. (2008). Improving fluid intelligence with training on working memory. *Proceedings of the National Academy of Sciences of the United States of America, 105*(19), 6829–6833. doi:10.1073/pnas.0801268105 PMID:18443283

Jean, L., Bergeron, M.-È., Thivierge, S., & Simard, M. (2010). Cognitive intervention programs for individuals with mild cognitive impairment: Systematic review of the literature. *The American Journal of Geriatric Psychiatry, 18*(4), 281–296. doi:10.1097/JGP.0b013e3181c37ce9 PMID:20220584

Jolles, D. D., & Crone, E. A. (2012). Training the developing brain: A neurocognitive perspective. *Frontiers in Human Neuroscience*, 6. PMID:22509161

Jolles, D. D., van Buchem, M. A., Crone, E. A., & Rombouts, S. A. R. B. (2013). Functional brain connectivity at rest changes after working memory training. *Human Brain Mapping, 34*(2), 396–406. doi:10.1002/hbm.21444 PMID:22076823

Kanaan, S. F., McDowd, J. M., Colgrove, Y., Burns, J. M., Gajewski, B., & Pohl, P. S. (2014). Feasibility and efficacy of intensive cognitive training in early-stage Alzheimer's disease. *American Journal of Alzheimer's Disease and Other Dementias, 29*(2), 150–158. doi:10.1177/1533317513506775 PMID:24667905

Karbach, J., & Kray, J. (2009). How useful is executive control training? Age differences in near and far transfer of task-switching training. *Developmental Science, 12*(6), 978–990. doi:10.1111/j.1467-7687.2009.00846.x PMID:19840052

Lawlor-Savage, L., & Goghari, V. M. (2014). Working memory training in schizophrenia and healthy populations. *Behav Sci (Basel), 4*(3), 301–319. doi:10.3390/bs4030301 PMID:25379283

Lee, G. Y., Yip, C. K., Yu, E., & Man, D. (2013). Evaluation of a computer-assisted errorless learning-based memory training program for patients with early Alzheimer's disease in Hong Kong: A pilot study. *Clinical Interventions in Aging, 8*, 623. PMID:23766638

Majerus, S., Cowan, N., Peters, F., Van Calster, L., Phillips, C., & Schrouff, J. (2014). Cross-Modal Decoding of Neural Patterns Associated with Working Memory: Evidence for Attention-Based Accounts of Working Memory. *Cereb Cortex*. doi:10.1093/cercor/bhu189 PMID:25146374

Majerus, S., D'Argembeau, A., Perez, T. M., Belayachi, S., Van der Linden, M., Collette, F., & Maquet, P. et al. (2010). The commonality of neural networks for verbal and visual short-term memory. *Journal of Cognitive Neuroscience*, *22*(11), 2570–2593. doi:10.1162/jocn.2009.21378 PMID:19925207

McNab, F., Varrone, A., Farde, L., Jucaite, A., Bystritsky, P., Forssberg, H., & Klingberg, T. (2009). Changes in cortical dopamine D1 receptor binding associated with cognitive training. *Science*, *323*(5915), 800–802. doi:10.1126/science.1166102 PMID:19197069

Morales, J., Padilla, F., Gomez-Ariza, C. J., & Bajo, M. T. (2015). Simultaneous interpretation selectively influences working memory and attentional networks. *Acta Psychologica*, *155*, 82–91. doi:10.1016/j.actpsy.2014.12.004 PMID:25577491

Nystrom, L. E., Braver, T. S., Sabb, F. W., Delgado, M. R., Noll, D. C., & Cohen, J. D. (2000). Working memory for letters, shapes, and locations: fMRI evidence against stimulus-based regional organization in human prefrontal cortex. *NeuroImage*, *11*(5), 424–446. doi:10.1006/nimg.2000.0572 PMID:10806029

Olesen, P. J., Westerberg, H., & Klingberg, T. (2004). Increased prefrontal and parietal activity after training of working memory. *Nature Neuroscience*, *7*(1), 75–79. doi:10.1038/nn1165 PMID:14699419

Organization, World Health. (2012). *Dementia: a public health priority*. World Health Organization.

Petersen, S. E., & Posner, M. I. (2012). The attention system of the human brain: 20 years after. *Annual Review of Neuroscience*, *35*(1), 73–89. doi:10.1146/annurev-neuro-062111-150525 PMID:22524787

Rämä, P., Sala, J. B., Gillen, J. S., Pekar, J. J., & Courtney, S. M. (2001). Dissociation of the neural systems for working memory maintenance of verbal and nonspatial visual information. *Cognitive, Affective & Behavioral Neuroscience*, *1*(2), 161–171. doi:10.3758/CABN.1.2.161 PMID:12467111

Ravizza, S. M., Delgado, M. R., Chein, J. M., Becker, J. T., & Fiez, J. A. (2004). Functional dissociations within the inferior parietal cortex in verbal working memory. *NeuroImage*, *22*(2), 562–573. doi:10.1016/j.neuroimage.2004.01.039 PMID:15193584

Rosario Rueda, M., Pozuelos, J., & Cómbita, L. (2015). Cognitive Neuroscience of Attention From brain mechanisms to individual differences in efficiency. *AIMS Neuroscience*, *2*(4), 183-202. doi: 10.3934/Neuroscience.2015.4.183

Rueda, M., Rothbart, M. K., McCandliss, B. D., Saccomanno, L., & Posner, M. I. (2005). Training, maturation, and genetic influences on the development of executive attention. *Proceedings of the national Academy of Sciences of the United States of America, 102*(41), 14931-14936.

Siegelbaum, S. A., & Kandel, E. R. (1991). Learning-related synaptic plasticity: LTP and LTD. *Current Opinion in Neurobiology, 1*(1), 113–120. doi:10.1016/0959-4388(91)90018-3 PMID:1822291

Strenziok, M., Parasuraman, R., Clarke, E., Cisler, D. S., Thompson, J. C., & Greenwood, P. M. (2014). Neurocognitive enhancement in older adults: Comparison of three cognitive training tasks to test a hypothesis of training transfer in brain connectivity. *NeuroImage, 85*(Pt 3), 1027–1039. doi:10.1016/j.neuroimage.2013.07.069 PMID:23933474

Tang, Y.-Y., Ma, Y., Fan, Y., Feng, H., Wang, J., Feng, S., & Li, J. et al. (2009). Central and autonomic nervous system interaction is altered by short-term meditation. *Proceedings of the National Academy of Sciences of the United States of America, 106*(22), 8865–8870. doi:10.1073/pnas.0904031106 PMID:19451642

Tang, Y.-Y., Ma, Y., Wang, J., Fan, Y., Feng, S., Lu, Q., & Fan, M. et al. (2007). Short-term meditation training improves attention and self-regulation. *Proceedings of the National Academy of Sciences of the United States of America, 104*(43), 17152–17156. doi:10.1073/pnas.0707678104 PMID:17940025

Tang, Y.-Y., & Posner, M. I. (2009). Attention training and attention state training. *Trends in Cognitive Sciences, 13*(5), 222–227. doi:10.1016/j.tics.2009.01.009 PMID:19375975

Thorell, L. B., Lindqvist, S., Nutley, B., & Sissela, B. (2009). Training and transfer effects of executive functions in preschool children. *Developmental Science, 12*(1), 106–113. doi:10.1111/j.1467-7687.2008.00745.x PMID:19120418

Todd, J., Fougnie, D., & Marois, R. (2005). Visual short-term memory load suppresses temporo-parietal junction activity and induces inattentional blindness. *Psychological Science, 16*(12), 965–972. doi:10.1111/j.1467-9280.2005.01645.x PMID:16313661

Todd, J., & Marois, R. (2004). Capacity limit of visual short-term memory in human posterior parietal cortex. *Nature, 428*(6984), 751–754. doi:10.1038/nature02466 PMID:15085133

Woods, C. L., Cook, M., Orrell, M., & Spector, A. (2003). Cognitive rehabilitation and cognitive training for early-stage Alzheimer's disease and vascular dementia. Cochrane Database Syst Rev, 4.

KEY TERMS AND DEFINITIONS

Alzheimer's Disease: Alzheimer's is a type of dementia that causes problems with memory, thinking and behavior. Symptoms usually develop slowly and become worse over time, becoming severe enough to interfere with daily tasks.

Attention Network: Attention is the ability to attend to some objectives and ignore others. There are three basic concepts in the attention system: alerting, orienting and executive control.

Training: Training is teaching, or developing in oneself or others, any skills and knowledge that relate to specific useful competencies. Training has the specific goals of improving one's capability, capacity, productivity and performance.

Working Memory: Working memory (WM) is the ability to store and manipulate information for short periods of time. It is an important predictor of scholastic aptitude and a critical bottleneck underlying higher-order cognitive processes, including controlled attention and reasoning.

Chapter 8
Cognitive and Neural Mechanisms Involved in Interactions between Touch and Emotion

Zhilin Zhang
Beijing Institute of Technology, China

Qiang Huang
Beijing Institute of Technology, China

Tianyi Yan
Beijing Institute of Technology, China

Jinglong Wu
Beijing Institute of Technology, China

ABSTRACT

Touch has been described as the most fundamental means of contact with the world and the most primitive modality among all sensory systems. In the past, the study of emotional communication has focused almost exclusively on facial and vocal channels but has ignored the channel for the sense of touch. However, the latest studies have documented that the sense of touch can convey at least six emotions, and its accuracy rate is comparable to that of facial expressions and vocal communication. Moreover, there is also mounting evidence indicating that the modality of touch encompasses two dimensions, which provide not only its well-recognized discriminative input from glabrous skin to sensory cortex but also an affective input from hairy skin to the insular cortex because a type of low-threshold mechanosensitive receptor that innervates hairy skin has been shown to convey emotions via C fibers. In light of recent advances in our research, this chapter aims to illustrate the cognitive and neural mechanisms that underlie interactions between touch and emotion.

DOI: 10.4018/978-1-5225-0925-7.ch008

INTRODUCTION

Recently, research has indicated that the sense of touch can convey at least six emotions and that its accuracy rate is comparable to that of facial expressions and vocal communications. Here, I summarize the current state of knowledge on the elaborate mechanisms that facilitate the formation of communication via touch. First, I describe behavioral results related to touch-communicated emotions. Next, I show that in agreement with physiological evidence, there is a class of low-threshold mechanosensitive C fibers that innervate hairy skin and that these neurons represent the neurobiological substrate for affective touch. Then, I present evidence that touch communicates distinct emotions and that this process requires several neural mechanisms, some of which are concerned to emotional processing and others that are involve in a specialized tactile perception system. Finally, I highlight factors that I believe are related to the neural bases of interactions between touch and emotion.

BACKGROUND

With the rapid aging of our population, human-robot emotional interactions are becoming a topical issue related to the process of helping the elderly and sick and performing medical rehabilitation as well as social services (Figure 1). However, humans would rather choose a more emotional animal than a cold machine companion. The emotional interactions between robots and humans that occur via the sense of touch seem to be an impenetrable barrier not only in the field of brain science but also in the field of humanoid robots. Recently, a growing amount of evidence has indicated that the sense of touch has another dimension and that it provides not only its well-recognized discriminative input to the brain but also an affective input (McGlone, Wessberg, & Olausson, 2014). This result will hopefully promote the development of methods to integrate the senses and new research in the brain sciences, provide theoretical and technological support for research into emotional interactions between human beings and robots, and drive the brain sciences and other industries related to advanced robots to thrive in the world.

Touch and Emotion

Happy, sad, fearful, anxious, elated, smitten, disappointed, angry, pleased, disgusted, excited, shameful, guilty, and infatuated are just some of the terms we use to describe our emotions. Emotions can be roughly described by the process of evaluating such an event, which includes the process of becoming aware of a feeling. Emotions are often intertwined with mood, temperament, personality, disposition, and motivation

Figure 1. (a) The aging population of China, including the increasing proportion of elderly people. (b) Humanoid robots can communicate emotions to people via face, voice, and touch modalities.

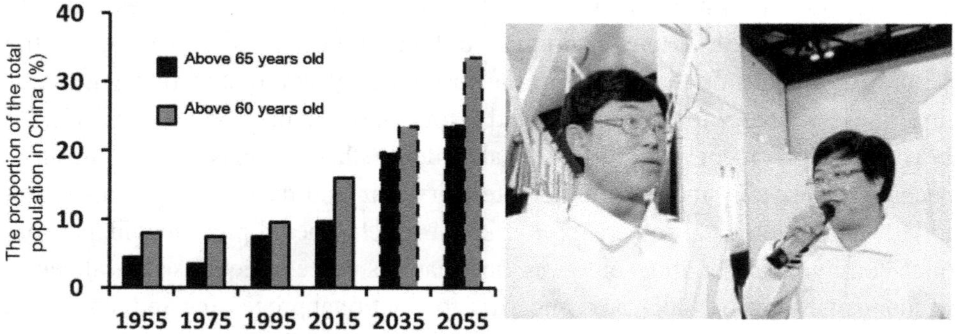

(a) (b)

(Damasio, 1994). However, emotions are complex. There is currently no unified and strict definition for this term that could be used around the world. Previously, researchers adopted two primary approaches to unifying our definition of emotion. First, basic emotions attempt to examine the universality of facial expression and define a finite set of human emotions (Ekman & Friesen, 1971). However, another way to approach the categorization of emotions is to describe them not as discrete states but as reactions to events in the world that vary along a continuum. Obviously, these basic and dimensional approaches make it difficult to converge all of our emotional experiences. The question of how we can scientifically research "emotion" has been plaguing us for many years.

Since the development of the field of neuroscience, humans have obtained a new understanding of the brain and emotions. However, the notion that a network of brain structures underlies emotional behavior has been very influential (Damasio, 2000). Since James Papez (1937) first proposed a circuit theory of the brain and emotions, MacLean's theory that the limbic system is the "emotional" brain has been generally accepted (Maclean, 1949). However, it remains difficult to determine criteria to use to define which structures and pathways should be included in the limbic system. For example, the hippocampus may be part of both the limbic system and systems involved in non-emotional processes (Scoville & Milner, 1957). Hence, the view that emotion is a unitary concept or that it is governed by a single neural system is inaccurate. When an individual performs different emotional tasks or scenes, we expect different neural systems to be involved. These systems include brain regions that may only be responsible for emotional processes and also a number of brain regions with multiple functions. Understanding the involvement of these different regions is crucial to our investigation into the cognitive neuroscience of emotion.

Early attempts at investigating the existence and localization of cortical circuits that govern emotion in humans have relied exclusively on experiments involving the facial and vocal channels. These studies have ignored the sense of touch. In these experiments, subjects have been scanned either while watching affective pictures or while listening to an emotional voice. Despite the sense of touch being the first sense we acquire and the fact that it is described as our most fundamental means of contact with the world, its role in communicating emotion has received much less attention than the roles of facial and vocal displays of emotion (Geldard, 1960). Some would even say that touch is thought to merely amplify the intensity of emotional displays by the face and voice (Knapp & Hall, 1997). Although probing our ability to nonverbally communicate emotions has been difficult to accomplish until recently, the idea that people can impart and interpret emotional content via another nonverbal modality, touch, has been demonstrated by Hertenstein. Indeed, we appear to be wired to interpret touch by our fellow humans. However, in relation to affective touch, there is still much work to do.

Since these early studies, the cognitive and neural mechanism of the interaction between touch and emotion has been widely investigated in humans and nonhuman primates using various tasks and techniques. These studies have aimed to integrate information from various domains to ascertain which neural circuits underlie the interaction between touch and emotion. Here, I summarize the current state of knowledge relating to the elaborate mechanisms that facilitate the development of communication via touch. First, I describe the behavioral results of touch that communicates emotions. Next, I show that in agreement with this physiological evidence, a class of low-threshold mechanosensitive C fibers innervates hairy skin, and these fibers represent the neurobiological substrate for affective emotion. Then, I present evidence showing that touch communicates distinct emotions and that this process requires several neural mechanisms, some of which are concerned with emotional processing and others that involve a specialized tactile perception system. Finally, I suggest factors that I believe are likely to be related to the neural bases of the interaction between touch and emotion.

The Behaviors of Interactions Between Emotion and Touch

The sense of touch helps us to discriminate the location of a stimulus on the skin surface, to explore objects haptically and to identify and manipulate objects. It also contributes to an integrated sense of our own body (Thompson & Hampton, 2011). However, research into the wide-ranging functions of touch leave out a very essential fact: touch can also be emotional. Hertenstein's early work documented that touch plays a role in emotional communication among humans (Hertenstein, Verkamp, Kerestes, & Holmes, 2006). As they stated, the game pat-a-cake, which is composed solely of tactile stimulation, is capable of generating positive emotions (Wolff, 1961). Subsequently, Gewirtz (1992) used two sets of stimuli to investigate infant preferences and showed that young infants who received touch displayed more smiles and vocalizations and spent less time crying than did infants who received no touch (Gewirtz & Peláez-Nogueras, 1992). Although touch is capable of generating positive emotions and modulating negative emotions, it is also capable of generating negative emotions (Peláez-Nogueras, Field, Hossain, & Pickens, 1996). An earlier study indicated that static touch (simply laying a hand on an infant's abdomens with little pressure) was less reinforcing and generated more negative emotional displays than other stimuli that involved dynamic tactile stimulation (Brossard & Decarie, 1968). Touch is clearly central to the communication of emotion and particularly the hedonics of emotion. Therefore, we need to construct reliable coding systems to further investigate the qualities and parameters of tactile stimulation.

The study of how touch communicates emotions was advanced by Hertenstein's landmark work on emotion and behavior coding (Hertenstein, Keltner, App, Bulleit, & Jaskollka, 2006). When encoders were asked to think and make contact with the decoder's bare arm from the elbow to the end of the hand to signal each emotion, all of the tactile displays were recorded by the researchers, including the specific type of touch and the intensity and duration of each emotion. Of the well-studied emotions, anger, fear, and disgust were decoded more significantly than happiness and surprise. Participants were more inclined to interpret attempts to communicate prosocial emotions (love, gratitude, sympathy) than self-focused emotions (embarrassment, envy, pride). However, these observations could be linked to those that were obtained in behavioral studies, in which different types of touch have been shown to indicate responses to different emotions in tests involving unacquainted dyads that were performed without visual cues. In another study, the subjects were divided into female-female, male-male, and male-female groups. Anger was communicated at greater-than-chance levels only when a male comprised at least one member of a communicating dyad. Sympathy was communicated at greater-than-chance levels only when a female comprised at least one member of the dyad. Happiness was communicated only if females comprised the entire dyad. Therefore, gender asymmetries also play a role in the accuracy of communicating distinct emotions via touch (Hertenstein & Keltner, 2011).

Another study provided more degrees of freedom to communicate various emotions by allowing encoders to touch the other member of the dyad anywhere on the body that was appropriate. This study also advanced our knowledge by developing precise descriptions of emotion-specific signals (Hertenstein, Holmes, McCullough, & Keltner, 2009). It provided evidence showing that touch communicates at least eight emotions: anger, fear, happiness, sadness, disgust, love, gratitude, and sympathy with accuracy rates that ranged from 50% to 70%. Touch communications showed more negatively valenced (anger, fear, sadness, disgust) and positive emotions (happiness, gratitude, sympathy, love) than communications inferred by the face and voice. Moreover, the authors also documented specific tactile behaviors that were associated with each emotion and located where and what percentage of the time the decoder's body was contacted by the encoder when emotions were accurately decoded (Table 1). For example, fear was communicated by holding the other, squeezing, and contact without movement, whereas sympathy was communicated by holding the other, patting, and rubbing.

A more recent study investigated touch's ability to increase emotion in communal relationships (Simao & Seibt, 2015). The authors proposed that a brief, friendly touch to the shoulder increases feelings of gratitude. One possible reason that was suggested was that a friendly touch on the shoulder was probably perceived as a responsive gesture because the receiver may have perceived it as signaling for attention, care, and consideration (Capraiello & Reis, 2010). Another similarity to a responsive gesture is intentionally responding to a partner's needs by benefitting him or her (Algoe, Haidt, & Gable, 2008). Nevertheless, the link between touch and gratitude was mediated by communal feelings rather than by liking or by positive effects. Therefore, touch signals the intention to initiate or maintain a communal relationship, thus confirming and reinforcing the existence of a communal feeling (Okun, et al, 2015). Although these experiments indicate that some features of communication between emotion and touch are similar in humans, the specific cognitive mechanism that underlies these processes remained unclear. Next, I pro-

Table 1. Behaviors, durations, intensities and locations of tactile displays that were associated with each of the emotions

Emotions	Behaviors	Duration Time (s)	Intensity of Tactile Displays	Location of Decoder's Body
Anger	Shake, Push	4.5±5.1	Strong	Arm
Fear	Shake, Squeeze	7.6±8.5	Moderate	Forearm
Happiness	Shake, Swing	5.8±3.7	Strong	Forearm, Hand
Sadness	Contact, Hug, Nuzzle	6.4±4.3	Light	Arm, Hand
Disgust	Push	5.8±7.0	Moderate	Forearm
Love	Hug	5.3±4.7	Moderate	Back
Gratitude	Shake	6.0±4.6	Moderate	Hand
Sympathy	Pat, Hug, Rub	6.4±5.6	Light	Arm, Forearm, Hand, Back

pose a set of underlying neural mechanisms that are involved in the communication of distinct motions by touch. I then provide suggestions for a more careful and detailed interpretation of these proposals.

The Neuropsychology of the Interaction Between Touch and Emotion

Since it was initially shown that there is a link between touch and emotions, the neuronal pathway underlying the interaction between emotion and touch has been a topic of investigation both at the level of peripheral neurophysiology and at the level of the brain. Four sub-modalities are often described to involve low-pressure mechanoreceptors (LTMs), including pressure/vibration, temperature, itch, and pain. These modalities share their anatomical locations in the skin with receptors that encode thermal and chemical stimuli (Figure 2) (Griffin, McArthur, & Polydefkis, 2001). Each channel generates distinct sensory/perceptual qualities that are performed by classes of stimulus-specific neurons that project in defined anatomical pathways to the cerebral cortex (Mountcastle, 2005).

Historically, researchers have viewed touch as generally subserving a primarily discriminative role (Johansson, Landstrom, & Lundstrom, 1982). However, micro-neurography experiments have demonstrated that there is a population of unmyelin-

Figure 2. Four types of mechanoreceptors are located in the skin

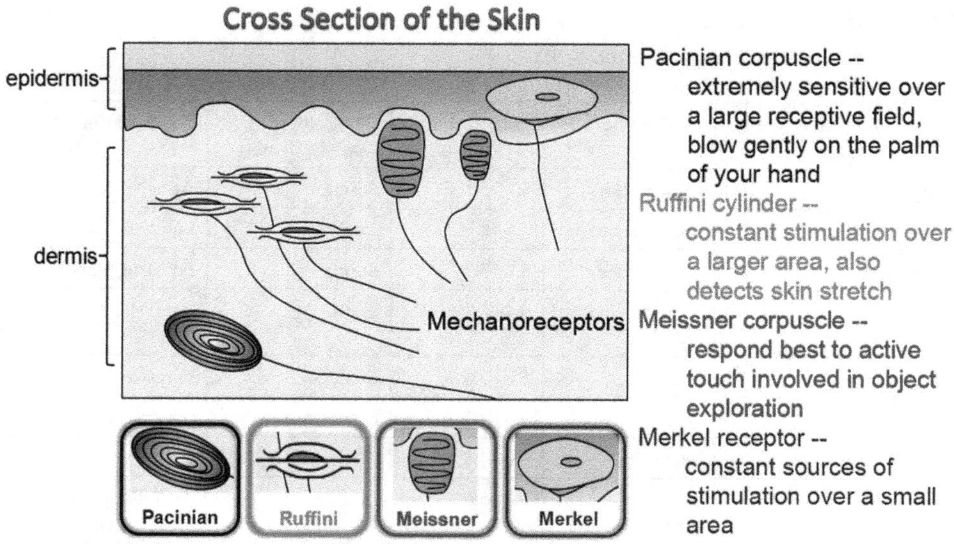

ated C-tactile afferents that respond optimally to emotional touch. The high degree of arborization of these C fibers is distributed in the infraorbital nerve, the supraorbital nerve, the arm and the leg (Vallbo, Olausson, & Wessberg, 1999). Interestingly, C-tactile afferents have never been recorded from nerves innervating the palmar skin of the hands. Information from neurophysiological experiments concluded that C-tactile afferents respond to very low indentation forces in the range of 0.3-2.5 mN with high frequency responses (50-100 impulses/s^{-1}) to innocuous stimuli, such as gentle stroking with a soft brush (Wessberg, Olausson, Fernstrom, & Vallbo, 2003). As has been shown in humans, C-tactile afferents showed an inverted U-shaped relationship between brushing velocity and firing frequency, with the highest responses recorded between 1 and 10 cm/s^{-1} (Cole, et al., 2006). Another fundamental process during temperature modulation involves the transformation of C-tactile afferents. These afferents discharge preferentially in response to slowly moving stimuli at a neutral (typical skin) temperature, rather than at cooler or warmer stimulus temperatures (Ackerley, et al., 2014). In fact, C-tactile afferents are not only velocity-tuned but also temperature-tuned.

Another study focused on animals during handling or maternal contact. These contacts resulted in more adaptive stress responses that reduced the effects of impaired cognitive ability or other stress-related diseases (Meaney, et al., 1991). An abundant amount of evidence indicates that handling and maternal contact increases glucocorticoid receptor expression, leading animals to exhibit adaptive and appropriate responses rather than prolonged responses to stress (Liu, et al., 1997; Meaney, Aitken, van-Berkel, Bhatnagar, & Sapolsky, 1988). In addition, handling appears to increase sensitivity to negative feedback from glucocorticoids in rats, perhaps because it causes an increase in receptor sites. Increased sensitivity to glucocorticoids is necessary to inhibit the release of more glucocorticoids, which exacerbates the stress response (Meaney, Aitken, Bodnoff, Bhatnagar, & Sapolsky, 2013; Francis, Caldji, Champagne, Plotsky, & Meaney, 1999).

Although microneurography has provided valuable insights into the electrophysiological properties of C-tactile afferents, little is known about what stimulus would adequately replicate the gentle, low-force stroking of hairy skin, which is a stimulus that is not in the nociceptor range. Depending on the principles of the Darwinian theory of evolution, any stimulus that is associated with a reward or punishment should be linked to the simple purpose of survival. The functional significance of a nociceptive system to survival remains unequivocal. Therefore, McGlone and colleagues (2010) proposed a similar duality for touch in which discriminative touch is mediated by myelinated fast-conducting Aβ nerves, while affective touch is mediated by C-tactile afferents that are activated only when touching stimulus has the appropriate properties for an adequate stimulus (Björnsdotter, Morrison, & Olausson, 2010). A more direct molecular neurobiology result was shown in electrode recordings that were obtained from the nerves of awake human volunteers while their tactile receptive fields were stimulated using a soft brush. However, this result also supports the notion that intact C-tactile afferent pathways are likely to be necessary for the normal evaluation of touch pleasantness on hairy skin, in addition to the notion that C-tactile afferents may operate as selectors that are activated in parallel with Aβ afferents. Importantly, these two systems are not separate, despite being at least partly dissociable. There are therefore undoubtedly sensory discriminative and motivational affective pathways for touch interactions (Morrison & Downing, 2010).

The Neuroimaging of Interaction Between Touch and Emotion

It is clear from recent investigations at the level of peripheral neurophysiology that C-tactile afferents transmit the affective properties of touch. This is also a topic for studies of the brain (Loken, Wessberg, Morrison, McGlone, & Olausson 2009; McGlone, Loken, & Wessberg, 2007). Brain imaging experiments have investigated the existence and localization of cortical circuits that communicate emotions by touch in humans. Some studies using functional Magnetic Resonance Imaging (fMRI) have focused on selected neuroanatomical regions of interest (ROI) during emotion interactions that involve the sense of touch. Other studies have used electroencephalograms (EEGs) to examine activity in cortical processing networks, and these have found that activation is associated with tactile-guided emotion in many additional areas.

Which neural pathways are involved during affective touch? In 2008, McCabe et al. used fMRI to investigate brain responses to the communication of emotion by touch (McCabe, Rolls, Bilderbeck, & McGlone, 2008). When participants were asked to apply moisturizing lotion to the hairy skin but not to the glabrous skin of the palm, increases were observed in regional cerebral blood flow in many cortical and subcortical areas, including motor and premotor areas, and in the mid-orbitofrontal cortex. In another study, subjects underwent fMRI to compare the effects of stroking at a C-tactile afferent optimal velocity (3 cm/s) to stroking at a non-C-tactile afferent optimal velocity (30 cm/s). C-tactile afferent stroking resulted in higher rates of regional cerebral blood flow in extensive regions of the posterior insula that are associated with somatic and multimodal responses than the rates provoked by non C-tactile afferent touching in the same areas (Bolognini, Rossetti, Fusaro, Vallar, & Miniussi, 2014).

Early attempts to use brain imaging to identify the functional anatomy underlying the generation of goal-directed arm movements during spontaneous facial self-touch gestures in humans used EEG. However, the changing dynamics of theta waves indicated that spontaneous self-touch gestures play a role in emotional processes, primarily in stressful situations (Grunwald, Weiss, Mueller, & Rall, 2014). Moreover, being touched by another person influences our readiness to empathize with and support that person. Event-related potential experiments have indicated that touch sensitizes ongoing cognitive and emotional processes and that this sensitization is mediated by bottom-up somatosensory processing. Moreover, touch seems to be perceived as a stronger sensory cue than tone (Gallese, 2003). However, when using single trial classification techniques, beta-power significantly distinguished between pleasant and unpleasant stimulation on a single trial basis with high accuracy (Singh, et al., 2014).

Other studies have focused on brain responses to the unpleasant emotion of pain, and the results of these studies have suggested that feeling and seeing pain may share neural processes (Morrison, Lloyd, di Pellegrino, & Roberts, 2004). When participants were asked to observe the painful experiences of others, brain areas coding the unpleasant aspects of pain contributed to an observer's representation of the other's pain (Jackson, Meltzoff, & Decety, 2005). Compared to the control group, pain-related motivational affective regions were more activated in the anterior and mid-cingulate cortex, anterior insula, motor and sensory cortex (Avenanti, Minio-Paluello, Bufalari, & Aglioti, 2006; Cheng, et al., 2007). However, there is currently no consensus regarding the exact location and existence of overlapping cingulate activity between felt and seen pain, which vary between individuals (Morrison, Loken, & Olausson, 2010).

Soft brush stroking on hairy skin activates the somatosensory areas SI and SII in addition to the posterior contralateral insular cortex. The insular cortex is classically considered to be a specific region for affective processes, and it is considered a gateway from sensory systems to emotional systems, especially in the posterior contralateral insular cortex (Craig, 2008). Olausson also demonstrated that when similar soft brushing stimuli were applied to Aβ-deafferented subjects, no activity was observed in somatosensory areas, whereas the posterior insular region was activated (Olausson, et al., 2002). Importantly, when brain activity was compared in response to touching either C-tactile afferent on hairy skin or glabrous skin, higher levels of cortical activity were observed in the posterior insular cortex and mid-anterior orbitofrontal cortex when the C-tactile afferents were touched than when the glabrous skin was touched (Gordon, et al., 2013). In fact, stimulation of unmyelinated C-tactile afferents evoked significant fMRI deactivation in the somatosensory cortex, probably because more emotional areas, mainly those related to emotion-related paralimbic cortical systems, were activated. In experiments addressing this issue, the posterior superior temporal sulcus, the medial prefrontal cortex and the dorso-anterior cingulate cortex have also been implicated in processing C-tactile afferent-targeted touch (Kramer, et al., 2007).

Although the contributions of tactile Aβ afferents and C-tactile afferents to emotional processing have not been widely explored, there is some evidence to support the notion that Aβ afferents may well underpin pleasant sensations. Studies in which similar touch stimuli were applied to the palm, where C-tactile afferents are lacking, showed fMRI responses in a target area for insular afferents in the orbitofrontal cortex, which is involved in complex emotional evaluations (Rolls, et al., 2003). Therefore, we hypothesize that glabrous skin can communicate emotions and that it is involved in secondary reinforcement mechanisms that involve low-threshold mechanoreceptors signaling in a pattern that is typical of tactile processing (McGlone, et al., 2012).

A growing amount of neurobiological evidence indicates that touch is more than a sensory input for discriminating what is on the skin. Instead, the gentle touch that is often observed during nurturing and social interactions reflects the presence of an evolutionary mechanism that is mediated via C-tactile afferents that project strongly to emotional systems but little or not at all to the discriminative cognitive systems that promote physical contact in specific contexts (Figure 3). In fact, growing up cannot occur without physical contact with others, and touching provides us with much more of a benefit than we appreciate throughout life.

Figure 3. Schematic model of affective and discriminative pathways involved in touch in the skin

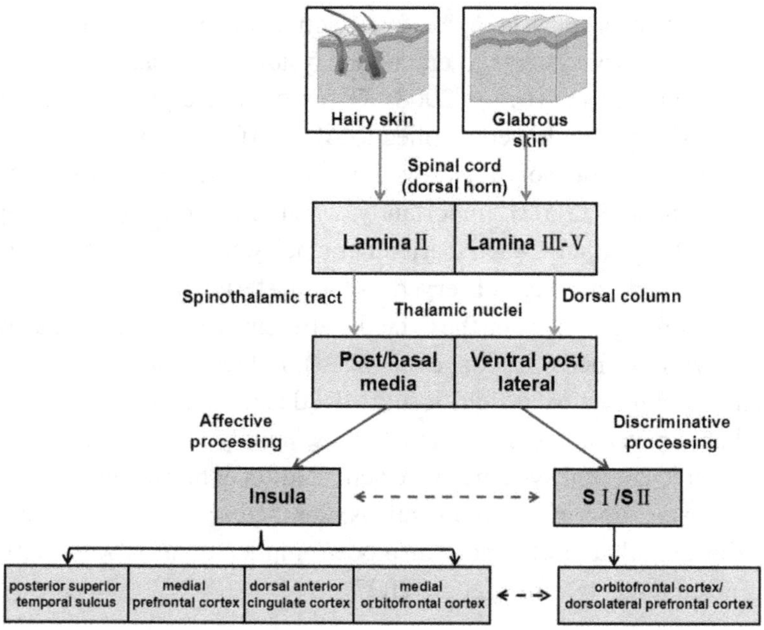

FUTURE RESEARCH DIRECTIONS

Because there is an urgent demand for improving human-robot emotional interactions that can help the elderly and sick and assist in medical rehabilitation and social services, some pivotal problems strike us as particularly important for understanding how the human brain actively facilitates multisensory integration and its attention for visual, audio and touch perception and how this information can be used in human-robot emotional interaction. How do we allocate limited attention? How do we integrate multisensory information (Figure 4)?

The results of this research will hopefully promote the development of methods to integrate the senses, improve research into brain science, provide theoretical and technological support for research into the emotional interactions between humans and robots, and drive brain science and related industries to develop advanced robots that can thrive in the world.

CONCLUSION

The development of fMRI has coincided with improvements in designs that may help researchers to address many of the problems involving in conducting emotion-centered studies. Earlier research and theories tended to view emotion as separate from cognition, implying that they could be studied and understood separately. However, all emotions have unique and defining characteristics that can be studied along with more “cognitive” behaviors. Ideally, a coordinated series of neuroimaging experiment should be performed to explore the interaction between emotion

Figure 4. Multisensory brain cognitive mechanisms involved in multisensory integration and attention

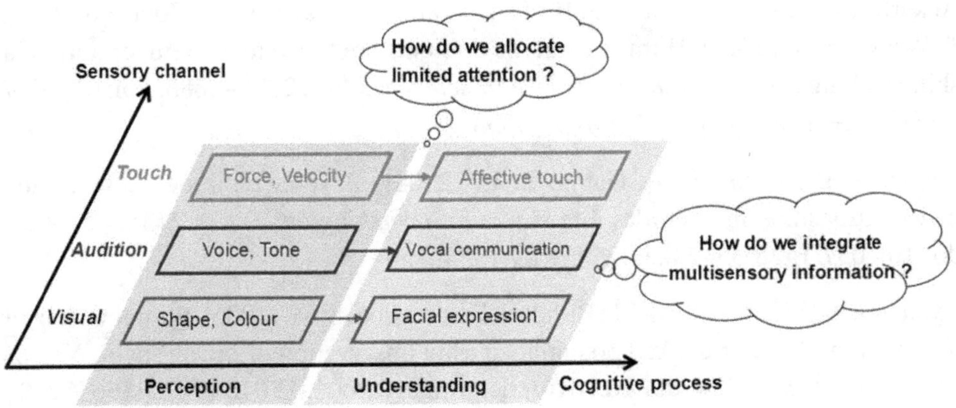

and touch. In addition, MRI-compatible systems now make it possible to perform electrophysiological and possibly kinematic recordings while subjects perform various tasks during scanning.

Some progress has been made in characterizing the cognitive neuroscience of emotion and the neural substrates that underlie it. Nonetheless, much remains unknown, and many important issues have yet to be addressed. The "affective touch hypothesis" implies that the essential role of the C-tactile afferents system is to provide or support emotional, hormonal, and behavioral responses to skin-to-skin contact with conspecifics. However, it is too difficult to quantitatively define the kind of behavior that is related to each emotion. In addition, the intensity and even the quality of the emotional response that is evoked by a particular stimulus is highly dependent on contextual factors. Therefore, an emerging shift in our approach to studying the cognitive neuroscience of emotion is movement toward an emphasis on the study of neural structures to investigations of neural systems.

Finally, we have learned that the sense of touch makes unique contributions to emotional communication and affective styles. Only through careful and thoughtful experimentation that uses converging techniques involving both the brain and behavior might we come to understand the neural systems underlying the interactions between emotion and touch.

ACKNOWLEDGMENT

This work was supported by the Chinese National Natural Science Foundation (Grants 61473043 and 61305142).

REFERENCES

Ackerley, R., Backlund-Wasling, H., Liljencrantz, J., Olausson, H., Johnson, R. D., & Wessberg, J. (2014). Human C-tactile afferents are tuned to the temperature of a skin-stroking caress. *The Journal of Neuroscience*, *34*(8), 2879–2883. doi:10.1523/JNEUROSCI.2847-13.2014 PMID:24553929

Algoe, S. B., Haidt, J., & Gable, S. L. (2008). Beyond reciprocity: Gratitude and relationships in everyday life. *Emotion (Washington, D.C.)*, *8*(3), 425–429. doi:10.1037/1528-3542.8.3.425 PMID:18540759

Avenanti, A., Minio-Paluello, I., Bufalari, I., & Aglioti, S. M. (2006). Stimulus-driven modulation of motor-evoked potentials during observation of others' pain. *NeuroImage*, *32*(1), 316–324. doi:10.1016/j.neuroimage.2006.03.010 PMID:16675270

Björnsdotter, M., Morrison, I., & Olausson, H. (2010). Feeling good: On the role of C fiber mediated touch in interoception. *Experimental Brain Research, 207*(3-4), 149–155. doi:10.1007/s00221-010-2408-y PMID:20963582

Bolognini, N., Rossetti, A., Fusaro, M., Vallar, G., & Miniussi, C. (2014). Sharing social touch in the primary somatosensory cortex. *Current Biology, 24*(13), 1513–1517. doi:10.1016/j.cub.2014.05.025 PMID:24954046

Brossard, L., & Decarie, T. (1968). Comparative reinforcing effects of eight stimulations on the smiling responses of infants. *Journal of Child Psychology and Psychiatry, and Allied Disciplines, 9*(1), 51–59. doi:10.1111/j.1469-7610.1968.tb02207.x PMID:5729746

Capraiello, P. A., & Reis, H. T. (2010). Perceived partner responsiveness minimizes defensive reactions to failure. *Social Psychological & Personality Science, 2*(4), 365–372. doi:10.1177/1948550610391914

Cheng, Y., Lin, C. P., Liu, H. L., Hsu, Y. Y., Lim, K. E., Hung, D., & Decety, J. (2007). Expertise modulates the perception of pain in others. *Current Biology, 17*(19), 1708–1713. doi:10.1016/j.cub.2007.09.020 PMID:17900903

Cole, J., Bushnell, M. C., McGlone, F., Elam, M., Lamarre, Y., Vallbo, A., & Olausson, H. (2006). Unmyelinated tactile afferents underpin detection of low-force monofilaments. *Muscle & Nerve, 34*(1), 105–107. doi:10.1002/mus.20534 PMID:16518853

Craig, A. D. (2008). *In handbook of emotions* (3rd ed.). New York, NY: Guilford Press.

Damasio, A. R. (Ed.). (1994). *Descartes' error: emotion, reason, and the human brain*. New York, NY: Vintage Press.

Damasio, A. R. (2000). Eighth C.U. Ariëns Kappers Lecture. The fabric of the mind: A neurobiological perspective. *Progress in Brain Research, 126*, 457–467. doi:10.1016/S0079-6123(00)26029-9 PMID:11105662

Ekman, P., & Friesen, W. V. (1971). Constants across cultures in the face and emotion. *Journal of Personality and Social Psychology, 17*(2), 124–129. doi:10.1037/h0030377 PMID:5542557

Francis, D. D., Caldji, C., Champagne, F., Plotsky, P. M., & Meaney, M. J. (1999). The role of corticotropin-releasing factor--norepinephrine systems in mediating the effects of early experience on the development of behavioral and endocrine responses to stress. *Biological Psychiatry, 46*(9), 1153–1166. doi:10.1016/S0006-3223(99)00237-1 PMID:10560022

Gallese, V. (2003). The manifold nature of interpersonal relations: The quest for a common mechanism. *Philosophical Transactions of the Royal Society of London. Series B, Biological Sciences, 358*(1431), 517–528. doi:10.1098/rstb.2002.1234 PMID:12689377

Geldard, F. A. (1960). Some neglected possibilities of communication. *Science, 131*(3413), 1583–1588. doi:10.1126/science.131.3413.1583 PMID:13827173

Gewirtz, J. L., & Peláez-Nogueras, M. B. (1992). Skinner's legacy to human infant behavior and development. *The American Psychologist, 47*(11), 1411–1422. doi:10.1037/0003-066X.47.11.1411 PMID:1482005

Gordon, I., Voos, A. C., Bennett, R. H., Bolling, D. Z., Pelphrey, K. A., & Kaiser, M. D. (2013). Brain mechanisms for processing affective touch. *Human Brain Mapping, 34*(4), 914–922. doi:10.1002/hbm.21480 PMID:22125232

Griffin, J. W., McArthur, J. C., & Polydefkis, M. (2001). Assessment of cutaneous innervation by skin biopsies. *Current Opinion in Neurology, 14*(5), 655–659. doi:10.1097/00019052-200110000-00016 PMID:11562579

Grunwald, M., Weiss, T., Mueller, S., & Rall, L. (2014). EEG changes caused by spontaneous facial self-touch may represent emotion regulating processes and working memory maintenance. *Brain Research, 1557*, 111–126. doi:10.1016/j.brainres.2014.02.002 PMID:24530432

Hertenstein, M. J., Holmes, R., McCullough, M., & Keltner, D. (2009). The communication of emotion via touch. *Emotion (Washington, D.C.), 9*(4), 566–573. doi:10.1037/a0016108 PMID:19653781

Hertenstein, M. J., & Keltner, D. (2011). Gender and the communication of emotion via touch. *Sex Roles, 64*(1-2), 70–80. doi:10.1007/s11199-010-9842-y PMID:21297854

Hertenstein, M. J., Keltner, D., App, B., Bulleit, B. A., & Jaskollka, A. R. (2006). Touch communicates distinct emotions. *Emotion (Washington, D.C.), 6*(3), 528–533. doi:10.1037/1528-3542.6.3.528 PMID:16938094

Hertenstein, M. J., Verkamp, J. M., Kerestes, A. M., & Holmes, R. M. (2006). The communicative functions of touch in humans, nonhuman primates, and rats: A review and synthesis of the empirical research. *Genetic, Social, and General Psychology Monographs, 132*(1), 5–94. doi:10.3200/MONO.132.1.5-94 PMID:17345871

Jackson, P. L., Meltzoff, A. N., & Decety, J. (2005). How do we perceive the pain of others? A window into the neural processes involved in empathy. *NeuroImage, 24*(3), 771–779. doi:10.1016/j.neuroimage.2004.09.006 PMID:15652312

Johansson, R. S., Landstrom, U., & Lundstrom, R. (1982). Responses of mechanoreceptive afferent units in the glabrous skin of the human hand to sinusoidal skin displacements. *Brain Research*, *244*(1), 17–25. doi:10.1016/0006-8993(82)90899-X PMID:6288178

Knapp, M. L., & Hall, J. A. (Eds.). (1997). *Nonverbal communication in human interaction*. Boston, MA: Harcourt Brace College Press.

Kramer, H. H., Lundblad, L., Birklein, F., Linde, M., Karlsson, T., Elam, M., & Olausson, H. (2007). Activation of the cortical pain network by soft tactile stimulation after injection of sumatriptan. *Pain*, *133*(1-3), 72–78. doi:10.1016/j.pain.2007.03.001 PMID:17449179

Liu, D., Diorio, J., Tannenbaum, B., Caldji, C., Francis, D., & Freedman, A. et al.. (1997). Maternal care, hippocampal glucocorticoid receptors, and hypothalamic-pituitary-adrenal responses to stress. *Science*, *277*(5332), 1659–1662. doi:10.1126/science.277.5332.1659 PMID:9287218

Loken, L. S., Wessberg, J., Morrison, I., McGlone, F., & Olausson, H. (2009). Coding of pleasant touch by unmyelinated afferents in humans. *Nature Neuroscience*, *12*(5), 547–548. doi:10.1038/nn.2312 PMID:19363489

Maclean, P. D. (1949). Psychosomatic disease and the visceral brain; recent developments bearing on the Papez theory of emotion. *Psychosomatic Medicine*, *11*(6), 338–353. doi:10.1097/00006842-194911000-00003 PMID:15410445

McCabe, C., Rolls, E. T., Bilderbeck, A., & McGlone, F. (2008). Cognitive influences on the affective representation of touch and the sight of touch in the human brain. *Social Cognitive and Affective Neuroscience*, *3*(2), 97–108. doi:10.1093/scan/nsn005 PMID:19015100

McGlone, F., Olausson, H., Boyle, J. A., Jones-Gotman, M., Dancer, C., Guest, S., & Essick, G. (2012). Touching and feeling: Differences in pleasant touch processing between glabrous and hairy skin in humans. *The European Journal of Neuroscience*, *35*(11), 1782–1788. doi:10.1111/j.1460-9568.2012.08092.x PMID:22594914

McGlone, F., Vallbo, A. B., Olausson, H., Loken, L., & Wessberg, J. (2007). Discriminative touch and emotional touch. *Journal of Experimental Social Psychology*, *61*(3), 173–183. PMID:17974312

McGlone, F., Wessberg, J., & Olausson, H. (2014). Discriminative and affective touch: Sensing and feeling. *Neuron*, *82*(4), 737–755. doi:10.1016/j.neuron.2014.05.001 PMID:24853935

Meaney, M. J., Aitken, D. H., Bodnoff, S. R., Bhatnagar, S., & Sapolsky, R. M. (2013). Early postnatal handling alters glucocorticoid receptor concentrations in selected brain regions. *Behavioral Neuroscience, 127*(5), 637–641. doi:10.1037/a0034187 PMID:24128353

Meaney, M. J., Aitken, D. H., van-Berkel, C., Bhatnagar, S., & Sapolsky, R. M. (1988). Effect of neonatal handling on age-related impairments associated with the hippocampus. *Science, 239*(4841 Pt 1), 766–768. doi:10.1126/science.3340858 PMID:3340858

Meaney, M. J., Mitchell, J. B., Aitken, D., Bhatnagar, S., Bodnoff, S. R., Iny, L. J., & Sarrieau, A. (1991). The effects of neonatal handling on the development of the adrenocortical response to stress: Implications for neuropathology and cognitive deficits in later life. *Psychoneuroendocrinology, 16*(1-3), 85–103. doi:10.1016/0306-4530(91)90072-2 PMID:1961847

Morrison, I., & Downing, P. E. (2007). Organization of felt and seen pain responses in anterior cingulate cortex. *NeuroImage, 37*(2), 642–651. doi:10.1016/j.neuroimage.2007.03.079 PMID:17588777

Morrison, I., Lloyd, D., di Pellegrino, G., & Roberts, N. (2004). Vicarious responses to pain in anterior cingulate cortex: Is empathy a multisensory issue? *Cognitive, Affective & Behavioral Neuroscience, 4*(2), 270–278. doi:10.3758/CABN.4.2.270 PMID:15460933

Morrison, I., Loken, L. S., & Olausson, H. (2010). The skin as a social organ. *Experimental Brain Research, 204*(3), 305–314. doi:10.1007/s00221-009-2007-y PMID:19771420

Mountcastle, V. B. (2005). *The sensory hand*. Cambridge, MA: Harvard University Press.

Okun, M., Steinmetz, N. A., Cossell, L., Iacaruso, M. F., Ko, H., Barthó, P., & Harris, K. D. et al. (2015). Diverse coupling of neurons to populations in sensory cortex. *Nature, 521*(7553), 511–515. doi:10.1038/nature14273 PMID:25849776

Olausson, H., Lamarre, Y., Backlund, H., Morin, C., Wallin, B. G., Starck, G., & Bushnell, M. C. et al. (2002). Unmyelinated tactile afferents signal touch and project to insular cortex. *Nature Neuroscience, 5*(9), 900–904. doi:10.1038/nn896 PMID:12145636

Peláez-Nogueras, M., Field, T. M., Hossain, Z., & Pickens, J. (1996). Depressed mothers' touching increases infants' positive affect and attention in still-face interactions. *Child Development, 67*(4), 1780–1792. doi:10.2307/1131731 PMID:8890507

Rolls, E. T., O' Doherty, J., Kringelbach, M. L., Francis, S., Bowtell, R., & McGlone, F. (2003). Representations of pleasant and painful touch in the human orbitofrontal and cingulate cortices. *Cerebral Cortex, 13*(3), 308–317. doi:10.1093/cercor/13.3.308 PMID:12571120

Scoville, W. B., & Milner, B. (1957). Loss of recent memory after bilateral hippocampal lesions. *Journal of Neurology, Neurosurgery, and Psychiatry, 20*(1), 11–21. doi:10.1136/jnnp.20.1.11 PMID:13406589

Simao, C., & Seibt, B. (2015). Friendly touch increases gratitude by inducing communal feelings. *Frontiers in Psychology, 6*, 815. doi:10.3389/fpsyg.2015.00815 PMID:26124737

Singh, H., Bauer, M., Chowanski, W., Sui, Y., Atkinson, D., Baurley, S., & Bianchi-Berthouze, N. et al. (2014). The brain's response to pleasant touch: An EEG investigation of tactile caressing. *Frontiers in Human Neuroscience, 8*, 893. doi:10.3389/fnhum.2014.00893 PMID:25426047

Thompson, E. H., & Hampton, J. A. (2011). The effect of relationship status on communicating emotions through touch. *Cognition and Emotion, 25*(2), 295–306. doi:10.1080/02699931.2010.492957 PMID:21432672

Vallbo, A. B., Olausson, H., & Wessberg, J. (1999). Unmyelinated afferents constitute a second system coding tactile stimuli of the human hairy skin. *Journal of Neurophysiology, 81*(6), 2753–2763. PMID:10368395

Wessberg, J., Olausson, H., Fernstrom, K. W., & Vallbo, A. B. (2003). Receptive field properties of unmyelinated tactile afferents in the human skin. *Journal of Neurophysiology, 89*(3), 1567–1575. doi:10.1152/jn.00256.2002 PMID:12626628

Wolff, P. H. (1961). Observations on the early development of smiling. *Determinants of Infant Behavior, 2,* 113-138.

ADDITIONAL READING

Bloom, F., Nelson, C. A., & Lazerson, A. (2001). *Brain, mind and behavior* (3rd ed.). New York, NY: Worth Publishers.

Bullock, T. H. (1984). Comparative neurosceince holds promise for a quiet revolution. *Science, 225*(4661), 473–478. doi:10.1126/science.6740319 PMID:6740319

Churchland, P. S. (1986). *Neurophilosophy: Toward a unified science of mind/brain.* Cambridge, MA: MIT Press.

D'esposito, M., Zarahn, E., & Aguirre, G. K. (1999). Event-related functional MRI: Implications for cognitive psychology. *Psychological bulletion, 125, 155-164.*

Gazzaniga, M. S. (2000). Cerebral specialization and interhemispheric communication: Does the corpus callosum enable the human condition? Bran, 123, 1293-1326.

Gazzaniga, M. S. (2005). *The ethical brain.* New York, NY: Dana Press.

Georgopoulos, A. P. (1995). *The Cognitive Neurosciences.* Cambridge, MA: MIT Press.

Hellige, J. B. (1993). *Hemispheric asymmetry: What' s right and what' left.* Cambridge, MA: Harvard University Press.

Hillyard, S. A. (1993). Electrical and magnetic brain recordings: Contributions to cognitive neuroscience. *Current Opinion in Neurobiology, 3*(2), 710–717. doi:10.1016/0959-4388(93)90213-I PMID:8513235

Ivry, R. B., & Rovertson, L. C. (1998). *The two sides of perception.* Cambridge, MA: MIT Press.

Jacob, F. (1977). Evolution and tinkering. *Science, 196*(4295), 1161–1166. doi:10.1126/science.860134 PMID:860134

Jeannerod, M. (1997). *The cognitive neuroscience of action.* Cambridge, MA: Blackwell Science Publishers.

Johnson, M. H. (1997). *Developmental cognitive neuroscience.* Cambridge, MA: Blackwall Science Press.

Kandel, E. R., Schwartz, J. H., & Jessell, T. M. (1995). *Essentials of neural science and behavior.* Norwalk, CT: Appleton and Lange Publishers.

Kass-Simon, G., & Farnes, P. (1990). *Women of science: righting the record.* Bloomington, IN: Indiana University Press.

Lindzey, G. (Ed.). (1936). *History ofpsychology in autobiography* (Vol. III). Worcester, MA: Clark University Press.

Merzenich, M. M., & Kaas, J. H. (1980). *Principles of organization of sensory-perceptual systems of mammals.* New York, NY: Academic Press.

Michael, S. G., Richard, B. I., & George, R. M. (2013). *Cognitive neuroscience: The biology of the mind* (4th ed.). New York, NY: W. W. Norton & Company Ltd. Press.

Passingham, R. (1993). *The friontal lobes and voluntary action.* New York, NY: Oxford University Press.

Pinkers, S. (1997). *How the mind works.* New York, NY: W. W. Norton Publishers.

Ponser, M. I., & Raichle, M. E. (1994). *Images of mind.* New York: W. H. Freeman Publishers.

Raichle, M. E. (1998). Behind the scenes of functional brain imaging: A historical and physiological perspective. *Proceedings of the National Academy of Sciences of the United States of America, 95*(3), 765–772. doi:10.1073/pnas.95.3.765 PMID:9448239

Rapp, B. (2001). *The handbook of cognitive neuropsychology: What deficits reveal about the human mind. Philadephia.* Psychology Press.

Rosenbaum, D. A. (1991). *Human motor control.* San Diego, CA: Academic Press.

Shaw, P., Greenstein, D., Lerch, J., Clasen, L., Lenroot, R., Gogtay, N., & Giedd, J. et al. (2006). Intellectual ability and cortical development in children and adolescents. *Nature, 440*(7084), 676–679. doi:10.1038/nature04513 PMID:16572172

Shepherd, G. M. (1988). *Neurobiology* (2nd ed.). New York, NY: Oxford University Press.

Shepherd, G. M. (1992). *Fundations of the neuron doctrine.* New York, NY: Oxford University Press.

Wilson, E. O. (1975). *Sociobiology, the new synthesis.* Cambridge, MA: Belknap Press of Harvard University Press.

KEY TERMS AND DEFINITIONS

Affective Touch: The affective dimension of touch pertains to the hedonic valence of tactile sensation.

Brain Cognitive Mechanism: A set of informational processes that occurs in the brain.

Discriminative Touch: Discriminative touch is a sensory modality that allows a subject to sense and localize touch.

EEG: An electrophysiological monitoring method to record electrical activity in the brain.

Emotional Interaction: The emotional communication between a human and a computer/robot.

fMRI: A functional neuroimaging procedure that uses MRI technology to measure brain activity by detecting changes associated with blood flow.

Multisensory Integration: The study of how information from different sensory modalities, such as sight, sound, touch, smell, self-motion and taste, are integrated by the nervous system.

Chapter 9
Effects of Visual Contrast on Inverse Effectiveness in Audiovisual Integration

Fengxia Wu
Okayama University, Japan

Weiping Yang
Hubei University, China & Okayama University, Japan

Xiaoyu Tang
Liaoning Normal University, China & Okayama University, Japan

Satoshi Takahashi
Okayama University, Japan

Yanna Ren
Okayama University, Japan

Jinglong Wu
Okayama University, Japan

ABSTRACT

Bimodal audiovisual signals can be detected more quickly and accurately than unimodal visual signals or auditory signals. This beneficial effect is called audiovisual integration. Audiovisual integration has often been described according to the spatial principle, the temporal principle and the inverse effectiveness principle. Inverse effectiveness indicates that the largest audiovisual enhancements are inversely correlated with the strength of the response to unisensory component stimuli; thus, weaker stimuli generate greater enhancement when presented together. In addition, some studies have suggested that the visual contrast feature can modulate audiovisual integration and obtained an inverse relationship between visual contrast and audiovisual integration. This review aims to summarize previous studies and describe the relationship between visual contrast and inverse effectiveness by behavior, ERP and fMRI experimental methods. By summarizing previous studies, we have determined the direction of future work.

DOI: 10.4018/978-1-5225-0925-7.ch009

BACKGROUND

The visual system is the part of the central nervous system that gives an organism the ability to process visual information. The visual system is the most important channel that has contact with the environment. Eighty percent of the outside information received through the visual system is transferred to our brain. The visual system detects and interprets information from visible light to build a representation of the surrounding environment. Visual information has two types of attributes: spatial and non-spatial. Non-spatial attributes have several basic features, such as color, shape, spatial frequency, and contrast. Here, we aim to describe the contrast feature. Contrast is defined as different luminance or color that can help distinguish an object. In the real world, visual contrast perception is determined by different colors or brightness between the objects or the same field. The human visual system is the most sensitive in 3-4 cycles per degree; when we are detecting different contrasts, we can detect the lowest contrast difference compared with any other spatial frequency (Barghout-Stein, 1999). The contrast threshold is defined as the minimum contrast that can be detected. The reciprocal of the contrast threshold is equal to the contrast sensitivity, and the contrast sensitivity changes with spatial frequency. Various definitions of contrast luminance are used in different situations. In fact, the definitions of contrast represent a ratio of the type. Here, we introduce two types of different methods used to calculate contrast luminance. One method is called the Weber contrast. The Weber contrast is defined as formula (1):

$$C_W = (I - I_b) / I_b \tag{1}$$

In which I and I_b represent the luminance of the features and the background. Another method is called the Michelson contrast. Generally, we use this method to calculate visual contrast. The Michelson contrast is defined as formula (2):

$$C_M = (\max - \min) / (\max + \min) \tag{2}$$

The max and min are represented by the highest and lowest luminance in the picture. Some previous studies have shown that with increasing contrast, the response time decreases, but the accuracy increases. Moreover, some studies have shown that contrast sensitivity can vary according to disease (Heywood, Nicholas, & Cowey, 1996) and age (Benedek et al., 2010; Costa, Nogueira, Pereira, & Santos, 2013; Packer & Ginsburg, 2007; Pardhan, 2004; Silva, d'Almeida, Oliveiros, Mateus, & Castelo-Branco, 2014).

INTRODUCTION

Audiovisual Integration

We recognize an event by many different information channels (such as vision, hearing, tactile, smell), and this information helps us understand the world more naturally. Visual and auditory inputs are the main channels that help us recognize the world. Audiovisual integration plays an important role in everyday life. For example, when we see a movie in a theatre, the combined appearance of a scary sound and a scary picture can make the event scarier than the sound or picture alone. Thus, when we receive auditory information and visual information together, we can rapidly detect and correctly identify the event. How does this phenomenon occur? Why does auditory information increase this scary atmosphere? Some previous studies have explained this phenomenon by suggesting that a combined signal in the environment is often processed faster and more accurately than a unimodal signal presented alone (Calvert, 2001; Molholm et al., 2002). Bimodal audiovisual signals can be detected more quickly and accurately than unimodal visual or auditory stimuli (Miller, 1982) (see Figure 1). This visual and auditory beneficial effect is called audiovisual integration.

Figure 1. Reaction times and hit rates for visual (V), auditory (A) and audiovisual (AV) modalities. For reaction times, audiovisual modality is faster than visual or auditory modality. For the hit rate, the audiovisual modality is more accurate than visual or auditory modalities. The benefit of audiovisual modality is called audiovisual integration.

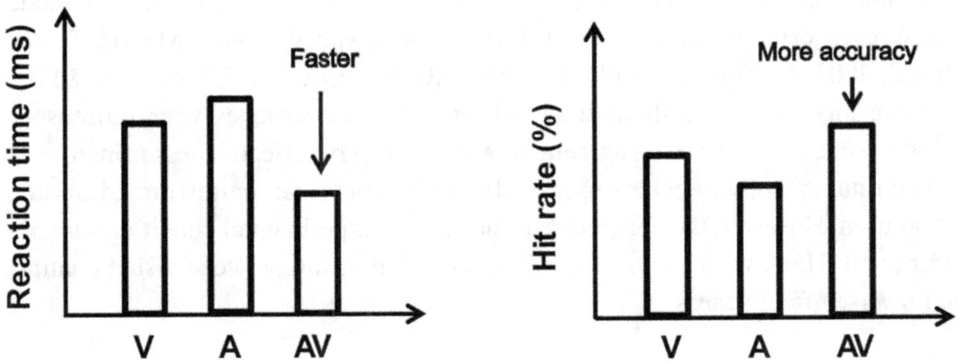

Principles of Audiovisual Integration

For several years, researchers have defined, described, and interpreted audiovisual integration by three simple principles. The spatial principle describes how the enhancement of audiovisual integration is stronger when the constituent unisensory visual and auditory stimuli are presented from the same location (Meredith & Stein, 1986). The temporal principle demonstrates that the facilitation of audiovisual integration is stronger when the unimodal visual and auditory stimuli are presented simultaneously (Meredith, Nemitz, & Stein, 1987). The principle of inverse effectiveness describes an inverse relationship between audiovisual integration enhancement and the strength of the responses to the unisensory stimuli (Meredith & Stein, 1983). However, the generality of the inverse effectiveness rule has also been questioned on the grounds that previous studies sampled an insufficient or incorrect range of stimulus intensities to critically test this hypothesis (Holmes, 2007). A number of studies have reported that not all results are inconsistent with this inverse effectiveness rule (Lakatos, Chen, O'Connell, Mills, & Schroeder, 2007; Ross, Saint-Amour, Leavitt, Javitt, & Foxe, 2007). However, for simplicity and clarity, we focus only on the explanation of inverse effectiveness according to the audiovisual integration study.

Inverse Effectiveness

Originally, inverse effectiveness was described by single-neuron studies in the superior colliculus (SC) of cats (Barry E Stein & Meredith, 1993). Those studies reported that maximal audiovisual response enhancements occur when the constituent unisensory stimuli is minimally responsible for evoking responses. They had detailed a basic set of principles for audiovisual integration. However, because of the tools involved and other various reasons, the neurophysiological basis for this finding in humans remains unknown. Nonetheless, human behavioral, ERP and fMRI studies have found an inverse relationship between stimulus intensity and the magnitude of the bisensory redundant signals effect (Corneil, Van Wanrooij, Munoz, & Van Opstal, 2002; Diederich & Colonius, 2004; Rach, Diederich, & Colonius, 2011). These results showed that the audiovisual interaction was strongest when unisensory responsiveness was weak, in agreement with the inverse effectiveness principle. A growing number of studies have proposed the effects of visual contrast on audiovisual integration. However, the concrete parameters and experimental conditions are not clear at all. Here, we focus on describing the relationship between visual contrast and inverse effectiveness.

INVERSE EFFECTIVENESS BY VISUAL CONTRAST FEATURE

Inverse effectiveness is a basic principle of audiovisual integration and has been well known as a stimulus feature. In this section, we describe the effect of the visual contrast feature on inverse effectiveness using behavioral and neural correlate methods (see Table 1).

Effect of the Visual Contrast Feature on Behavioral Inverse Effectiveness

Behavioral research on the law of inverse effectiveness typically intends to show that multisensory integration is the strongest with the weakest responses or worst performance in unisensory conditions. Recently, studies focusing on multisensory integration processing between auditory and visual stimuli reported that the presentation of bisensory stimuli with low contrast leads to stronger behavior facilitation than with high contrast (Molholm et al., 2002; Talsma, Doty, & Woldorff, 2007). Some recently published articles have claimed to find behavioral evidence to support the law of inverse effectiveness (Rach et al., 2011; Serino, Farnè, Rinaldesi, Haggard, & Làdavas, 2007). Stefan Rach reported an article about audiovisual integration

Table 1. Inverse effectiveness of audiovisual integration

Study	Task	Contrast	Behavioral Integration Effect	Correlated Brain Area	Times
Stefan Rach, 2011	Detection	C_d: 80%, 90%	RT:80% > 90%	-	-
Ryan A, 2009	2AFC	C: 55%, 65%, 75%, 85%, 95%	-	STS: 55% *, 65% *	-
Toemme Noesselt, 2010	Detection	C_d: 60%, 85%	d': 60% **, H: 60% *	STS: 18%*, Thalamic: 18% * Sensory-specific cortices: 18% *,	-
Daniel Senkowski, 2011	Detection	C: 10%, 50%, 90%	RT: 10% **, 50% **, 90% ** Racemodal: 10% **	Right anterior: 10% *, Left posterior: 10% *	40-60 ms
Ryan A, 2012	2AFC	C: 72.5%, 85%, 97.5%	Racemodal: 72.5% **, 85% **, 97.5% *	Occipital, Vertex, Right Temporo-parietal	P1-N1 -P2

Note: 2AFC: two-alternative forced choice task; C: the size of the contrast; C_d: the hit rate is X%, the contrast is calculated by the hit rate; H: hit rate; RT: reaction times; d': sensitivity index; STS: superior temporal sulcus.

according to the contrast feature in 2011. Their experiment involved eight types of visual and auditory intensities and three types of conditions. The participants were instructed to use both visual modality and auditory modality. The results revealed that the magnitude of audiovisual integration was better when the visual intensity was weak (0.0045 mcd) than when the visual intensity was strong (0.0106 mcd). Moreover, two similar behavioral results were found in other experiments. Holmes found that the co-occurrence of a sound enhanced human detection sensitivity for lower but not for higher-contrast visual targets (Holmes, 2007). Another result was obtained by Serino. His experiment indicated that the redundant target effect was exceeded based on the probability summations of unisensory response time, which is indicative of integrative audiovisual processing, but only for low intensity stimuli (Serino et al., 2007). These audiovisual integration study results are in line with the principle of inverse effectiveness.

Nevertheless, several different analytical methods utilizing the same data have produced effects that are either consistent with or in disagreement with inverse effectiveness (Ross et al., 2007). When audiovisual integration is considered an enhancement relative to unisensory baselines, the audiovisual integration gain is in accord with inverse effectiveness in behavioral studies. However, when audiovisual integration is expressed as absolute enhancements, both in numbers and audiovisual gains in correct performance, then audiovisual integration may not specifically agree with inverse effectiveness. Therefore, if we desire to research the principle of inverse effectiveness, we must be aware of the analysis method used.

Effect of the Visual Contrast Feature on Neural Correlative Inverse Effectiveness

For brain activity studies, researchers often use transcranial magnetic stimulus (TMS), single neuron, event-related potential (ERP), functional magnetic resonance imaging (fMRI) and magnetoencephalography (MEG) methods to measure neural correlate brain activity. Here, we discuss neural correlate brain activity through event-related potential and functional magnetic resonance imaging methods.

ERP is a basic measure method used to test brainneural activity and to detect brain activity by detecting the changes in brain waves produced by events. Compared with behavioral procedures, ERP can provide a continuous measure between the stimulus and response. This continuous measure can easily determine which stage is affected by the specific experimental operation. Some audiovisual integration effects were found by ERP experimental methods in previous studies, such as inverse effectiveness effects. Audiovisual modality is not only helpful in audiovisual integration, but it also can obtain an inverse relationship between stimulus intensity and audiovisual integration. This result has been demonstrated by Senkowski (Senkowski, Saint-Amour, Hofle, & Foxe, 2011). In that study, the participants had to detect all sensory modalities and make a speeded button response with their right index finger. Both visual and auditory stimuli have three contrasts (low, middle or high), but the results suggested that audiovisual integration evoked brain activity elicited by low contrast 40-60 ms earlier in the left posterior and right anterior; these results were not observed for middle contrast or high contrast. This result showed that audiovisual processing in early evoked brain activity follows the principle of the visual contrast feature. The other study also showed an inverse relationship between the visual contrast feature and audiovisual integration with audiovisual speech (Ryan A Stevenson et al., 2012). In this study, participants had to complete a two-alternative forced choice (2AFC) task to identify the word that they heard or saw by pressing a button with either the left or right hand. Their results suggested that the P1 and P1-N1 components exhibited less multisensory gains relative to the summed unisensory components with reduced salience, whereas the N1-P2 amplitude exhibited greater audiovisual gains as salience was reduced, consistent with the principle of inverse effectiveness.

FMRI is a neuroimaging technique available to research the neural mechanisms of the audiovisual perceptual process in humans. This technique measures brain activity by detecting changes associated with blood flow. Unlike single-unit recording methods, fMRI is a noninvasive method based on populations of thousands of neurons. Neural mechanism research was previously limited to animals, such as monkeys or cats, by single-unit recording methods before this technique appeared. The groundbreaking fMRI method verifies many principles of audiovisual processing at the level of single neurons and improves our understanding of audiovisual mechanisms (B. E. Stein & Stanford, 2008), such as the principle of inverse effectiveness. The first evidence that neural activation in the human brain area follows the law of inverse effectiveness, based on fMRI measures, was provided at the superior temporal sulcus (STS) brain area by Ryan (R. A. Stevenson & James, 2009; Tang, Wu, & Shen, 2015). Before this experiment, neuronal inverse effectiveness had never been shown in humans. Some previous studies have demonstrated that STS is a site where audiovisual integration occurs in non-human primates (Hikosaka, Iwai, Saito, & Tanaka, 1988). Subsequently, this STS brain area has been found in humans (Bushara, Grafman, & Hallett, 2001; Macaluso, George, Dolan, Spence, & Driver, 2004). There were two fMRI experiments in Ryan's study; they used an audiovisual method and speech stimuli (talking heads) presented at varied levels of signal strength. Using a decreasing stimulus property, they obtained bold activation with the audiovisual stimulus. They found that the bi-modal neurons produced activity was greater than the maximum activity produced by either unisensory stimulus. In addition, in the high (75%, 85%, and 95%) contrast strength conditions, the simulated audiovisual activation clearly does not exceed the additive criterion (the sum of A and V is bigger than the audiovisual stimulus). However, for low (55 and 65%) contrast strength conditions, the simulated audiovisual activation was obviously stronger than the sum of A and V. Thus, bold activation may exceed the additive criterion when degraded stimuli are used, although neurons in audiovisual regions decrease their impulse counts when stimuli are less salient. The experiments reported strongly suggest that human STS respond in an inversely-effective manner. These results show that this pattern of neural activation in human STS is inversely effective. This inverse effectiveness based on simulated audiovisual bold activation was also found by Toemme. In their studies, they used a co-occurring sound with low or high visual contrast to study the effect of sound compared with visual stimuli. Compared with high contrast, low visual contrast events can result in stronger activity in sensory-specific cortices and STS. For this fMRI result, visual and auditory thalamic nuclei were more activated when a sound co-occurred with a lower visual contrast.

AGING EFFECTS ON INVERSE EFFECTIVENESS

The aging population is a serious problem for the future world and will result in dramatic effects on social services. Normal aging is accompanied with many sensory and cognitive changes. These changes may lead to impairments in communication, balance, action and memory. Moreover, these changes will cause difficulty in performing basic activities in daily life, and many diseases are caused by aging, such as Alzheimer's disease, cerebral arteriosclerosis, senile psychosis, etc. Therefore, we recognize that research on the elderly population is increasingly important. Cognitive changes with aging highlight a new field that requires further research. Although many studies have investigated audiovisual integration, few studies have evaluated the effects of aging on audiovisual integration processing.

Several early studies showed mixed results regarding the audiovisual process between older and younger adults (Cienkowski & Carney, 2002; Helfer, 1998; Stine, Wingfield, & Myers, 1990). Stine and Colleagues (1990) reported that although memory for new events with audiovisual stimuli is better than with auditory stimuli alone in younger adults, this improvement with audiovisual conditions was not found in older adults. However, some other articles have shown that audiovisual interactions were significantly greater in older adults relative to younger adults, even when adjusting for age-related differences in processing speed ((Salthouse & Czaja, 2000; Salthouse, Hancock, Meinz, & Hambrick, 1996; Salthouse & Lichty, 1985). Peiffer obtained similar results using a simple reaction time task (Peiffer, Mozolic, Hugenschmidt, & Laurienti, 2007). In this experiment, they found that older adults have greater audiovisual enhancement than younger adults. Even with aging, the reaction times were increased in both unisensory conditions and audiovisual conditions. This result suggests that other mechanisms beyond inverse effectiveness may be necessary to explain the age-related enhancement.

The existing literature on audiovisual processing in aging shows that there is not yet a clear explanation for why older adults have greater audiovisual integration than younger adults. The mechanisms underlying age-related enhancements in audiovisual integration are not clear at all. Some researchers have proposed this as a new brain function being exploited in older adults. If this hypothesis is correct, further neural correlative studies are necessary. To our knowledge, there have been no conclusive studies on the relationship between stimulus properties and audiovisual gains in older adults. The evidence for inverse effectiveness as a source of enhanced audiovisual integration in older adults is not yet clear. In other words, no conclusion has been reached about the relationship between inverse effectiveness and aging.

FUTURE RESEARCH DIRECTIONS

We aimed to explain some of the recent evidence showing that inverse effectiveness occurs in a richly interconnected brain system as a result of visual contrast. It is obvious from the discussion above that the field of audiovisual integration is at an intermediate stage of development. However, it is not clear whether this principle is effect by aging or other factors. Although there are many outstanding issues, it is important to note that the progress in this field has been impressive, although the best understanding is yet to come. With the advancements in experimental technologies and methodologies, we will continue to understand the mechanisms of audiovisual integration in greater detail.

CONCLUSION

In summary, this review describes a very brief summary of visual contrast feature effects on audiovisual integration and has focused on the behavioral and neural correlate basis of audiovisual processing in humans. We found that the effects of visual contrast on audiovisual integration were followed by inverse effectiveness.

ACKNOWLEDGMENT

This study was supported in part by the JAPAN SOCIETY FOR THE PROMOTION OF SCIENCE (JSPS) KAKENHI, grant numbers: 25249026 and 25303013;

a Grant-in-Aid for Strategic Research Promotion from Okayama University; and the National Natural Science Foundation of China (NSFC61473043).

REFERENCES

Barghout-Stein, L. (1999). *On differences between peripheral and foveal pattern masking*. Berkeley, CA: University of California.

Benedek, K., Janaky, M., Braunitzer, G., Rokszin, A., Keri, S., & Benedek, G. (2010). Parallel development of contour integration and visual contrast sensitivity at low spatial frequencies. *Neuroscience Letters*, *472*(3), 175–178. doi:10.1016/j.neulet.2010.02.001 PMID:20138967

Bushara, K. O., Grafman, J., & Hallett, M. (2001). Neural correlates of auditory-visual stimulus onset asynchrony detection. *The Journal of Neuroscience*, *21*, 300–304. PMID:11150347

Calvert, G. A. (2001). Crossmodal processing in the human brain: Insights from functional neuroimaging studies. *Cerebral Cortex*, *11*(12), 1110–1123. doi:10.1093/cercor/11.12.1110 PMID:11709482

Cienkowski, K. M., & Carney, A. E. (2002). Auditory-visual speech perception and aging. *Ear and Hearing*, *23*(5), 439–449. doi:10.1097/00003446-200210000-00006 PMID:12411777

Corneil, B. D., Van Wanrooij, M., Munoz, D. P., & Van Opstal, A. J. (2002). Auditory-visual interactions subserving goal-directed saccades in a complex scene. *Journal of Neurophysiology*, *88*, 438–454. PMID:12091566

Costa, T.L., Nogueira, R.M., Pereira, A.G., and Santos, N.A. (2013). Differential effects of aging on spatial contrast sensitivity to linear and polar sine-wave gratings. *Brazilian Journal of Medical and Biological Research, 46*, 855-860.

Diederich, A., & Colonius, H. (2004). Bimodal and trimodal multisensory enhancement: Effects of stimulus onset and intensity on reaction time. *Perception & Psychophysics*, *66*(8), 1388–1404. doi:10.3758/BF03195006 PMID:15813202

Helfer, K. S. (1998). Auditory and auditory-visual recognition of clear and conversational speech by older adults. *Journal of the American Academy of Audiology*, *9*, 234–242. PMID:9644622

Heywood, C. A., Nicholas, J. J., & Cowey, A. (1996). Behavioural and electrophysiological chromatic and achromatic contrast sensitivity in an achromatopsic patient. *Journal of Neurology, Neurosurgery, and Psychiatry*, *60*(6), 638–643. doi:10.1136/jnnp.60.6.638 PMID:8648330

Hikosaka, K., Iwai, E., Saito, H., & Tanaka, K. (1988). Polysensory properties of neurons in the anterior bank of the caudal superior temporal sulcus of the macaque monkey. *Journal of Neurophysiology*, *60*, 1615–1637. PMID:2462027

Holmes, N. P. (2007). The law of inverse effectiveness in neurons and behaviour: Multisensory integration versus normal variability. *Neuropsychologia*, *45*(14), 3340–3345. doi:10.1016/j.neuropsychologia.2007.05.025 PMID:17663007

Lakatos, P., Chen, C. M., O'connell, M. N., Mills, A., & Schroeder, C. E. (2007). Neuronal oscillations and multisensory interaction in primary auditory cortex. *Neuron*, *53*(2), 279–292. doi:10.1016/j.neuron.2006.12.011 PMID:17224408

Macaluso, E., George, N., Dolan, R., Spence, C., & Driver, J. (2004). Spatial and temporal factors during processing of audiovisual speech: A PET study. *NeuroImage*, *21*(2), 725–732. doi:10.1016/j.neuroimage.2003.09.049 PMID:14980575

Meredith, M. A., Nemitz, J. W., & Stein, B. E. (1987). Determinants of multisensory integration in superior colliculus neurons. I. Temporal factors. *The Journal of Neuroscience*, *7*, 3215–3229. PMID:3668625

Meredith, M. A., & Stein, B. E. (1983). Interactions among converging sensory inputs in the superior colliculus. *Science*, *221*(4608), 389–391. doi:10.1126/science.6867718 PMID:6867718

Meredith, M. A., & Stein, B. E. (1986). Spatial Factors Determine the Activity of Multisensory Neurons in Cat Superior Colliculus. *Brain Research*, *365*(2), 350–354. doi:10.1016/0006-8993(86)91648-3 PMID:3947999

Miller, J. (1982). Divided attention: Evidence for coactivation with redundant signals. *Cognitive Psychology*, *14*(2), 247–279. doi:10.1016/0010-0285(82)90010-X PMID:7083803

Molholm, S., Ritter, W., Murray, M. M., Javitt, D. C., Schroeder, C. E., & Foxe, J. J. (2002). Multisensory auditory-visual interactions during early sensory processing in humans: A high-density electrical mapping study. *Brain Research. Cognitive Brain Research*, *14*(1), 115–128. doi:10.1016/S0926-6410(02)00066-6 PMID:12063135

Packer, M., & Ginsburg, A. P. (2007). Contrast sensitivity and aging. *Ophthalmology, 114*(8), 1589, author reply 1589–1590. doi:10.1016/j.ophtha.2007.03.046 PMID:17678702

Pardhan, S. (2004). Contrast sensitivity loss with aging: Sampling efficiency and equivalent noise at different spatial frequencies. *Journal of the Optical Society of America. A, Optics, Image Science, and Vision, 21*(2), 169–175. doi:10.1364/JOSAA.21.000169 PMID:14763759

Peiffer, A. M., Mozolic, J. L., Hugenschmidt, C. E., & Laurienti, P. J. (2007). Age-related multisensory enhancement in a simple audiovisual detection task. *Neuroreport, 18*(10), 1077–1081. doi:10.1097/WNR.0b013e3281e72ae7 PMID:17558300

Rach, S., Diederich, A., & Colonius, H. (2011). On quantifying multisensory interaction effects in reaction time and detection rate. *Psychological Research, 75*(2), 77–94. doi:10.1007/s00426-010-0289-0 PMID:20512352

Ross, L. A., Saint-Amour, D., Leavitt, V. M., Javitt, D. C., & Foxe, J. J. (2007). Do you see what I am saying? Exploring visual enhancement of speech comprehension in noisy environments. *Cerebral Cortex, 17*(5), 1147–1153. doi:10.1093/cercor/bhl024 PMID:16785256

Salthouse, T. A., & Czaja, S. J. (2000). Structural constraints on process explanations in cognitive aging. *Psychology and Aging, 15*(1), 44–55. doi:10.1037/0882-7974.15.1.44 PMID:10755288

Salthouse, T. A., Hancock, H. E., Meinz, E. J., & Hambrick, D. Z. (1996). Interrelations of age, visual acuity, and cognitive functioning. *The Journals of Gerontology. Series B, Psychological Sciences and Social Sciences, 51*(6), 317–330. doi:10.1093/geronb/51B.6.P317 PMID:8931619

Salthouse, T. A., & Lichty, W. (1985). Tests of the neural noise hypothesis of age-related cognitive change. *Journal of Gerontology, 40*(4), 443–450. doi:10.1093/geronj/40.4.443 PMID:4008879

Senkowski, D., Saint-Amour, D., Hofle, M., & Foxe, J. J. (2011). Multisensory interactions in early evoked brain activity follow the principle of inverse effectiveness. *NeuroImage, 56*(4), 2200–2208. doi:10.1016/j.neuroimage.2011.03.075 PMID:21497200

Serino, A., Farnè, A., Rinaldesi, M. L., Haggard, P., & Làdavas, E. (2007). Can vision of the body ameliorate impaired somatosensory function? *Neuropsychologia, 45*(5), 1101–1107. doi:10.1016/j.neuropsychologia.2006.09.013 PMID:17101158

Silva, M. F., D'almeida, O. C., Oliveiros, B., Mateus, C., & Castelo-Branco, M. (2014). Development and aging of visual hemifield asymmetries in contrast sensitivity. *Journal of Vision (Charlottesville, Va.)*, 14. PMID:25326605

Stein, B. E., & Meredith, M. A. (1993). *The merging of the senses*. The MIT Press.

Stein, B. E., & Stanford, T. R. (2008). Multisensory integration: Current issues from the perspective of the single neuron. *Nature Reviews. Neuroscience*, *9*(4), 255–266. doi:10.1038/nrn2331 PMID:18354398

Stevenson, R. A., Bushmakin, M., Kim, S., Wallace, M. T., Puce, A., & James, T. W. (2012). Inverse effectiveness and multisensory interactions in visual event-related potentials with audiovisual speech. *Brain Topography*, *25*(3), 308–326. doi:10.1007/s10548-012-0220-7 PMID:22367585

Stevenson, R. A., & James, T. W. (2009). Audiovisual integration in human superior temporal sulcus: Inverse effectiveness and the neural processing of speech and object recognition. *NeuroImage*, *44*(3), 1210–1223. doi:10.1016/j.neuroimage.2008.09.034 PMID:18973818

Stine, E. A., Wingfield, A., & Myers, S. D. (1990). Age differences in processing information from television news: The effects of bisensory augmentation. *Journal of Gerontology*, *45*(1), 1–8. doi:10.1093/geronj/45.1.P1 PMID:2295777

Talsma, D., Doty, T. J., & Woldorff, M. G. (2007). Selective attention and audiovisual integration: Is attending to both modalities a prerequisite for early integration? *Cerebral Cortex*, *17*(3), 679–690. doi:10.1093/cercor/bhk016 PMID:16707740

Tang, X., Wu, J., & Shen, Y. (2015). The interactions of multisensory integration with endogenous and exogenous attention. *Neuroscience and Biobehavioral Reviews*, *61*, 208–224. doi:10.1016/j.neubiorev.2015.11.002 PMID:26546734

KEY TERMS AND DEFINITIONS

Audiovisual Integration: Bimodal audiovisual signals can be detected or discriminated more quickly and accurately than unimodal visual signals or auditory signals; this effect is called audiovisual integration.

Contrast: Contrast is the difference in luminance or color that can distinguish an object (image or display).

Inverse Effectiveness: Inverse effectiveness is an inverse relationship between audiovisual integration enhancement and the strength of stimuli. For example, compared to high visual contrast, low visual contrast can result in a stronger audiovisual integration effect.

Spatial Rule: Audiovisual integration is faster or stronger when the constituent unisensory stimuli appear from almost the same location.

Temporal Rule: Audiovisual integration is faster or stronger when the constituent unisensory stimuli appear almost simultaneously.

Chapter 10
The Status of Research into Intention Recognition

Luyao Wang
Beijing Institute of Technology, China

Chunlin Li
Capital Medical University, China

Jinglong Wu
Beijing Institute of Technology, China

ABSTRACT

In recent years, service robots have been widely used in many fields, especially for assisting the elderly and disabled. For example, the medical care of patients with Alzheimer's disease has become a worldwide problem. Existing service robots with some intelligence quotient can perform actions that are programmed by a human. However, the robot cannot understand human intentions or communicate with people naturally. Understanding the intent of the service object could allow the robot to provide better service. Therefore, the most critical component of human-computer interactions is intention recognition. There are currently many methods by which intention recognition can be achieved, such as EMG, EOG and EEG. In addition, emotion is one of the important factors during intention recognition, and this has been a breakthrough notion. This chapter summarizes the current status of research into intention recognition and gives a brief description of the relationship between emotion and intention. We hope to provide more ideas for optimizing human-computer interactions.

DOI: 10.4018/978-1-5225-0925-7.ch010

INTRODUCTION

In this chapter, we focus on the status of research into intention recognition.

In the first part, we provide an overview of the current research status of the field of intelligent robots, and we describe the key technologies related to improving robot intelligence in human-computer interactions. Intention recognition is one of the problems to be solved urgently.

In the second part, recent research using EMG, eye movements and EEG as human physiological electrical signals are introduced in detail. EMG studies focus on surface EMG signals, which can be acquired more directly. They contain information describing the state of muscle functions and a wealth of information about movement intention. We introduce the research results and the methods used to analyze surface EMG signals. Eye movement has a certain regularity and is primarily related to intention. The methods used for eye tracking mainly include Electro-OculoGraphy (EOG) and Video-OculoGraphy (VOG). Based on the above methods, further types of mature eye-trackers have been developed. EEG has good temporal resolution and can extract enough characteristics to perform intention recognition. A brain computer interface can be used to facilitate communication between the brain and the external environment. Its development is helpful for people aiming to understand and study the neural activity of the brain. The status of studies of intention recognition that are based on visual-evoked potentials, cortical slow potential, P300 signals and sensory motor rhythms is introduced in this paper. In recent years, research into emotion has provided new ideas to the field of intention recognition. The overall summary of this manuscript is described in Figure 1.

Figure 1. An overall summary of this chapter

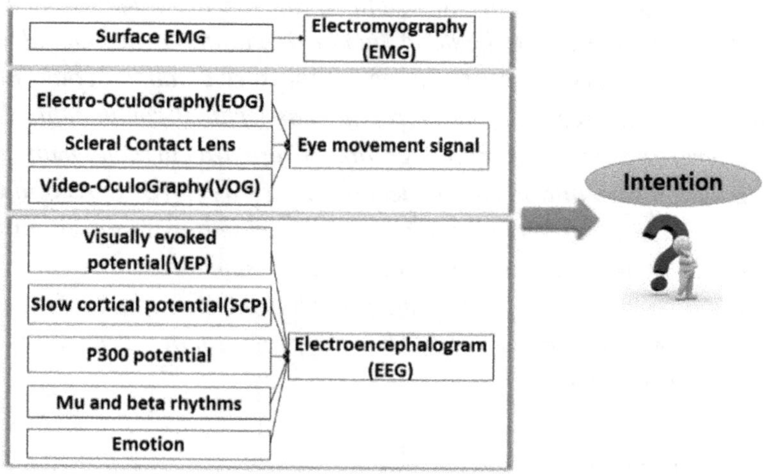

Finally, we summarize the above three research methods. Furthermore, we propose a multimodal fusion strategy that can be used to simulate the complex information processing functions of the human brain and achieve a deep recognition of intention.

BACKGROUND

With the progress of society, the development of intelligent robots is being paid more and more attention. The list of potential uses for such robots is continuously increasing, and applications have been suggested in many fields, including industrial, space, underwater, disaster relief, service, military, and especially medical fields. Because the number of elderly and disabled people in the world is increasing year by year, how to help them has become a serious social problem. With the development of human-robot interaction technologies, robots have played an increasingly important role in many fields. They are expected to provide multiple services for the elderly and disabled, such as travel, care and medical rehabilitation, all of which improve their quality of life and ensure the steady development of our society. For example, paralyzed patients can control the movement of a robot arm through EEG, which helps these patients during daily life activities (Alberts, 2012; Collinger, 2013 et al.).

Every country in the world has developed an intelligent service robots. A new range of application domains (e.g., domestic, entertainment, and health care) is driving the development of robots that can interact and cooperate with people as a partner rather than as a tool. These include Care-0-Bot II from Germany, which is a mobile home care system that helps the disabled and the elderly to live independently. The Hibernian VA-PAM-AID, Japanese RFID and Walking Helper navigation robot can help older people and children with amblyopia to walk independently. They are generally equipped with environmental sensors to achieve navigation and obstacle avoidance, and the working parameters can be set according to the user's walking habits. These robots use a man-machine interface for operation and information feedback. However, these service robots can only act according to procedures that were prepared by people, and they do not understand the intention of the people and are not capable of naturally communicating with people. These deficits greatly limit the scope of applications in which these robots can be used. It is expected that robots with a certain intelligent can understand people's intentions and satisfy the needs of different users. The question of how to make a robot that can understand human intentions is an important precondition for an ideal service robot (Breazeal, & Brooks, 2005). Therefore, there is important scientific significance and practical application value in studying robots that have the ability to understand human intentions (Severinson-Eklundh, Green, & Hüttenrauch, 2003).

To develop robots with ability to recognize intentions, the first important thing is to study the mechanisms underlying intention and methods that will facilitate intention recognition. There are currently many disciplines that study human intention, such as philosophy, economics, and political science. However, they involve only macro studies of human intention. Cognitive neuroscience studies aim to determine the mechanisms involved in cognitive activity in the brain. Human intentions involve mental activities that are generated by the brain, and these allow us to use cognitive neuroscience to obtain a deeper understanding of their mechanisms. These studies show that recognizing the intentions of others encompasses our ability to interpret their behavior in terms of mental states, to interact in social groups and to predict how others will feel, think and behave, and that these abilities are based on social cognition. Discourse comprehension, body language, facial expressions, eye gaze, and contact with objects are ways of expressing explicit intention. However, it is difficult to determine implicit intent (Rizzolatti, & Sinigaglia, 2008; Wang, Ling, & Yuan et al. 2010; Frith, 2002). Researchers around the world have been exploring the mechanism involved in intention and how intention can be identified through human physiological signals. Researchers have made substantial progress in identifying human intentions using electroencephalograph (EEG), Electro-Oculogram (EOG) and electromyography (EMG).

RESEARCH STATUS OF INTENTION RECOGNITION

The idea that social intelligence might be independent or dissociable from general intelligence comes from several sources (Baron-Cohen, 1999; Baron-Cohen, Tager-Flusberg, & Cohen, 2000). Intention as a kind of mental representation is very necessary to achieve a goal. It often comes in the form of ideas that are not put into action, and we can simply regard the intention as the attitude before doing something. However, intention recognition is a process of reasoning. In fact, it is the awareness and understanding of the intentions of others.

In the field of cognitive psychology, the intention is one's ideal before action (Carruthers, 2007). Human beings can express, predict and explain their intentions naturally. In Human–Computer Interaction, a human's explicit intent, such as "copying the file" or "closing the window", can be easily conveyed using the mouse or keyboard. Many works have solved the problem of identifying peoples' explicit intentions (Erol, Bebis, & Nicolescu, 2007; Jaimes, & Sebe, 2007). However, explicit intent may be disguised so that it does not reflect a person's true intentions. A system that can identify only explicit intentions could perform well under fixed conditions but not in a natural environment. Furthermore, implicit intention has been widely used in the field of network application and network security, which contains more intent information than explicit intent. However, people's implicit intention is usually very vague, and it is difficult to detect it directly. It is important to recognize the user's implicit intention to construct an efficient human-computer interaction system. Hence, various agent systems have been designed using their own methods to achieve this goal (Chen, Fan, & Huan, 2002; Spyrou, & Darzentas, 1996). Brain science research studies have noted that people's implicit intention is produced in the hippocampus (Anatoli, & Michael, 2002). In this chapter, we will introduce you to some methods of intention recognition, including EMG, eye movement tracking technique, and EEG, which can be used to speculate on people's implicit intentions.

Electromyography (EMG)

Electromyography (EMG) is an electrodiagnostic medicine technique for evaluating and recording electrical activity that is produced by skeletal muscles. Surface EMG is a hot research topic in many fields, such as rehabilitation medicine, biomedical Engineering, exercise physiology, and signal processing. Since Calvani confirmed the close relationship between muscle contractions and electrical power in 1791, many studies have been performed using EMG. In 1851, the German scholar Reymond first detected the electrical signal that is generated by human body muscle contractions, and he then put forward the concept of the action potential. In 1890, Marey first recorded electrical activity during a muscle contraction, which is referred to as EMG (Konrad, 2005).

The sEMG signal acquisition mode is more direct than the EEG signal, which not only reflects the electrical signal generated during muscle contraction but also contains information about movement intention. Using EMG as an input for a Human-Computer Interface has become common. sEMG contains a wealth of muscle state information, which can be used to determine the intention of the human body and the state of muscle function and to thereby accomplish a natural Human-Computer Interaction. Hence, with the development of signal processing technologies, the EMG technology has been widely used in fields including intelligent robots, rehabilitation medicine, and sports science.

Motion Intention Recognition System Based on sEMG

In 2008, Christan et al. presented a human-machine interface that controlled exoskeletons that utilized electrical signals from the muscles of the operator as the main means of transporting information. This machine was designed and constructed to verify the model and to investigate the interaction between the operator and the machine during experiments performed using force support during everyday movements (Fleischer, & Hommel, 2008). Then, in 2009, Raymond et al. from Hong Kong University designed a rehabilitation robot system that was based on EMG signals and a human-computer interaction for patients with stroke. The system used muscle activation from affected limbs as the control signal. The system was designed to train the wrist, elbow, knee and ankle joints while in vertical and horizontal positions (Tong, Leung, & Hu, 2009). To assist the elderly and disabled in performing daily living motions, the Japanese scholars Kiguchi et al. proposed using power-assist robots with a perception-assist. This robot assists not only the user's motion but also the user's interaction with the environment by applying a modifying force to the user's motion when necessary. Both EMG signals and EEG signals are measured at the same time to integrate the features of these signals when users are using the power-assist robot. EEG signals and EMG signals are used as the criteria for the effectiveness of the performed perception-assist (Kiguchi, &Hayashi, 2012).

Systems that use sEMG signal control based on pattern recognition have been widely used in the field of rehabilitation training, and these systems can identify a patient's motor intentions or assist them during treatment with a therapist. Most of these robots have used the design described in Figure 2.

sEMG is a very weak biological electrical signal, and it varies in different patients. It is therefore important to extract the sEMG signals and analyze them accurately and efficiently.

Figure 2. A motion intention recognition system based on sEMG

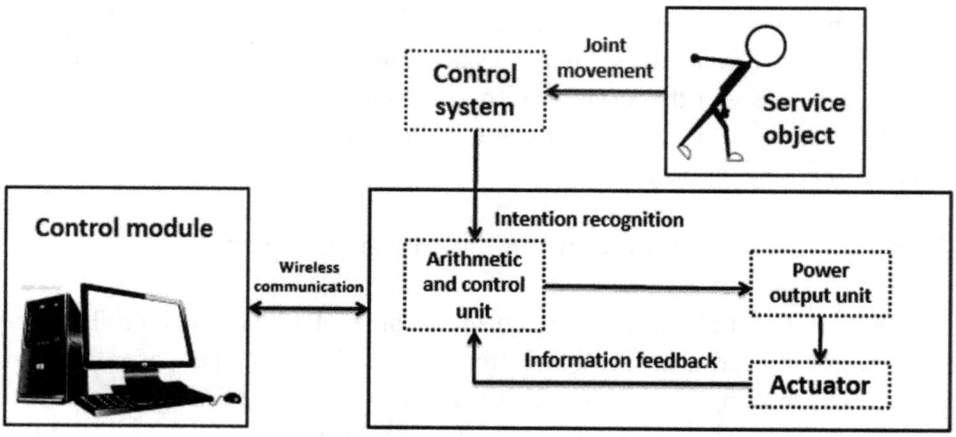

Analysius Methods for sEMG Signals

Research into human motion intention recognition using the detection method comes in basically two types: one is the use of the human body surface EMG signal as the means of detection, and the other is detecting the interaction between the limbs and the robot arm. The EMG signal has advantages, including the fact that it is non-invasive, can be used in real-time, and is simple to use. It uses a group of voltage signals that are related to time and that are the result of the synthesis of an action potential at the electrode. The pattern recognizes the EMG signal to extract the features of each movement and then classifies the EMG signal using an appropriate mapping method that is based on certain features. According to the characteristics of the EMG signal, the current EMG analysis methods can be divided into time-domain analysis methods, frequency-domain analysis methods and time-frequency analysis methods. Previous approaches for analyzing the aspects of the EMG signals that vary with time have used a linear prediction model. In addition, mean power frequency (MPF) and median frequency (MF) are common characteristic indexes that are used in frequency-domain analyses. Currently, the analysis method with the most potential is the time-frequency analysis method, which takes both time domain and frequency domain information into account.

Artificial neural networks have also played an important role in identifying EMG signals. Jung et al. proposed a method for classifying EMG patterns using the Yule-Walker algorithm and the LVQ. Experimental results showed that the success rate of the proposed classifier was approximately 78% (Jung, Kim, & Lee, 2007). In 2008, Daydamony et al. presented a computerized SEMG system. A HMM model was chosen to characterize the surface EMG signal. The results showed that four features were used to characterize each segment. It obtained an accuracy rate of 90% (Daydamony, Gayar, & Chadi, 2008). To increase its recognition accuracy, Qizhong Zhang et al. proposed a new recognition method that combined fuzzy entropy (FuzzyEn) with multi-scale analysis. The results showed that the MSFuzzyEn is effective and precise for classifying SEMG signals (Zhang, Xi, & Luo, 2014).

Eye Movement Signal

In addition to using EMG signals, eye movement signals have also been shown to be an effective input signal for intention control. Eye movements are arguably the most frequent of all human movements. The eyes are the windows of the soul, and through the eyes, we can explore many human psychological activities. Eye movement follows certain laws, and eye rotation and visual information are directly related to the interests of visual information. The EOG is one of very few methods of recording eye movements that does not require a direct attachment to the eye itself. Because eye movements can be controlled volitionally, to some degree, and tracked using modern technology with great speed and precision, they can now be used as a powerful input device, and they have been applied in many practical applications in human-computer interactions. In the application of this technology, eye movement replaced the hand operated mouse, allowing users to select icons and menus using a graphical user interface (Ding, Tong, & Li, 2006). Human-computer interaction systems that are based on eye movement signals not only allow people with disabilities to perform daily actions by controlling eye movement but also have uses that extend into the activities of normal people, including games and other recreational activities.

At present, the eye tracking technique is being applied in many fields. For example, it can be applied to usability analysis tests of software and websites to help researchers to understand user behavior and usability problems. It also helps development researchers to explain the transition of human cognition, perception, and social behavior during the progress of human development from infancy to adulthood. In ophthalmology, visual researchers use eye tracking techniques to analyze eye movement behavior, visual perception and visual impairment. The trend toward using eye tracking technology in sports research also continues to grow. Scientific research institutes that study sports are leading the development of eye tracking techniques as a standard research method for improving the performance of athletes and their visual search skills. In addition, eye tracking technology has also been widely used in the field of medicine. For example, during surgical operations, a probe can be automatically extended to the exact point that the doctor is watching on the screen under the control of the computer, thus avoiding the error and shaking of a manual probe.

Eye Movement Data Associated with Intention

Data associated with eye movements mainly include fixation times, glance duration, diversion duration, saccade, pupil diameter, and blinking. Pupil diameter is the most sensitive index. Some studies have found that pupil diameter increases to 0.6 mm when a simple memory test is performed, and after the experiment, it is restored to its starting size. This shows that pupil diameter can be used to detect mental workload (Kahneman, & Beatty, 1977). When people look at a certain point, it can cause cognitive activity and the pupil's size to fluctuate. Based on the above research, researchers presented a kind of evaluation method that was based on the relationship between pupil responses and cognitive activity. This was called the "cognitive activity index" (Marshall, 2000). Iqbal, Zheng et al. investigated how well pupil size correlates with the mental workload that was demanded during interactive tasks that were representative of daily computer-based tasks that users often perform. Their results showed that a more difficult task demands longer processing time, induces higher subjective ratings of mental workload, and reliably evokes a greater pupillary response during a corresponding subtasks than during a less difficult task. Based on these results, pupil size can provide a reliable measure of mental workload during interactive tasks that are required by an attention manager (Iqbal, Zheng, &Bailey, 2004).

Methods for Measuring Ocular Movements

Over time, the methods used to measure eye movement data have been increasingly improved. The original research method was to directly observe the eye movement of the subject using the naked eye. Scholars have also explored the situation of eye movement using mechanical recordings (Morimoto, & Mimica, 2005). However, these two methods involve many human factors, and the recording method is very complex, which results in less accurate experimental results, and it has therefore been eliminated. Researchers later explored the use of optical methods to record eye movement data, such as using reflected light (Yarbus, 1967) or the Purkinje image tracking method. The tracker Dual Purkinje Image (DPI) was designed based on the second method. In the 1960s, Robinson pioneered the electromagnetic induction method to monitor the movements of the eyes (Robinson, 1963), but this method is mainly used for animal eye movement research because it requires a coil to be placed in the eyes, which causes discomfort and damage to the subjects and is easily affected by human eye secretions. The early eye movement research methods mentioned above are simple and intuitive, but there are common shortcomings that mean that they cannot be used to study eye movement characteristics. Another disadvantage is that the accuracy is too low, so that results do not reflect true eye movement characteristics. With the rapid development of electronic and computer technologies, research into eye movements has become more intelligent, more objective and more accurate.

In the 1980s, the first eye tracker method was published in which the eye was placed in a fixed position to obtain the gaze direction of the subject. By the 1990s, the eye tracker could be placed in a hat or headband that could be worn by the user while maintaining a fixed position. Gaze direction was obtained by calculating the information obtained from the eye movement apparatus with respect to the position of the subject. Modern eye trackers use infrared light to directly determine the subject's pupil position. Compared to other parts of the eye, the retina can reflect longer wavelengths of infrared light. The pupil position can therefore be determined without the need for special image recognition technology, allowing us to obtain a more accurate assessment of the direction of the subject's gaze. There are currently three types of eye tracking devices: Electro-OculoGraphy (EOG), Scleral Contact Lens, and Video-OculoGraphy (VOG) (Duchowski, 2007).

There are many ways in which eye movement can be measured, and some are more accurate than EOG, but most of them are far more expensive in addition to being inconvenient and uncomfortable for the user. The EOG method is noninvasive, low-cost and easy to use. Compared to EEG, EOG signals are easier to capture, and the mechanism and mode of EOG are much clearer than those of EEG. Less training is needed than for a brain computer interface, and they have many practical applications in human-computer interactions (Ding, Tong, & Li, 2006), as shown in Figure 3. However, this method can easily make the subject feel uncomfortable over long-term use, and it is therefore not suitable for fixation point measurements. Scleral Contact Lenses are one of the most accurate methods for measuring eye movements. However, it is intrusive because it must be worn in the eyes. Video-OculoGraphy (VOG) analyzes eye movement information generally through a camera that is sued to capture the image on the human eye (Figure 4). The system is not connected to the human body, so the experimental subjects are often not aware of the existence of the eye movement monitoring system. With the rapid development of image processing technology, an increasing number of people favor this type of non-contact and completely natural eye movement monitoring technology. However, these methods can measure eye movements but cannot measure the fixation point. Pupil-corneal reflex-based VOG can capture eye images using a fixed camera. According to the principle of the dark pupil and bright pupil, the pupil in the eye image is extracted, and the relative positions of the eye and the camera are corrected using the corneal reflection method. The data relating the corneal reflex point is hen used to determine the relative positions of the eyeball and the camera to determine the fixation point.

Figure 3. Schematic diagram of EOG

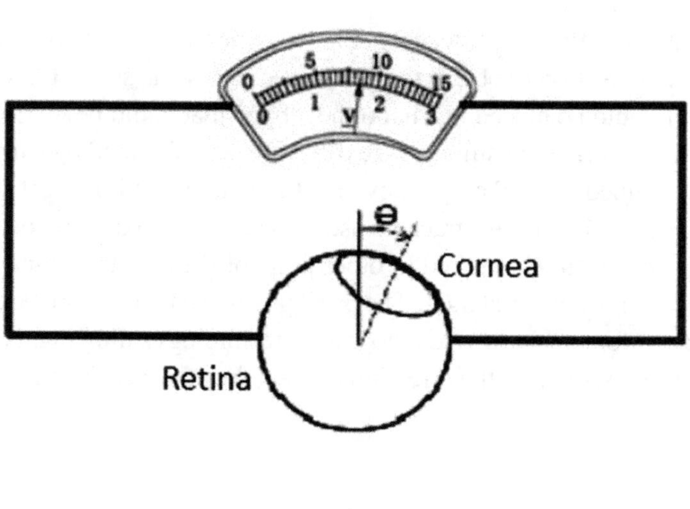

Figure 4. An eye tracking process based on VOG

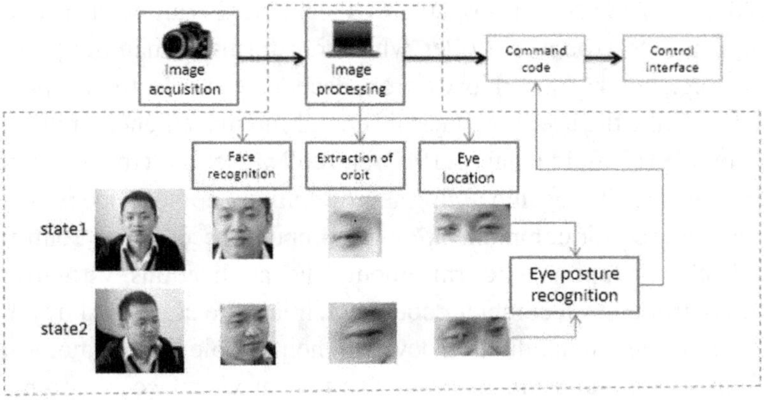

In eye tracking technology, it is generally believed that what people see is what they want. This is why it is important to explore the idea that people's ideas at a particular time can be determined by observing their eye movements.

Electroencephalogram (EEG)

In early 1924, the German neurologist H. Berger identified a potential difference in the human scalp that resulted from brain activity that was called an electroencephalogram (EEG). He then began to use more invasive methods to collect brain waves. Electroencephalography (EEG) is an electrophysiological monitoring method that is used to record the electrical activity of the brain. It measures voltage fluctuations resulting from ionic currents within the neurons of the brain. A number of recent studies have found neural correlates for when subjects decide to initiate a movement. Despite the relatively poor spatial sensitivity of EEG, it possesses multiple advantages. First, it has very high temporal resolution that is on the order of milliseconds rather than seconds. Second, it is typically noninvasive. In recent years, people have published many studies of intention recognition based on EEG signals. With regard to non-invasive EEG studies, the earliest evidence of the neural correlates of voluntary movement intention was discovered by Kornhuber and Deecke (Kornhuber, & Deecke, 1965), who identified a slow, negative potential as early as 1.5 s before the execution of a movement.

At present, brain–computer interface (BCI) technologies are mainly used to identify human intention using EEG signals (Figure 5). A BCI, sometimes called a mind-machine interface (MMI) or brain–machine interface (BMI), is a direct communication pathway between the brain and an external device. BCI, also known as a brain-machine interface, is a system that allows a person to control a computer or other electronic device using only his or her brainwaves, with no movement required (Sandro, 2000). Currently, non-invasive BCI technologies allow the user to deliver mental commands to a robot controller, which transforms them into appropriate motor actions—e.g., left, right, and forward are decoded from electroencephalography (EEG) signals while the user imagines different limb movements. Phillip Kennedy (who later founded Neural Signals in 1987) and colleagues built the first intracortical brain–computer interface by implanting neurotrophic-cone electrodes into monkeys.

BCIs can be used for communication or computer access or to control devices such as a wheelchair or prosthetic arm, among other applications. Virtually anything that can be controlled by a computer could potentially be controlled by a BCI. BCI is being examined as a rehabilitation device to help people re-gain motor skills that are lost from stroke and a prosthetic device that may replace or compensate for motor skills that will never return. In the transportation and military fields, we can use brain machine interfaces to achieve autonomous driving. Children can play electronic games using a brain computer interface technology to achieve an unprecedented form of leisure and entertainment. The combination of a brain computer interface and a device that controls a robot not only opens up a new way to achieve better daily care for the elderly and disabled but also provides a new method for normal people to communicate. Another important significance and value of brain computer interface technology is that it can provide a new information output channel for the brain. In this way, BCI systems can achieve communication between the brain and the external environment, which would be helpful for allowing people to understand and study the complex neural activity of the brain. Research in brain cognitive science could thereby be greatly enriched and developed.

To identify the intentions of others using explicit information, such as a speaker's words or body language or contact with an object, could lead to a large deviation. The question of how we can obtain a brain signal and understand other people's implicit intentions using non-destructive EEG technology is the key scientific problem that prevents us from realizing human-robot interactions that are based on a brain computer interface.

Figure 5. The composition of a BCI system

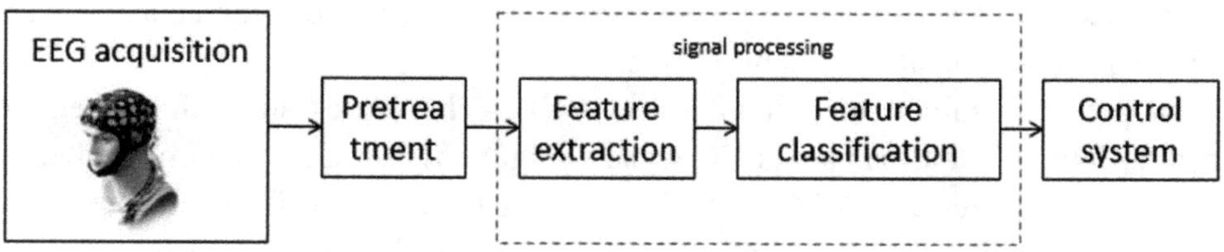

The BCI system explains the user's intentions by analyzing active signals from brain, which contains a large number of signals that are synchronized with cognitive behavior. In the field of BCI research, it is necessary to extract and classify the EEG signal correctly and to then send each type of signal to the robot to achieve the purpose of controlling the robot. Some of the physiological phenomena that are associated with signals that could be used as the control signals for the BCI system have been used by humans to explain a user's intention, and these include visual-evoked potential (VEP), slow cortical potentials (SCP), P300 potentials and mu and beta rhythms. In addition, emotion is one of the important factors in intention recognition, and it has therefore received an extensive amount of attention in recent years. They are translated in real-time into commands that operate a computer display or other device.

Visually-Evoked Potential (VEP)

The terms visually-evoked potential (VEP), visually-evoked response (VER) and visually-evoked cortical potential (VECP) are equivalent. They refer to electrical potentials that are initiated by brief visual stimuli that are then recorded from the scalp that overlies the visual cortex. VEP waveforms are extracted from the electroencephalogram (EEG) using signal averaging. VEPs are used primarily to measure the functional integrity of the visual pathways from the retina via the optic nerves to the visual cortex of the brain. VEPs better quantify the functional integrity of the optic pathways than scanning techniques such as magnetic resonance imaging (MRI). Depending on the frequency of the visual stimuli, visual-evoked potentials can be divided into steady-state visual-evoked potentials (SSVEP) and transient visual-evoked potentials (TVEP). BCI systems that are based on VEPs have a high rate of information transmission, are convenient to prepare and involve a small amount of user training. However, the user must be glued to the screen and must keep the eye fixed at one point, which causes users or patients to feel tired.

Slow Cortical Potentials (SCP)

Slow cortical potentials are negative or positive polarizations of the electroencephalogram (EEG) that have a low frequency (below 1Hz) and that last from 300 ms to several seconds. When the brain is excited, the cortex will generate a negative slow potential, whereas the cortex itself will generate a positive slow potential. Birbaumer and his colleagues showed that people can learn to control SCPs and to thereby control the movement of an object on a computer screen. This demonstration is the basis for a BCI that is referred to as a "thought translation device" (TTD) (Wolpaw, Birbaumer, & Mc Farland, 2002). Lew et al. investigated the feasibility of detecting the intention to perform a reaching movement before the actual execution of the movement in single trials using human EEG readings. Their SCP approach yielded a high detection rate close to the movement onset (sensitivity) and below the random detection level during the non-movement period (specificity). In addition, movement intention was detected approximately 500 ms before actual onset (Lew, Chavarriaga, & Silvoni, 2012).

P300 Potential

The P300 is a positive component of the event-related potential (ERP) that peaks at 300 ms or more (up to 900 ms) after a stimulus. It is considered to be an endogenous potential because its occurrence is not linked to a physical attribute of a stimulus but is instead linked to a person's reaction to it. The presence, magnitude, topography and timing of this signal are often used as metrics of cognitive function during decision-making processes. Interestingly, P300 responses are also observed when trains of regular stimuli are interrupted by stimulus omissions, which emphasizes the endogenous nature of this component. The amplitude of the P300 increases with the lower probability and higher discriminability of the target. In later research, the P300 is commonly investigated using "oddball" paradigms, in which occasional relevant ("target") stimuli must be detected in a train of frequent irrelevant "nontarget" or "standard" stimuli (Farwell, & Donchin, 1988). Because the P300 signal does not require training to produce, it is widely used in BCI systems.

Mu and Beta Rhythms

Motor imagery is a cognitive-perceptive process that involves the mental performance of movements that are not accompanied by any kind of peripheral (muscular) activity. Many studies of healthy subjects have shown that imaginary movements produce the activation of structures that are activated during the performance of voluntary movements (Lotze, & Cohen, 2006). These waves can therefore be used during the neurorehabilitation of patients with profound past-stroke pareses because existing methods of motor training that are based on the active use of the paralyzed limb are inappropriate for this category of patients. This type of training can also be used in patients with mild motor impairments to train them to achieve better movement planning and greater accuracy of execution (Rupp, & Cemer, 2004_. Motor imagery could play an important role in EEG-based communications, and mu and beta rhythms could be used as independent control signals. People learned to control an 8-12 Hz mu rhythm and/or an 18-25 Hz beta rhythm in EEGs that were recorded over sensorimotor cortex, and they used these abilities to control a cursor on a video screen. Rasmussenet al. let users directly control a BCI by modulating the magnitude of these rhythms by switching between motor imagery tasks. This study showed that users were able to achieve a reasonable level of control over a two-target BCI program within a very short time after the initial screening (Rasmussen, Acharya, & Thakor, 2006).

There are many mirror neurons in our brains. This system consists of a class of neurons that was first studied in the 1990s in macaque monkeys. Studies have found that these sets of neurons fire when monkeys perform simple tasks and also when the monkeys view others performing the same simple tasks. This suggests they play a role in mapping others' movements into the brain while not actually physically performing the movements. Tests in both monkeys (using invasive measuring techniques) and humans have found that mirror neurons fire during basic motor tasks and that they also have components that address intention. There is evidence for an important role for mirror neurons in humans, and mu waves and beta waves may represent a mechanism for the high level coordination of those mirror neurons.

Although the results of these studies have been positive, specific modes of connection and functional brain activities change as intentions vary, and the changes in functional brain activity that are related to intention also vary between individuals. Therefore, it is very difficult to find a model that accurately reflects intention. The study of implicit intention recognition using EEG is still in the primary stage.

Emotion and Intention

Emotions play an essential role in many aspects of our daily lives, including decision making, perception, learning, rational thinking and behavior. Without the ability to process emotions, computers and robots cannot communicate with humans in a natural way. Emotions are complex. According to some theories, they are a state of feeling that results in physical and psychological changes that influence our behavior. One goal of research into the cognitive neuroscience of emotions is to identify and understand the neural systems that underlie different emotional states and processes. Emotional penetration is in all aspects of intention connected to other cognition process. In 1937, James Papez proposed a circuit theory of the brain and emotion in which he suggested that emotional responses involve a network of brain regions that include the hypothalamus, anterior thalamus, cingulated gyrus, and hippocampus. In Damasio's experiments, normal participants and patients with prefrontal damage and decision-making defects performed a gambling task in which behavioral, psychophysiological, and self-account measures were obtained in parallel. They found that the ability of patients with prefrontal damage to identify intent was diminished (Damasio, 1994; Bechara, Damasio, & Tranel, 1997). Many studies supported the notion that the anterior cingulate cortex is also involved in interaction between emotions and intentions, but the specific neural mechanisms are still unknown (Smith, & Jonides, 1999).

Assessing emotions is key to understanding human beings. Therefore, emotion classifications provide a substantial step towards aiding people, such as the disabled, using brain-computer interfaces. Previous studies have indicated that there is a strong correlation between EEG and emotion, and visual-evoked EEG signals can be used as an effective method for emotion recognition. Mu Li et al. utilized smile and cry facial expression figures to evoke emotions from subjects, and the validity of the stimulus was tested using SAM. They received 93.5%±6.7%, and 93.0%±6.2% classification accuracies in 10 subjects for 3 s length and 1 s length trials using CSP, SVM and sophisticated frequency band selection strategies. Their results indicate that the ERD/ERS activities in gamma band EEG can be used to classify happiness and sadness with high temporal resolution. However, their study used still pictures as the source of stimulation and a single signal. There is therefore a large gap between this application and its usefulness in a natural environment.

Murugappan et al. decomposed raw EEG signals into three different frequency bands (alpha, beta, and gamma) using Discrete Wavelet Transform (DWT). They then used two simple pattern classification methods to classify emotional states. The results indicated that one of the proposed features (ALREE) gave a maximum average classification rate of 83.26% using KNN and 75.21% using LDA compared to the rates for conventional features. The results of this study provide a framework methodology that can be used to determine the dynamic mechanisms underlying human emotional changes and brain structures.

FUTURE RESEARCH DIRECTIONS

All of the above methods are intended to identify intention using a single approach that affects the accuracy of system. This is not only because the amount of information that is collected is limited but also because of the characteristics, performance and scope of use of the restrictions. Multimodal information fusion technology can be used. With the acquisition of a variety of signals (e.g., EEG signals and eye movement signals) and the integration of information processing methods (e.g., multi-feature extraction and multi classifier fusion), we can collection intention information from multiple aspects and multiple channels. This process simulates the functions involved in complex information processing in the human brain, in which more reliable and abundant information can be obtained. Although information with different foci are not expressed in the same manner, we can bring them together using some of the necessary links. Redundant and complementary parts can be used to improve the fault tolerance and reliability of the system, thereby reducing ambiguity resulting from a lack of certain information that leads to an understanding of intention.

At present, research into multi-modal signal fusion methods is mainly focused on image, voice and other signals and less focused on physiological signals. This is a key problem when constructing robust multimodal brain computer interaction systems using different modal characterizations and related structures. In addition, most of the existing multimodal fusion methods require the user to input the same signal during the training and testing processes. Whether a model that uses a multimodal joint probability distribution that is obtained using a deep learning network to learn higher order correlations between different modes can still get achieve good performance during its practical application in the environment is an important question that needs to be researched.

CONCLUSION

Psychological research suggests that understanding the intentions of others may be a prerequisite for a higher-level understanding of other people's minds or theory of mind. In recent years, service robots have been widely used in many fields, such as assisting the elderly and the disabled. This trend has led to an increasing demand for robots that have intention recognition ability. People expect robots can identify their intentions to get better services or control them more convenient. Some recent studies have shown that robots can get people's intention by transferring electrical signals from bioelectrical signal, such as EMG, eye movement and EEG. However, it is not yet known how we can extract more physiological signals about intentions and then accurately classify them. At the end of this chapter, we hope multimodal information fusion technology can be used in intention recognition. Through this process, robots can not only identify human explicit intentions but they can also identify human implicit intentions.

ACKNOWLEDGMENT

This study was supported by the National Natural Science Foundation of China (61473043).

REFERENCES

Alberts, B. (2012). The breakthroughs of 2012. *Science*, *388*(6114), 1511. doi:10.1126/science.1234108 PMID:23258851

Anatoli, G., & Michael, E. H. (2002). A model of hippocampal circuitry mediating goal-driven navigation in a familiar environment. *Neurocomputing*, *44*, 423–427.

Baron-Cohen, S., Ring, H., Wheelwright, S., Bullmore, E. T., Brammer, M. J., Simmons, A., & Williams, S. C. R. (1999). Social intelligence in the normal and autistic brain: An fMRI study. *The European Journal of Neuroscience*, *11*(6), 1891–1898. doi:10.1046/j.1460-9568.1999.00621.x PMID:10336657

Baron-Cohen, S., Tager-Flusberg, H., & Cohen, D. J. (2000). *Understanding the minds: perspectives from developmental cognitive neuroscience*. Oxford University Press.

Bechara, A., Damasio, H., Tranel, D., & Damasio, A. R. (1997). Deciding advantageously before knowing the advantageous strategy. *Science*, *275*(5304), 1293–1295. doi:10.1126/science.275.5304.1293 PMID:9036851

Breazeal, C., & Brooks, R. (2005). Robot emotion: A functional perspective. In J. Fellous (Ed.), *Who needs emotions* (pp. 271–310). Oxford, UK: Oxford University Press. doi:10.1093/acprof:oso/9780195166194.003.0010

Carruthers, P. (2007). The illusion of conscious will. *Synthese*, *159*(2), 197–213. doi:10.1007/s11229-007-9204-7

Chen, Z., Fan, L., Huan, L., Liu, Y., Ma, W. Y., & Liu, W. Y. (2002). User Intention Modelling in Web Applications Using Data Mining. *Internet and Web Information Systems Journal Kluwer Academic Publishers*, *5*, 181–192.

Collinger, J. L., Wodlinger, B., Downey, J. E., Wang, W., Tyler-Kabara, E. C., Weber, D. J., & Schwartz, A. B. et al. (2013). High-performance neuroprosthetic control by an individual with tetraplegia. *Lancet*, *381*(9866), 557–564. doi:10.1016/S0140-6736(12)61816-9 PMID:23253623

Damasio, A. R. (Ed.). (1994). *Descartes' Error: Emotion, Reason, and the Human Brain*. New York: Vintage Press.

Daydamony, E. M., Gayar, M. E., & Chadi, F. (2008). A computerized system for SEMG signals analysis and classifieation.*25th National Radio Science Conference* (pp. 1-7). Tanta: IEEE. doi:10.1109/NRSC.2008.4542388

Ding, Q. P., Tong, R. K., & Li, G. (2006). Development of an EOG (electro-oculography) based human-computer interface. In *Engineering in Medicine and Biology Society 27th Annual International Conference* (pp. 6829-6831). Shanghai: IEEE.

Duchowski, A. (2007). *Eye tracking methodology: Theory and practice*. Springer.

Erol, A., Bebis, G., Nicolescu, M., Boyle, R. D., & Twombly, X. (2007). Vision-based hand pose estimation: A review. *Computer Vision and Image Understanding, 108*(1-2), 52–73. doi:10.1016/j.cviu.2006.10.012

Farwell, L. A., & Donchin, E. (1988). Talking off the top of your head: Toward a mental prosthesis utilizing event-related brain potentials. *Electroencephalography and Clinical Neurophysiology, 70*(6), 510–523. doi:10.1016/0013-4694(88)90149-6 PMID:2461285

Fleischer, C., & Hommel, G. A. (2008). A human-exoskeleton interface utilizing electromyography. *IEEE Transactions on Robotics, 24*(4), 872–882. doi:10.1109/TRO.2008.926860

Frith, C. (2002). Attention to action and awareness of other minds. *Consciousness and Cognition, 11*(4), 481–487. doi:10.1016/S1053-8100(02)00022-3 PMID:12470618

Iqbal, S. T., Zheng, X. S., & Bailey, B. P. (2004). Task-evoked pupillary response to mental workload in human-computer interaction. *Conference on Human factors in computing systems* (pp. 1477-1480). Association for Computing Machinery. doi:10.1145/985921.986094

Jaimes, A., & Sebe, N. (2007). Multimodal human–computer interaction: A survey. *Computer Vision and Image Understanding, 108*(1-2), 116–134. doi:10.1016/j.cviu.2006.10.019

Jung, K. K., Kim, J. W., Lee, H. K., Chung, S. B., & Eom, K. H. (2007). EMG pattern classification using spectral estimation and neural network.*SICE Annual Conference* (pp. 1108-1111). IEEE.

Kahneman, D., & Beatty, J. (1977). Pupil diameter and load on memory. *Science, 154*(3756), 1583–1585. doi:10.1126/science.154.3756.1583 PMID:5924930

Kiguchi, K., & Hayashi, Y. (2012). A study of EMG and EEG during perception-assist with an upper-limb power-assist robot. *IEEE International Conference on Robotics and Automation* (vol. 162, pp. 2711-2716). IEEE. doi:10.1109/ICRA.2012.6225027

Konrad, P. (2005). *The abc of emg: A practical introduction to kinesiological electromyography*. Noraxon INC.

Kornhuber, H. H., & Deecke, L. (1965). Changes in the brain potential in voluntary movements and passive movements in man: Readiness potentials and reafferent potentials. *Pflügers Archiv für die Gesamte Physiologie des Menschen und der Tiere*, *284*, 1–17. doi:10.1007/BF00412364 PMID:14341490

Lew, E., Chavarriaga, R., Silvoni, S., & Millán, J. (2012). Detection of self-paced reaching movement intention from EEG signals. *Frontiers in Neuroengineering, 5.*

Lotze, M., & Cohen, L. G. (2006). Volition and imagery in neurorehabilitation. *Cognitive and Behavioral Neurology*, *19*(3), 135–140. doi:10.1097/01.wnn.0000209875.56060.06 PMID:16957491

Marshall S. P. (2000). *Method and apparatus for eye tracking and monitoring pupil dilation to evaluate cognitive activity*. US: US6090051.

Morimoto, C. H., & Mimica, M. R. M. (2005). Eye gaze tracking techniques for interactive applications. *Computer Vision and Image Understanding*, *98*(1), 4–24. doi:10.1016/j.cviu.2004.07.010

Rasmussen, R. G., Acharya, S., & Thakor, N. V. (2006). Accuracy of a Brain-Computer Interface in Subjects with Minimal Training.*Proceedings of the IEEE 32nd Annual Northeast Bioengineering Conference* (pp. 167-168). IEEE. doi:10.1109/NEBC.2006.1629805

Rizzolatti, G., & Sinigaglia, C. (2008). Further reflections on how we interpret the actions of others. *Nature*, *455*(7213), 589. doi:10.1038/455589b PMID:18833249

Robinson, D. A. (1963). *A method of measuring eye movements using a scleral search coil in a magnetic field. In Transactions on Biomedical Engineering* (pp. 137–145). IEEE.

Rupp, R., & Cemer, H. J. (2004). NeuroProstheties of the upper extremity-elinieal applieation in spinal cord injury and future perspectives. *Bio/Technology*, *49*, 93–98. PMID:15171589

Sandro, M. I. (2000). Neural engineering: Real brains for real robots. *Nature*, *408*, 305–306. PMID:11099027

Severinson-Eklundh, K., Green, A., & Hüttenrauch, H. (2003). Social and collaborative aspects of interaction with a service robot. *Robotics and Autonomous Systems*, *42*(3-4), 223–234. doi:10.1016/S0921-8890(02)00377-9

Smith, E. E., & Jonides, J. (1999). Storage and Executive Processes in the Frontal Lobes. *Science*, *283*(5408), 1657–1661. doi:10.1126/science.283.5408.1657 PMID:10073923

Spyrou, T., & Darzentas, J. (1996). Intention Modelling: Approximating Computer User Intentions for Detection and Prediction of Intrusions. In *Information Systems Security* (pp. 319–335). London: Chapman & Hall, Ltd. doi:10.1007/978-1-5041-2919-0_28

Tong, R. K. Y., Leung, W. W. F., Hu, X. L., & Song, R. (2009). Interactive robot-assisted training system using continuous EMG signals for stroke rehabilitation. *Proceedings of the 3rd International Convention on Rehabilitation Engineering & Assistive Technology: No.* 20. New York: ACM. doi:10.1145/1592700.1592723

Wang, Y. W., Ling, C. D., Yuan, B., Huang, L., Zhang, W. X., & Shen, D. L. (2010). Person perception precedes theory of mind: An event related potential analysis. *Neuroscience*, *170*(1), 238–246. doi:10.1016/j.neuroscience.2010.06.055 PMID:20603189

Wolpaw, J. R., Birbaumer, N., Mc Farland, D. J., Pfurtscheller, G., & Vaughan, T. M. (2002). Brain–computer interfaces for communication and control. *Clinical Neurophysiology*, *113*(6), 767–791. doi:10.1016/S1388-2457(02)00057-3 PMID:12048038

Yarbus, A. L. (1967). *Eye movements and vision*. New York: Plenum Press. doi:10.1007/978-1-4899-5379-7

Zhang, Q. Z., Xi, X. G., & Luo, Z. Z. (2014). A Pattern Recognition Method for Surface Electromyography Based on Nonlinear Features. *Journal of Electronics & Information Technology*, *35*(9), 2054–2058. doi:10.3724/SP.J.1146.2012.01325

KEY TERMS AND DEFINITIONS

Cognitive Neuroscience: An academic field that explores questions related to how psychological/cognitive functions are produced by neural circuits in the brain.

Electroencephalogram (EEG): An electrophysiological monitoring method to record the electrical activity of the brain.

Emotion and Attention: Emotional penetration of all aspects of intention and their connection with other cognitive processes.

Eye Tracking Technique: Includes Electro-OculoGraphy (EOG), Scleral Contact Lens, and Video-OculoGraphy (VOG).

Intention Recognition: Recognizing others' intentions based on social cognition, such as interpreting others' behaviors, interacting in social groups, and predicting how others will feel, think and behave.

Multimodal Information Fusion Technology: We can collect information related to intention from multiple aspects and multiple channels.

Surface Electromyography (EMG): An electrodiagnostic medical technique used to evaluate and record the electrical activity that is produced by skeletal muscles.

Chapter 11
Research on Current Situations for Functional Classification of Timing

Zhihan Xu
Okayama University, Japan

Qiong Wu
Okayama University, Japan

Chunlin Li
Capital Medical University, China

Yujie Li
Central China Normal University, China

Hongbin Han
Peking University, China

Dehua Chui
Peking University, China

Satoshi Takahashi
Okayama University, Japan

Jinglong Wu
Okayama University, Japan

ABSTRACT

Time is a fundamental variable that must be quantified by organisms to survive. Depending on the previous functional definition, timing can be divided into explicit timing and implicit timing. For an explicit timing task, the estimation of the stimulus duration is given in the form of perceptual discrimination (perceptual timing) or a motor response (motor timing). For implicit timing, participants can subconsciously (exogenous) or consciously (endogenous) establish temporal expectation. However, the ability of humans to explicitly or implicitly direct attention in time varies with age. Moreover, specific brain mechanisms have been suggested for temporal processing of different time scales (microseconds, hundreds of milliseconds, seconds to minutes, and circadian rhythms). Furthermore, there have been numerous research studies on the neural networks involved in explicit timing during the measurement of sub-second and supra-second intervals.

DOI: 10.4018/978-1-5225-0925-7.ch011

FUNCTIONAL CLASSIFICATION OF TIMING

Temporal processing is crucial for human behavior and cognition. It allows us to determine what is occurring in our environment and when to respond to events. The ability to direct attention to task-relevant information can enhance our behavioral performance. Temporal orienting selective attention is central for optimizing performance by biasing the neural processing of relevant information and suppressing irrelevant items (Moran & Desimone, 1985). Coull and Nobre (2008) suggested that tasks used temporal cues might be divided on the basis of whether the cue is explicitly or implicitly processed. Explicit timing is engaged when the participants make a deliberate estimate of a discrete duration. Implicit timing is engaged, even without a specific instruction to time, whenever sensorimotor information is temporally structured and can be used to predict the duration of future events. In explicit timing, the subjects are instructed to pay attention to the duration of a stimulus. In contrast, implicit timing requires the participants to perform tasks in which timing is important but not the main focus of the task (J. Coull & Nobre, 2008). For example, in a collision judgment task, participants must judge the speed of one or more objects that are moving and then predict the future location of the objects. Thus, this temporal processing focuses on collision judgment; however, time is not central to the task. The critical distinction between explicit timing and implicit timing is whether the task instructions require the participants to afford an overt estimate of duration.

Explicit Timing

In explicit timing, subjects must provide an overt estimate of the inter-stimulus interval (ISI) or the stimulus duration. One form of this estimation is perceptual timing (perceptual discrimination), in which subjects discriminate whether one ISI or stimulus duration is shorter or longer than another (J. T. Coull, Cheng, & Meck, 2011). For example, in the temporal discrimination task, subjects compare a new duration (t2) with a duration (t1) that was previously stored in the reference or working memory; the subject then determines which duration is longer (Figure 1a). Another form of explicit timing is motor timing (motor production), in which subjects represent the ISI or timed duration with a delayed, sustained, or periodic motor act. For example, the task most commonly used to examine motor timing is the temporal reproduction task and the paced finger tapping task. In the temporal reproduction task, subjects reproduce the standard target sensory stimulus duration (t) by producing a sustained motor response whose duration (te) corresponds to the standard duration (Figure 1b). In the paced finger tapping task. During the synchronization phase, the subjects press the button simultaneously with the sensory presented stimulus that occurs at a regular ISI. During the continuation phase, subjects depend on the temporal information they learned during the synchronization phase to reproduce a motor representation of the timed ISI without the sensory pacing stimulus. Above all cases, the task goal is to provide an accurate prediction of elapsed duration. Furthermore, the basal ganglia (BG), cerebellum, supplementary motor area, and prefrontal cortex have all been linked to explicit timing (Livesey, Wall, & Smith, 2007).

Implicit Timing

Implicit timing is engaged when the sensory stimuli or motor responses can be used to achieve non-temporal task goals. For example, we can depend on the velocity parameters of an oncoming car to estimate when the car will reach us and then identify whether we can cross the road safely. In this condition, sensory stimuli are used to achieve a non-temporal goal (cross the road safely) rather than make an overt estimate of elapsing time (whether one car is faster than the other). In this example, temporal expectation is subconscious and incidentally induced as the by-product of the rhythmic or constant temporal dynamics of the stimuli themselves (exogenous). However, temporal expectation can also be engaged consciously and deliberately by informative pre-cue or regular temporal intervals (endogenous). For example, the task most commonly used for exogenous temporal expectation is the spatiotemporal

Figure 1. Explicit timing tasks. (a) Temporal discrimination task. The subjects compare the probe sensory stimulus (duration t2) with the target stimulus (duration t1) that has been previously stored in the working memory then discriminate between the two durations. (b) Temporal reproduction task. The subjects reproduce the standard target sensory stimulus duration (t) by producing a sustained motor response whose duration (te) corresponds to the standard duration.

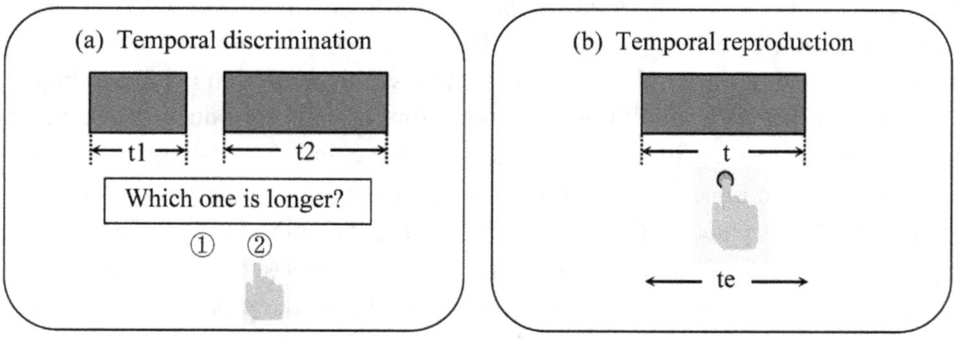

trajectory task. In this task, subjects unintentionally use the constant speed of the moving sensory stimulus to estimate its final location and then determine whether the two stimuli will collide (Figure 2a). For endogenous temporal expectation, a temporal pre-cues task is normally used. First, the subjects learn the temporal associations between the pre-cue and inter-stimulus intervals (ISI): a small circle indicates a short (t1) ISI, and a large circle indicates a long (t2) ISI. Finally, the subjects deliberately use the pre-cue to estimate when the target will appear (Figure 2b). In both exogenous and endogenous cases, temporal expectations are incurred to improve the speed and accuracy of non-temporal task goals (J. T. Coull & Nobre, 1998). Furthermore, implicit timing preferentially engages the left inferior parietal cortex (supramarginal gyrus) (M. Wiener, P. E. Turkeltaub, & H. B. Coslett, 2010).

AGE-REALTED CHANGES IN TEMPORAL PROCESSING

Infants can perceive temporal deviants in rhythmic auditory sequences (Trainor, 2012), and they show evidence of scalar timing for duration discrimination (Brannon, Suanda, & Libertus, 2007). By 3 years of age, children have the same fundamental properties of time perception as adults, although their accuracy of making duration judgments is reduced (Droit-Volet, Clement, & Wearden, 2001). By 7 years

Figure 2. Implicit timing tasks. (a) Spatio-temporal trajectories task. The subjects unintentionally use the constant speed of the moving sensory stimulus to estimate its final location and then determine whether the two stimuli will collide. (b) Temporal pre-cue task. The subjects learn the temporal associations between the pre-cue and inter-stimulus intervals (ISI); a small circle indicates a short (t1) ISI, and a large circle indicates a long (t2) ISI. Finally, the subjects deliberately use the pre-cue to estimate when the target will appear.

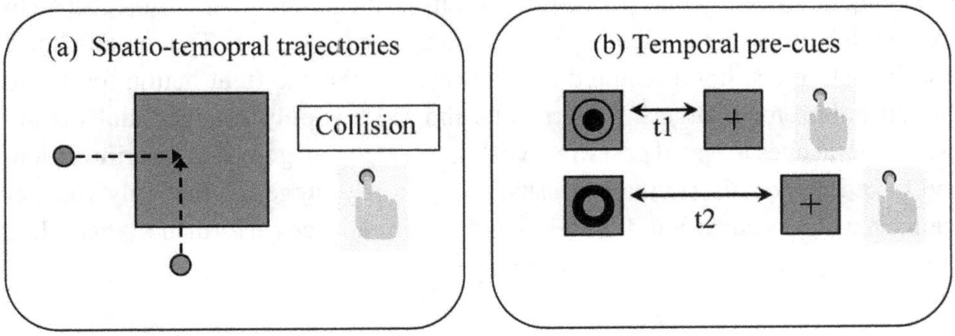

of age, children can discriminate the correct temporal order of two acoustic events (Berwanger, Wittmann, von Steinbuchel, & von Suchodoletz, 2004). The ability of temporal expectation improves precisely during childhood (Droit-Volet & Wearden, 2001) and is suggested to be associated with the development of sustained attention, working memory, cognitive flexibility and speed information processing (Zelanti & Droit-Volet, 2011).

Recently, Katherine (2015) used symbolic ("endogenous") spatial and temporal cues to instruct subjects to predict when (Time) and/or where (Space) targets will appear. All of the subjects performed a modified version of the spatial and temporal orienting task (J. T. Coull & Nobre, 1998). In the space endogenous cue condition, either the left or the right side of a central clock face would brighten, indicating that the target would most likely appear in either the left or right side of the box, respectively. In the time endogenous cue condition, either a short or long inner line of the hand of the clock would brighten, indicating that the target would most likely appear either sooner (short line, 500ms) or later (long line, 1100ms). Their results confirmed previous studies stating that adults have the ability to utilize both spatial and temporal cues to speed behavior; the responses were significantly slower for invalid cue targets in either space or time. Children's responses were also significantly slower when the spatial cues were invalid, given the evidence of their use of spatial cues to optimize behavior. By contrast, children's responses were not slowed by invalid temporal cues, suggesting that they could not use the temporal cue to voluntarily orient attention in time (Kopf et al., 2015).

Theodore and Peter (2011) suggest that older adults also cannot use temporal cues to orient attention in time, similar to children. In that study, the subjects were instructed to respond as quickly and accurately as possible to a target (x or +), which appeared after a fore-period indicated by the letter S (short for 600ms), L (long for 1400ms), or N (neutral for 600 or 1400ms). Furthermore, the responses were contingent on three different task conditions. In the detection condition, the subjects had to press two buttons simultaneously using their left and right thumbs to respond to either target (x or +). In the go/no-go discrimination condition, the subjects had to press both buttons simultaneously only when the target was a +. The forced-choice discrimination condition required the subjects to press the right button for + and the left button for x targets. Their results showed that only younger adults could use temporal cues to speed performance during detection, go/no-go discrimination, and forced-choice discrimination tasks. Overall, they suggested that only younger adults, not older adults, could use temporal cues to enhance performance, regardless of task complexity (Zanto et al., 2011).

TIMESCALES OF TEMPORAL PROCESSING

Timescales

Based on the relevant timescales and assumed underlying neural mechanisms, Mauk and Buonomano (2004) categorized temporal processing into four different types of timescales (Figure 3): microseconds (Carr, 1993; Covey & Casseday, 1999), milliseconds (Buonomano & Karmarkar, 2002), seconds (Gibbon, Malapani, Dale, & Gallistel, 1997), and circadian rhythms (King & Takahashi, 2000).

Figure 3. Timescales of temporal processing. Different behaviors and neural mechanisms are involved in microseconds, hundreds of milliseconds, seconds to minutes, and circadian rhythms.

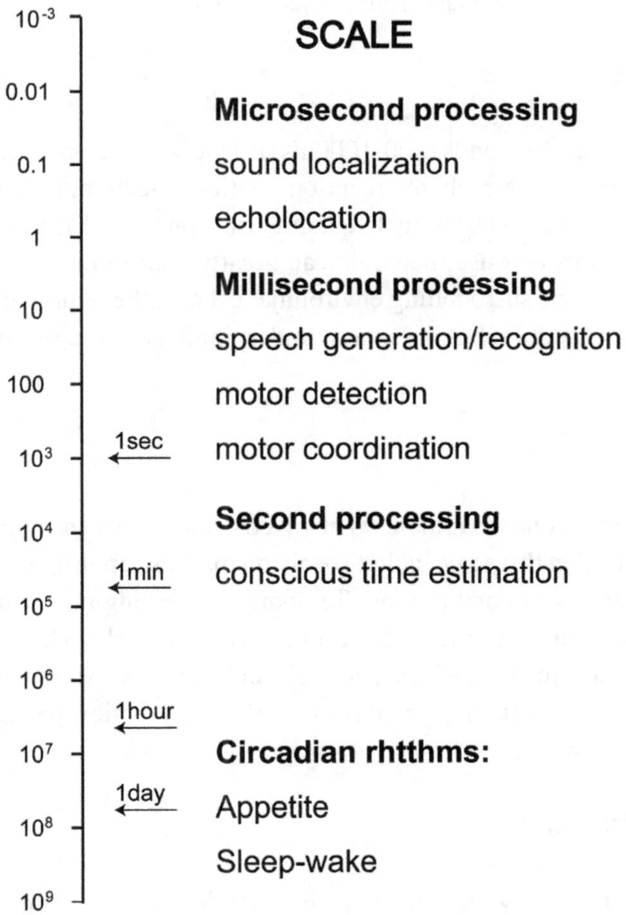

Microseconds

Microseconds have been connected with binaural hearing and echolocation. Binaural hearing, along with frequency cues, allows humans and other animals determine the direction and origin of sounds. It is particularly useful for our ability to localize sounds and to determine the meaning and content of those sounds. Microsecond scale binaural hearing is involved when using the auditory system to determine the difference in time of sound reaching each ear, which is called interaural delay. The sound will arrive in the near ear approximately 600-700μs earlier; this is the natural interaural time difference (ITD). Furthermore, to determine the spatial source of a sound, the neurons that tune for different ITDs are critical for encoding small time differences in the binaural input. Echolocation is that echolocation animals emit calls into the environment and listen to the echoes of those calls that return from various objects near them. They use these echoes to locate and identify nearby objects. A single echolocation call can last from 200μs to 10 ms.

Milliseconds

Interval timing in milliseconds (200-1000ms) is involved in a broad range of behaviors, such as music and speech, interception, motion detection, motor coordination and collision avoidance. The ability to quantify time on the millisecond scale is very complex. Organisms that use this scale can greatly control the onset or the offset time depending on the surrounding environment. Thus, the temporal processing of this scale is very flexible, but the neural underpinnings of the milliseconds range are still unclear.

Seconds

Interval timing in seconds to minutes is involved in conscious and cognitive control. Behaviors involved in this scale include decision marking, multiple-step arithmetic, motor performance and conditioning. Temporal processing in seconds to minutes serves as the contextual framework with the external world. Thus, the timing on this scale is highly influenced by attention and memory. Moreover, the natural underpinning of this scale has been associated with attention processes, working memory and movement.

Circadian Rhythms

A circadian rhythm is any biological process that displays an endogenous, entrainable oscillation of approximately 24 hours. These 24-hour rhythms are driven by a circadian clock, and they have been widely observed in plants, animals, fungi, and cyanobacteria. The circadian clock that synchronizes internal time with the external cycle for light to dark is in the hypothalamic suprachiasmatic nuclei (SCN). Therefore, the SCN controls the rhythms of feeding, activity and resting (Mauk & Buonomano, 2004).

SUB-SECOND AND SUPRA-SECOND TIME PERCEPTION

Many previous studies have suggested that different systems are used to measure time at sub-second and supra-second perceptions. Different ranges of time intervals are associated with different types of behavior and perception. For example, the measurement of a few hundred milliseconds (i.e., sub-second) is crucial for the coordination of muscles during movement (Hore, Wild, & Diener, 1991), speech perception and production (Diehl, Lotto, & Holt, 2004), music recognition, and dancing (Janata & Grafton, 2003; Phillips-Silver & Trainor, 2005), whereas the measurement of a few seconds (i.e., supra-seconds) is involved in conscious time estimation and decision making (Buhusi & Meck, 2005; Mauk & Buonomano, 2004). Furthermore, many previous pharmacological studies have shown that distinct neural systems were involved in measuring sub-second and supra-second intervals. It has been suggested that ethanol impairs discrimination under sub-second intervals; however, discrimination under intervals is not influenced (Rammsayer & Vogel, 1992). By contrast, it has also been suggested that remoxipride and benzodiazepines impair discrimination under supra-second intervals, but not sub-second intervals (Rammsayer, 1994, 1997, 1999). Furthermore, several neuroimaging studies have suggested that a different neural network is involved in the time perception of sub-second and supra-second intervals (Jahanshahi, Jones, Dirnberger, & Frith, 2006; Lewis & Miall, 2003; Morillon, Kell, & Giraud, 2009; M. Wiener, P. Turkeltaub, & H. B. Coslett, 2010).

Viviane and Nathalie (2005) measured short (450ms) and long (1300ms) sub-second intervals in a temporal discrimination task. In this study, the subjects were first trained to discriminate standard durations from nonstandard durations for the two conditions of 450 and 1300ms. The nonstandard durations for the 450ms standard interval consisted of shorter (325ms) and longer (575ms) intervals, and the nonstandard durations for the 1300ms interval consisted of shorter (975ms) and longer (1,625ms) intervals. All of the intervals were represented as two brief light-emitting diode (LED) flashes. The subjects discriminated standard/nonstandard intervals by pressing the right/left buttons. The letter "C" indicated that the interval between the two LED flashes was 450/325–575ms (sub-second condition).

The letter "L" indicated that the interval was 1,300/975– 1,625ms (supra-second condition). The control trials with the letters "C" or "L" required no estimation. The subjects pressed one of the two buttons at random. Finally, the results showed that the presupplementary motor area (preSMA), the prefrontal and parietal cortices, the anterior cingulate, and the basal ganglia were involved in the temporal discrimination trials, regardless of the duration. Moreover, only a subset of the regions within this network, including the preSMA, the anterior cingulate cortex, the right inferior frontal gyrus, the bilateral premotor cortex, and the right caudate nucleus, yielded increased activation with increasing time. They proposed that the caudate-preSMA circuit, the anterior cingulate, and the premotor-inferior frontal regions may be crucial for the clock mechanism, decision making and the maintenance of temporal information, respectively.

Masamichi and Moona (2014) used structural magnetic resonance imaging (MRI) and a VBM analysis with a temporal discrimination task in which thresholds were determined for sub-second (700ms) and supra-second (3.5 sec) durations. In this experiment, the subjects were instructed to discriminate the duration of two consecutively appearing stimuli that were separated by 1.5 sec with their right index finger or middle finger by pressing two keys, J or K, respectively. The J key indicated that the first stimulus was longer, whereas the K key indicated that the second stimulus was longer. The standard duration for the sub-second task was 700ms and that of the supra-second task was 3.5 sec. Finally, the results showed that individual differences in regional GM volume were suggested to determine an individual's ability to discriminate durations. Different brain areas were linked with the ability to estimate sub-second and supra-second intervals. The bilateral anterior cerebellum was associated with the sub-second interval, according to the idea that the cerebellum is crucial for temporal discrimination in the sub-second range. The right IPL was linked with the supra-second durations, in line with the idea that the capacity of attention and working memory support temporal discrimination in the supra-second range. This study provided a dissociable neuroanatomical correlation of sub-second and supra-second time perceptions (Hayashi, Kantele, Walsh, Carlson, & Kanai, 2014).

FUTURE RESEARCH DIRECTIONS

In summary of the published studies of temporal processing for sub-second and supra-second intervals (Figure 4), most of the studies investigated dissociable neu-

Figure 4. Published studies investigating temporal processing

Study	Contrast	Duration(ms)
Masamichi et al.,2014	Temporal discrimination	700,3500
Shih et al.,2009	Temporal discrimination	100,450
Bueti et al.,2008	Temporal reproduction	300,600,900,1200
Livesey et al.,2007	Temporal discrimination	1000,1500
Steven et al.,2007	Paecd finger tapping	750,1500,3500
Marjan et al.,2006	Temporal reproduction	500,2000
Jahanshahi et al.,2006	Temporal reproduction	500,2000
Viviane et al.,2005	Temporal discrimination	450,1300
Bengtsson et al.,2005	Paecd finger tapping	375,750,1125
Pouthas et al.,2005	Temporal discrimination	450,1300
Coull et al.,2004	Temporal discrimination	540,1080,1620
Lewis et al.,2003	Temporal discrimination	600,3000
Katja et al.,1998	Paecd finger tapping	600,5000
Penhune et .,al.,1998	Paecd finger tapping	250,750

roanatomical correlates of sub-second and supra-second intervals in explicit timing tasks (temporal discrimination task/temporal reproduction task/paced finger tapping task). However, it is unclear whether the source of this variability is the same in the different tasks and task goals (explicit vs implicit timing). Furthermore, future studies are required to investigate the dissociable neuroanatomical correlates of sub-second and supra-second intervals in implicit timing tasks (temporal expectation task).

REFERENCES

Berwanger, D., Wittmann, M., von Steinbuchel, N., & von Suchodoletz, W. (2004). Measurement of temporal-order judgment in children. *Acta Neurobiologiae Experimentalis, 64*(3), 387–394. PMID:15283480

Brannon, E. M., Suanda, S., & Libertus, K. (2007). Temporal discrimination increases in precision over development and parallels the development of numerosity discrimination. *Developmental Science, 10*(6), 770–777. doi:10.1111/j.1467-7687.2007.00635.x PMID:17973794

Buhusi, C. V., & Meck, W. H. (2005). What makes us tick? Functional and neural mechanisms of interval timing. *Nature Reviews. Neuroscience, 6*(10), 755–765. doi:10.1038/nrn1764 PMID:16163383

Buonomano, D. V., & Karmarkar, U. R. (2002). How do we tell time? *The Neuroscientist, 8*(1), 42–51. doi:10.1177/107385840200800109 PMID:11843098

Carr, C. E. (1993). Processing of temporal information in the brain. *Annual Review of Neuroscience, 16*(1), 223–243. doi:10.1146/annurev.ne.16.030193.001255 PMID:8460892

Coull, J., & Nobre, A. (2008). Dissociating explicit timing from temporal expectation with fMRI. *Current Opinion in Neurobiology, 18*(2), 137–144. doi:10.1016/j.conb.2008.07.011 PMID:18692573

Coull, J. T., Cheng, R. K., & Meck, W. H. (2011). Neuroanatomical and neurochemical substrates of timing. *Neuropsychopharmacology, 36*(1), 3–25. doi:10.1038/npp.2010.113 PMID:20668434

Coull, J. T., & Nobre, A. C. (1998). Where and when to pay attention: The neural systems for directing attention to spatial locations and to time intervals as revealed by both PET and fMRI. *The Journal of Neuroscience, 18*(18), 7426–7435. PMID:9736662

Covey, E., & Casseday, J. H. (1999). Timing in the auditory system of the bat. *Annual Review of Physiology, 61*(1), 457–476. doi:10.1146/annurev.physiol.61.1.457 PMID:10099697

Diehl, R. L., Lotto, A. J., & Holt, L. L. (2004). Speech perception. *Annual Review of Psychology, 55*(1), 149–179. doi:10.1146/annurev.psych.55.090902.142028 PMID:14744213

Droit-Volet, S., Clement, A., & Wearden, J. (2001). Temporal generalization in 3- to 8-year-old children. *Journal of Experimental Child Psychology, 80*(3), 271–288. doi:10.1006/jecp.2001.2629 PMID:11583526

Droit-Volet, S., & Wearden, J. H. (2001). Temporal bisection in children. *Journal of Experimental Child Psychology*, *80*(2), 142–159. doi:10.1006/jecp.2001.2631 PMID:11529672

Gibbon, J., Malapani, C., Dale, C. L., & Gallistel, C. (1997). Toward a neurobiology of temporal cognition: Advances and challenges. *Current Opinion in Neurobiology*, *7*(2), 170–184. doi:10.1016/S0959-4388(97)80005-0 PMID:9142762

Hayashi, M. J., Kantele, M., Walsh, V., Carlson, S., & Kanai, R. (2014). Dissociable neuroanatomical correlates of subsecond and suprasecond time perception. *Journal of Cognitive Neuroscience*, *26*(8), 1685–1693. doi:10.1162/jocn_a_00580 PMID:24456398

Hore, J., Wild, B., & Diener, H. C. (1991). Cerebellar dysmetria at the elbow, wrist, and fingers. *Journal of Neurophysiology*, *65*(3), 563–571. PMID:2051195

Jahanshahi, M., Jones, C. R., Dirnberger, G., & Frith, C. D. (2006). The substantia nigra pars compacta and temporal processing. *The Journal of Neuroscience*, *26*(47), 12266–12273. doi:10.1523/JNEUROSCI.2540-06.2006 PMID:17122052

Janata, P., & Grafton, S. T. (2003). Swinging in the brain: Shared neural substrates for behaviors related to sequencing and music. *Nature Neuroscience*, *6*(7), 682–687. doi:10.1038/nn1081 PMID:12830159

King, D. P., & Takahashi, J. S. (2000). Molecular genetics of circadian rhythms in mammals. *Annual Review of Neuroscience*, *23*(1), 713–742. doi:10.1146/annurev.neuro.23.1.713 PMID:10845079

Kopf, A., Bicak, M., Kottmann, R., Schnetzer, J., Kostadinov, I., Lehmann, K., & Glockner, F. O. et al. (2015). The ocean sampling day consortium. *Gigascience*, *4*(1), 27. doi:10.1186/s13742-015-0066-5 PMID:26097697

Lewis, P. A., & Miall, R. C. (2003). Brain activation patterns during measurement of sub- and supra-second intervals. *Neuropsychologia*, *41*(12), 1583–1592. doi:10.1016/S0028-3932(03)00118-0 PMID:12887983

Livesey, A. C., Wall, M. B., & Smith, A. T. (2007). Time perception: Manipulation of task difficulty dissociates clock functions from other cognitive demands. *Neuropsychologia*, *45*(2), 321–331. doi:10.1016/j.neuropsychologia.2006.06.033 PMID:16934301

Mauk, M. D., & Buonomano, D. V. (2004). The neural basis of temporal processing. *Annual Review of Neuroscience*, *27*(1), 307–340. doi:10.1146/annurev.neuro.27.070203.144247 PMID:15217335

Moran, J., & Desimone, R. (1985). Selective attention gates visual processing in the extrastriate cortex. *Science, 229*(4715), 782–784. doi:10.1126/science.4023713 PMID:4023713

Morillon, B., Kell, C. A., & Giraud, A. L. (2009). Three stages and four neural systems in time estimation. *The Journal of Neuroscience, 29*(47), 14803–14811. doi:10.1523/JNEUROSCI.3222-09.2009 PMID:19940175

Phillips-Silver, J., & Trainor, L. J. (2005). Feeling the beat: Movement influences infant rhythm perception. *Science, 308*(5727), 1430. doi:10.1126/science.1110922 PMID:15933193

Rammsayer, T. H. (1994). Effects of practice and signal energy on duration discrimination of brief auditory intervals. *Perception & Psychophysics, 55*(4), 454–464. doi:10.3758/BF03205302 PMID:8036124

Rammsayer, T. H. (1997). Are there dissociable roles of the mesostriatal and mesolimbocortical dopamine systems on temporal information processing in humans? *Neuropsychobiology, 35*(1), 36–45. doi:10.1159/000119328 PMID:9018022

Rammsayer, T. H. (1999). Neuropharmacological evidence for different timing mechanisms in humans. *The Quarterly Journal of Experimental Psychology. B, Comparative and Physiological Psychology, 52*(3), 273–286. doi:10.1080/713932708 PMID:10467900

Rammsayer, T. H., & Vogel, W. H. (1992). Pharmacologic properties of the internal clock underlying time perception in humans. *Neuropsychobiology, 26*(1-2), 71-80.

Trainor, L. J. (2012). Predictive information processing is a fundamental learning mechanism present in early development: Evidence from infants. *International Journal of Psychophysiology, 83*(2), 256–258. doi:10.1016/j.ijpsycho.2011.12.008 PMID:22226901

Wiener, M., Turkeltaub, P., & Coslett, H. B. (2010). The image of time: A voxel-wise meta-analysis. *NeuroImage, 49*(2), 1728–1740. doi:10.1016/j.neuroimage.2009.09.064 PMID:19800975

Wiener, M., Turkeltaub, P. E., & Coslett, H. B. (2010). Implicit timing activates the left inferior parietal cortex. *Neuropsychologia, 48*(13), 3967–3971. doi:10.1016/j.neuropsychologia.2010.09.014 PMID:20863842

Zanto, T. P., Pan, P., Liu, H., Bollinger, J., Nobre, A. C., & Gazzaley, A. (2011). Age-related changes in orienting attention in time. *The Journal of Neuroscience*, *31*(35), 12461–12470. doi:10.1523/JNEUROSCI.1149-11.2011 PMID:21880908

Zelanti, P. S., & Droit-Volet, S. (2011). Cognitive abilities explaining age-related changes in time perception of short and long durations. *Journal of Experimental Child Psychology*, *109*(2), 143–157. doi:10.1016/j.jecp.2011.01.003 PMID:21334637

KEY TERMS AND DEFINITIONS

Explicit Timing: Explicit timing is engaged when the participants make a deliberate estimate of discrete duration.

fMRI: Functional magnetic resonance imaging is a technique for measuring and mapping brain activity that is noninvasive and safe.

Implicit Timing: Implicit timing is engaged even without a specific instruction to time, whenever sensorimotor information is temporally structured and can be used to predict the duration of future events.

Temporal Discrimination: Observation and recording of the elapsed time of an act, action, or process.

Temporal Expectation: The ability to select the precise moment for doing something for the optimum effect.

Time Perception: Time perception is a field of study within psychology and neuroscience that refers to the subjective experience of time, which is measured by someone's own perception of the duration of the indefinite and continuous unfolding of events.

Timescales: The span of time within which certain events occur or are scheduled to occur in relation to any broader period of time.

Chapter 12
MRI-Compatible Haptic Stimuli Delivery Systems for Investigating Neural Substrates of Touch

Jiabin Yu
Okayama University, Japan

Jiajia Yang
Okayama University, Japan

Zhiwei Wu
Okayama University, Japan

Jinglong Wu
Okayama University, Japan

ABSTRACT

Functional magnetic resonance imaging (fMRI) has been widely used to study human tactile perception. To reveal many unsolved problems to human tactile perception, developing complex and fMRI-compatible stimulation devices are crucial for tactile perception research. These stimulation devices, combined with functional magnetic resonance imaging (fMRI), can assist researchers in analyzing human brain activity. Through analyzing human brain activity, researchers can clarify how the human brain controls the body. Meanwhile, these device scan provide the best rehabilitation program for patients. This chapter presents previous fMRI-compatible stimulation devices, including texture stimulation, shape stimulation, vibrotactile stimulation, etc., which involve the hands, face, ears, legs and other parts of the body. In this chapter, we examine the design of the devices in greater detail. Finally, we summarize the characteristics of these devices and create an outlook for future fMRI-compatible devices.

DOI: 10.4018/978-1-5225-0925-7.ch012

INTRODUCTION

Functional magnetic resonance imaging is a functional neuroimaging technique that uses MRI technology to measure brain activity by detecting changes in oxygen levels in the blood (Huettel, S. A, et al., 2009). Neuronal activation and cerebral blood flow are coupled. When an area of the brain is activated and requires energy, blood flow to this region also increases. Therefore, the primary form of this technique depends on the principle of blood-oxygen-level dependent (BOLD) contrast (Huettel, S. A, et al., 2009), which was discovered by Seiji Ogawa.

This procedure is similar to MRI but uses the change in magnetization between oxygen-poor and oxygen-rich blood, which can be detected on the basis of differential magnetic susceptibility.Although this measure is always disturbed by noise from various sources, statistical methods are used to extract the underlying signal. Then, the activation in the brain can be presented graphically by color-coding the strength of activation across the brain; thus, this technique can localize activity to within millimeters.

When neurons are activated, they require more energy in the form of sugar and oxygen. This process is called the hemodynamic response, and blood will bring oxygen to the activated neurons. This technology uses a type of specialized brain scan to map neural activity in the brain by imaging changes in the hemodynamic response as a result of energy use by brain cells (Huettel, S. A, et al., 2009).

BACKGROUND

Since the early 1990s, fMRI has dominated brain mapping research because it does not require people to undergo surgery, shots, be exposed to ionizing radiation, etc. (Huettel, S. A, et al., 2009). During the late 19th century, Angelo Mosso invented the 'human circulation balance', which worked like a seesaw to measure blood flow changes in the brain (Sandrone S, et al., 2012).

However, although briefly mentioned by William James in 1890, the precise workings of this balance and the experiments remained unclear until the discovery of the original instrument as well as Mosso's reports by Stefano Sandrone and colleagues (Sandrone S, et al., 2014). In 1890, Charles Roy and Charles Sherrington first experimentally linked brain function to its blood flow at Cambridge University (Raichle, M. E, et al., 2000). In 1936, Linus Pauling and Charles Coryell discovered solutions to measure blood flow to the brain. They found that oxygen-depleted blood with dHb was attracted to a magnetic field, although less so than ferromagnetic elements, such as iron, whereas oxygen-rich blood with Hb was weakly repelled by magnetic fields. As Seiji Ogawaat At&T Ball labs recognized, this could be used to augment MRI, which merely evaluates the static structure of the brain, because the different magnetic properties of Hb and dHb that are caused by blood flow to the activated brain regions would cause measurable changes in the MRI signal (Huettel, S. A, et al., 2009). In 1990, Ogawa discovered BOLD, which is the MRI contrast of dHb. Ogawa, Thulborn et al. and colleagues scanned rodents in a strong magnetic field(7.0T) in a seminal 1990 study.

They changed the proportion of oxygen that the animals breathed to manipulate the blood oxygen level. As this proportion fell, a map of blood flow in the brain was observed via MRI. They verified this by placing test tubes with deoxygenated or oxygenated blood and creating separate images. Belliveau and others used the contrast agent Magnevist, a ferromagnetic substance remaining in the bloodstream after intravenous injection, to detect the regional activity in the brain at Harvard University. Although the agent remains in the blood for only a short time, it was not acceptable for human fMRI because any medically unnecessary injection is to some extent uncomfortable and unsafe (Huettel, S. A, et al.,2009).In 1992, three studies first evaluated fMRI using BOLD contrast in humans. Kenneth Kwong and colleagues studied activation in the visual cortex by using a gradient-echo Echo planar Imaging(EPI) sequence at a magnetic field strength of 1.5T. Ogawa and others used a higher field(4.0 T) to conduct their study and showed that the BOLD signal depended on T2* loss of magnetization. Bandettini and colleagues used EPI at 1.5 T to show activation in the primary motor cortex, a brain region that in humans is located in the dorsal portion of the frontal lobe (Huettel, S. A, et al., 2009).

APPLICATIONS OF FMRI IN TACTILE PERCEPTION

A Novel MRI-Compatible Tactile Stimulator for Cortical Mapping of Foot Sole Pressure Stimuli with fMRI (Ying Hao, et al., 2013)

Foot sole somatosensation plays an important role in controlling the human ability to stand and walk. Disease and aging often impair foot sole somatosensation, which consequently increases the risk of falling and decreases balance.

However, behavior research indicates that some older adults with foot sole somatosensory impairment can maintain their balance to a similar degree as their healthy counterparts (Manor B,et al.,2010).Furthermore, both perceptible and imperceptible foot sole vibratory stimulation during standing (Costa M, et al., 2007) and walking (Novak P, et al., 2006) reduce movement variability in older adults both with and without movement disorders. To identify the neural mechanisms underlying these adaptive capacities, the author developed and evaluated an MRI-compatible tactile stimulator capable of applying controlled patterns of pressure to the foot sole. Many devices have been developed to study the brain's response to foot sole somatosensory stimuli. These devices have similar features, such as low amplitude and high-frequency vibratory stimuli (Golaszewski SM, et al., 2002; Graham SJ, et al., 2001; Harrington GS, et al., 2000; Stippich C, et al., 1999). Regarding the foot sole, Gallach et al. (Gallasch E, et al., 2006) successfully mapped somatosensory cortical activation in response to mechanical vibration(i.e., 20-100 Hz oscillations with a maximum contact force of 20 N), which was produced by an electrically-driven magnetic actuator. However, the pressure beneath the foot during weight-bearing activities often meets or exceeds one's body weight and may vary considerably in frequency and amplitude. As an important first to enable the study of the brain's response to this type stimulus, the author developed an air-driven stimulation system that was capable of applying relatively high pressure stimuli to the foot sole with a programmable waveform and adjustable surface area over which the pressure is applied. The combination of this new tool with functional MRI (fMRI) will provide insight into the functional brain networks underlying this source of afferent feedback under different experimental conditions. This device can study the neural circuits underlying foot sole somatosensation and the mechanisms of neural adaption that optimize behavior in the presence of both acute and chronic alterations to this source of afferent feedback(Hao Y, et al., 2013). This device is capable of producing 1-DOF oscillations with a preset waveform, frequency(≤10 Hz),duty cycle (20-100%), force magnitude (5-500 N), and contacted surface area over which pressures are applied to the foot sole.

Image tests in a functional/anatomical/field map showed that the device is compatible with 3T MRI. The author used a typical block-designed 1 Hz sinusoidal simulation protocol on seven healthy young adults, and GRE-EPI images demonstrated that significant activation occurred contralaterally within the paracentral gyrus and primary somatosensory cortex and bilaterally within the secondary somatosensory cortex. Thus, the device also can study the functional brain networks that are involved in the perception and modulation of foot sole somatosensation and its relationship to motor control.

The device consists of an air compressor, an aluminum pneumatic actuator attached to a non-ferromagnetic support platform and a control unit (i.e., a microprocessor, proportional valve, 5-port air-operated valve and user-interface) (Figure 1). This device is produced by a linear pneumatic actuator consisting of a single-acting, single-rod air cylinder (CG1BN32-40-XC6, SMC, Tokyo, Japan). There are many reasons for choosing this actuator. Importantly, it consists of aluminum and is driven by air; thus, the device is non-ferromagnetic. Second, the device is capable of producing a linear output force ranging from 5 to 500N and is thus suitable for generating large pressure stimuli. Third, the device can rapidly generate pressures to the foot sole because the stroke movement speed is 40-1000 mm/s. There are several independent units that control the magnitude and frequency of the device applied to the foot sole. Specifically, the microprocessor(MSP430 F168, Texas Instruments, USA) controls the air flow to the pneumatic actuator by regulating the voltage input to two electronic air valves. The microprocessor also produces a trigger in/out(TTL level) signal to synchronize the system with the MR scanner. The author developed an interface by using C programming, which can allow the investigator to program the characteristics of foot stimulation. This interface consisted of four control buttons and a 16-character LCD display. During stimulation, the duty cycle, magnitude and frequency of force, which are determined by the voltage input, are displayed on the LCD screen. All of the components of the control unit are located outside the scanner

Figure 1. Force generation is regulated by a control unit located outside of the magnet room (c, lower panel) attached to the non-ferromagnetic actuator and platform (c, upper panel) via 4 m plastic air tubes

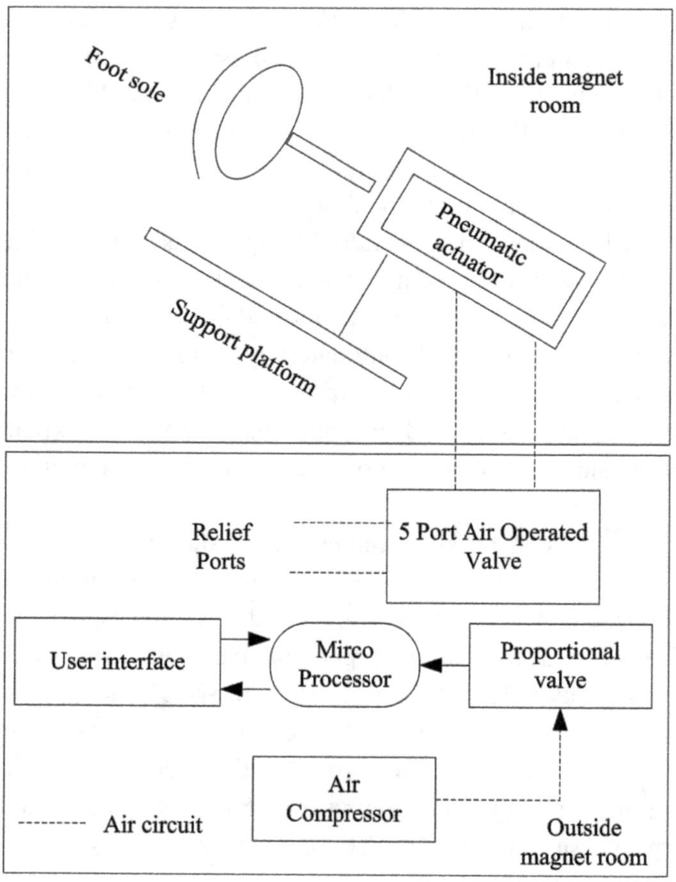

Table 1. MRI compatibility test on the phantom center ROI

Foot Stimulator Condition	Anatomic SNR (mean±SD)	Anatomic SNR (mean±SD)	Anatomic SNR (mean±SD)
Powered on	80±2	768±71	2013±15
Powered off	80±1	771±66	2018±15
Absent from room	79±1	764±65	2011±15

SNR=Signal-to-Noise Ratio; SFNR=Signal-to-Fluctuation-Noise Ratio

and are connected to the actuator inside by plastic air tubes. A plastic medical tube was attached to a support surface consisting of non-ferromagnetic plastic materials.

The reliability of a novel MRI-compatible tactile stimulator mainly depends on the compatibility of fMRI. The author used aphantom to test fMRI compatibility, which showed that the foot sole stimuli device did not affect image quality. The author compared the presence of the stimulation system (whether powered on or off) with the absence of the stimulation system within the tested ROI, and the SFNR of the functional images, the SNR of the anatomic images, and the mean and standard deviation of the magnetic field maps were virtually identical (Table 1).

Brain Activity During Stepping: A Novel MRI-Compatible Device (Hollnagel, C, et al., 2011)

There are few papers investigating the effect of supraspinal centers on the control of human locomotion. We can clarify these effects and improve the effects of locomotor training by analyzing brain activity. For the sake of these problems, an fMRI-compatible pneumatic robotic device has been developed that can generate freely programmable and passive leg movements, including knee, hip and ankle joint displacement.

Although few papers have dealt with this subject, there are many clinical experiments regarding this topic. After a spinal cord injury, a dysfunction of the neuronal circuits relevant for locomotion remains immobile over time (Dietz et al., 2009). Gait training with robotic gait orthoses, such as the LOKOMAT (Hocoma AG, Switzerland, Colombo et al., 2000), has been suggested to prevent such a neuronal dysfunction. However, neither the therapeutic effects of gait training or the treated mechanism of dysfunction on supraspinal and spinal neuronal circuits are fully elucidated. Therefore, developing these mechanisms can improve the therapeutic efficacy of gait training. Although training effects on spinal neuronal centers have been described (Dietz et al., 2002), training effects on supraspinal centers are unclear. We can assess brain activity during lower limb movement or gait and recognize the significance of specific brain regions by functional magnetic resonance imaging (fMRI). Developing an MR-compatible robotic device is vitally important, and the device can enable gait-like movements in a controlled and repetitive manner. However, there are several challenges to inserting a robotic device into the magnetic resonance scanner environment without disturbing the quality of the images. First, the device should not disturb the quality of the images and should not harm the technical scanner environment. Second, the supine posture yields unnatural gravitational effects to the feet and the trunk. Third, the fMRI scanner should also not disturb the functionality of the device. Forth, leg movements will be simplified compared with physiological gait because of the restricted space inside the scanner (Hollnagel, Brugger et al., 2011).

The devices have several key characteristics, including the coordinated trajectories of the knee, ankle and hip joints in the sagittal plane, as well as foot contact forces(Dietz and Duysens, 2000; Dietz et al., 1992). To result in a locomotion pattern in the relevant leg muscles, the pattern must remain similar regarding these characteristics(Dietz et al., 2002). In addition, to assure that the images will not be affected because of head motion, movement artifacts are necessary to limit head motion. Brain activity has been investigated with fMRI during multi-joint leg movements, such as during cycling (Christensen et al., 2000;Mehta et al., 2009). However, these approaches suffered from excessive head motion, and they did not consider appropriate foot loading. Several other groups have investigated brain activity during simplified gait-related movements. They focused on isolated joint movements, such as knee and ankle extension/flexion (Ciccarelli et al., 2005; Dobkin et al., 2004; Luft et al., 2005, 2002; MacIntosh et al., 2004; Sahyoun et al., 2004) or the imagination of walking (Bakker et al., 2007a; Jahn et al., 2004; Malouin et al., 2003; Sahyoun et al., 2004). Coordinated movement of several joints is very important to activate gait-like muscle activity and a realistic gait pattern in the legs (Ivanenko et al., 2002; Kawashima et al., 2005) with the associated nervous representations in the brain. Brain activity has been studied with positron single photon emission computed tomography (SPECT) and positron emission tomography (PET) during natural gait(Fukuyama et al., 1997; Hanakawa et al., 1999; la Fougère et al., 2010). Furthermore, brain activity has also been observed by applying near-infrared spectroscopy (NIRS) during gait (Miyai et al., 2006, 2001). Compared with SPECT and PET, this method can concurrently acquire brain activity without contrast medium during gait, but it has very poor spatial resolution(Bakker et al., 2007b). To combat this limitation, a Magnetic Resonance Compatible Stepper (MARCOS) has been constructed that can allow gait-like movements inside an fMRI scanner without affecting the quality of the image because of the magnetic field of the scanner(Hollnagel, Brugger et al., 2011).

Previous research has shown that the electromyographic activity of angular trajectories and leg muscles at the knee and hip maintain physiological relevance as long as the incorporated ground reaction forces are at least half the magnitude of the obtained body weight (Ivanenko et al., 2002; Kamibayashi et al., 2009), with sufficient hip joint excursions (Dietz et al., 2002). MARCOS can generate forces of up to 400N at the foot sole and can move the legs in an alternating manner (Figure 2). Furthermore, pneumatic actuators can easily be switched to a force-free state by connecting both cylinder chambers to the atmosphere, and it is important to maintain the safety of the patient. All of the ferromagnetic parts in the piston are replaced by aluminum and brass custom-made pieces, and the feet and knees of the subject are strapped to a modified pneumatic cylinder. The pneumatic cylinder at the foot produces a force in the way that the foot moves along the linear guide to generate the appropriate afferent input (Figure 2). At the hip, flexion can range from 0° and 40°, and flexion between 0°to 60° is possible at the knee. Optical encoders (Type MS20, RSF Elektronik AG, Schwerzenbach, Switzerland) with a ceramic scale and one foil potentiometer (MTP L22, Resenso, Ins., Switzerland) have been used to measure the position of each cylinder.

In task Alt-pas-F, a strong drift was detected during the first scan. Activity in the primary sensory/motor network (SMA, S1/M1, preSMA) was observed in all of the conducted tasks. Leg movement in MARCOS was restricted with a maximal

Figure 2. Principle sketch of MARCOS

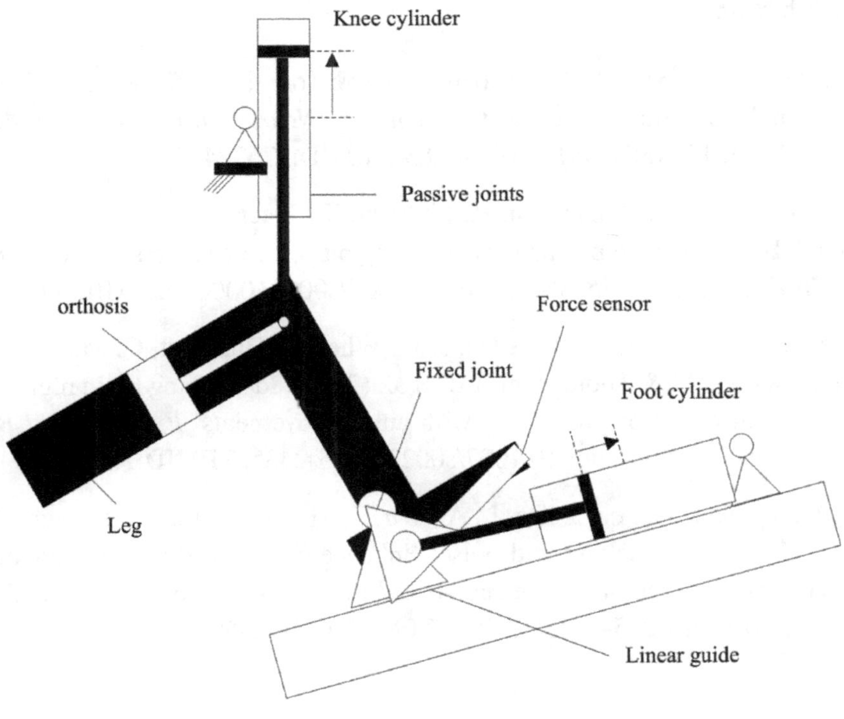

force error of 20 N and a maximal position error of 5 mm. Activity was restricted to the knee/lower-leg/upper-leg region within the human homunculus.

FUTURE RESEARCH DIRECTIONS

Future studies will utilize multiple, independently-controlled pneumatic actuators over larger surface areas of the body to accurately simulate pressure and optimize therapeutic protocols and approaches; this will allow us to learn about the functional brain networks involved in this critical source of afferent feedback and will afford deep insight into the cortical networks underlying human behavior in both disease and health.

ACKNOWLEDGMENT

This study was supported in part by the JAPAN SOCIETY FOR THE PROMOTION OF SCIENCE (JSPS) KAKENHI, grant numbers: 25249026 and 25303013; a Grant-in-Aid for Strategic Research Promotion from Okayama University.

REFERENCES

Bakker, M., Verstappen, C. C. P., Bloem, B. R., & Toni, I. (2007). Recent advances in functional neuroimaging of gait. *Journal of Neural Transmission*, *114*(10), 1323–1331. doi:10.1007/s00702-007-0783-8 PMID:17622483

Christensen, L. O. D., Johannsen, P., Sinkjaer, T., Petersen, N., Pyndt, H. S., & Nielsen, J. B. (2000). Cerebral activation during bicycle movements in man. *Experimental Brain Research*, *135*, 66–72. doi:10.1007/s002210000493 PMID:11104128

Ciccarelli, O., Toosy, A. T., Marsden, J. F., Wheeler-Kingshott, C. M., Sahyoun, C., Matthews, P. M., & Thompson, A. J. et al. (2005). Identifying brain regions for integrative sensorimotor processing with ankle movements. *Experimental Brain Research*, *166*(1), 31–42. doi:10.1007/s00221-005-2335-5 PMID:16034570

Costa, M., Priplata, A. A., Lipsitz, L. A., Wu, Z., Huang, N. E., Goldberger, A. L., & Peng, C. K. (2007). Noise and poise: Enhancement of postural complexity in the elderly with a stochastic-resonance-based therapy. *Europhysics Letters*, *77*(6), 68008. doi:10.1209/0295-5075/77/68008 PMID:17710211

Dietz, V., & Duysens, J. (2000). Significance of load receptor input during locomotion: A review. *Gait & Posture*, *11*(2), 102–110. doi:10.1016/S0966-6362(99)00052-1 PMID:10899663

Dietz, V., Gollhofer, A., Kleiber, M., & Trippel, M. (1992). Regulation of bipedal stance: Dependency on "load" receptors. *Experimental Brain Research*, *89*(1), 229–231. doi:10.1007/BF00229020 PMID:1601101

Dietz, V., Grillner, S., Trepp, A., Hubli, M., & Bolliger, M. (2009). Changes in spinal reflex and locomotor activity after a complete spinal cord injury: A common mechanism? *Brain*, *132*(8), 2196–2205. doi:10.1093/brain/awp124 PMID:19460795

Dietz, V., Muller, R., & Colombo, G. (2002). Locomotor activity in spinal man: Significance of afferent input from joint and load receptors. *Brain*, *125*(12), 2626–2634. doi:10.1093/brain/awf273 PMID:12429590

Dobkin, B. H., Firestine, A., West, M., Saremi, K., & Woods, R. (2004). Ankle dorsiflexion as an fMRI paradigm to assay motor control for walking during rehabilitation. *NeuroImage*, *23*(1), 370–381. doi:10.1016/j.neuroimage.2004.06.008 PMID:15325385

Fukuyama, H., Ouchi, Y., Matsuzaki, S., Nagahama, Y., Yamauchi, H., Ogawa, M., & Shibasaki, H. et al. (1997). Brain functional activity during gait in normal subjects: A SPECT study. *Neuroscience Letters*, *228*(3), 183–186. doi:10.1016/S0304-3940(97)00381-9 PMID:9218638

Gallasch, E., Golaszewski, S. M., Fend, M., Siedentopf, C. M., Koppelstaetter, F., Eisner, W., & Felber, S. R. et al. (2006). Contact force- and amplitude-controllable vibrating probe for somatosensory mapping of plantar afferences with fMRI. *Journal of Magnetic Resonance Imaging*, *24*(5), 1177–1182. doi:10.1002/jmri.20742 PMID:17031838

Golaszewski, S. M., Siedentopf, C. M., Baldauf, E., Koppelstaetter, F., Eisner, W., Unterrainer, J., & Felber, S. R. et al. (2002, September). Functional magnetic resonance imaging of the human sensorimotor cortex using a novel ibrotactile stimulator. *NeuroImage*, *17*(1), 421–430. doi:10.1006/nimg.2002.1195 PMID:12482095

Graham, S. J., Staines, W. R., Nelson, A., Plewes, D. B., & McIlroy, W. E. (2001). New devices to deliver somatosensory stimuli during functional MRI. *Magnetic Resonance in Medicine*, *46*(3), 436–442. doi:10.1002/mrm.1211 PMID:11550233

Hanakawa, T., Katsumi, Y., Fukuyama, H., Honda, M., Hayashi, T., Kimura, J., & Shibasaki, H. (1999). Mechanisms underlying gait disturbance in Parkinson's disease—a single photon emission computed tomography study. *Brain*, *122*(7), 1271–1282. doi:10.1093/brain/122.7.1271 PMID:10388793

Harrington, G. S., Wright, C. T., & Downs, J. R. (2000). A new vibrotactile stimulator for functional MRI. *Human Brain Mapping*, *10*(3), 140–145. doi:10.1002/1097-0193(200007)10:3<140::AID-HBM50>3.0.CO;2-0 PMID:10912593

Huettel, S. A., Song, A. W., &McCarthy, G. (2009). *Functional Magnetic Resonance Imaging* (2nd ed.). Sinauer.

Ivanenko, Y. P., Grasso, R., Macellari, V., & Lacquaniti, F. (2002). Control of foot trajectory in human locomotion: Role of ground contact forces in simulated reduced gravity. *Journal of Neurophysiology*, *87*, 3070–3089. PMID:12037209

Jahn, K., Deutschlander, A., Stephan, T., Strupp, M., Wiesmann, M., & Brandt, T. (2004). Brain activation patterns during imagined stance and locomotion in functional magnetic resonance imaging. *NeuroImage*, *22*(4), 1722–1731. doi:10.1016/j.neuroimage.2004.05.017 PMID:15275928

Kamibayashi, K., Nakajima, T., Takahashi, M., Akai, M., & Nakazawa, K. (2009). Facilitation of corticospinal excitability in the tibialis anterior muscle during robot-assisted passive stepping in humans. *The European Journal of Neuroscience*, *30*(1), 100–109. doi:10.1111/j.1460-9568.2009.06795.x PMID:19523098

Luft, A. R., Forrester, L., Macko, R. F., McCombe-Waller, S., Whitall, J., Villagra, F., & Hanley, D. F. (2005). Brain activation of lower extremity movement in chronically impaired stroke survivors. *NeuroImage*, *26*(1), 184–194. doi:10.1016/j.neuroimage.2005.01.027 PMID:15862218

Luft, A. R., Smith, G. V., Forrester, L., Whitall, J., Macko, R. F., Hauser, T.-K., & Hanley, D. F. et al. (2002). Comparing brain activation associated with isolated upper and lower limb movement across corresponding joints. *Human Brain Mapping*, *17*(2), 131–140. doi:10.1002/hbm.10058 PMID:12353246

MacIntosh, B. J., Mraz, R., Baker, N., Tam, F., Staines, W. R., & Graham, S. J. (2004). Optimizing the experimental design for ankle dorsiflexion fMRI. *NeuroImage*, *22*(4), 1619–1627. doi:10.1016/j.neuroimage.2004.03.035 PMID:15275918

Malouin, F., Richards, C. L., Jackson, P. L., Dumas, F., & Doyon, J. (2003). Brain activations during motor imagery of locomotor-related tasks: A PET study. *Human Brain Mapping*, *19*(1), 47–62. doi:10.1002/hbm.10103 PMID:12731103

Manor, B., Costa, M. D., Hu, K., Newton, E., Starobinets, O., Kang, H. G., & Lipsitz, L. A. et al. (2010). Physiological complexity and system adaptability: Evidence from postural control dynamics of older adults. *Journal of Applied Physiology (Bethesda, Md.)*, *109*(6), 1786–1791. doi:10.1152/japplphysiol.00390.2010 PMID:20947715

Mehta, J. P., Verber, M. D., Wieser, J. A., Schmit, B. D., & Schindler-Ivens, S. M. (2009). A novel technique for examining human brain activity associated with pedaling using fMRI. *Journal of Neuroscience Methods*, *179*(2), 230–239. doi:10.1016/j.jneumeth.2009.01.029 PMID:19428532

Miyai, I., Suzuki, M., Hatakenaka, M., & Kubota, K. (2006). Effect of body weight support on cortical activation during gait in patients with stroke. *Experimental Brain Research*, *169*(1), 85–91. doi:10.1007/s00221-005-0123-x PMID:16237521

Miyai, I., Tanabe, H. C., Sase, I., Eda, H., Oda, I., Konishi, I., & Kubota, K. et al. (2001). Cortical mapping of gait in humans: A near-infrared spectroscopic topography study. *NeuroImage*, *14*(5), 1186–1192. doi:10.1006/nimg.2001.0905 PMID:11697950

Novak, P., & Novak, V. (2006, May4). Effect of step-synchronized vibration stimulation of soles on gait in Parkinson's disease: A pilot study. *Journal of Neuroengineering and Rehabilitation*, *3*(1), 9. doi:10.1186/1743-0003-3-9 PMID:16674823

Raichle, M. E., Toga, A. W., & Mazziotta, J. C. (2000). *Brain mapping: the systems*. London: Academic Press.

Sahyoun, C., Floyer-Lea, A., Johansen-Berg, H., & Matthews, P. M. (2004). Towards an understanding of gait control: Brain activation during the anticipation, preparation and execution of foot movements. *NeuroImage*, *21*(2), 568–575. doi:10.1016/j.neuroimage.2003.09.065 PMID:14980558

Sandrone, S., Bacigaluppi, M., Galloni, M. R., Cappa, S. F., Moro, A., Catani, M., & Martino, G. et al. (2014). Weighing brain activity with the balance: Angelo Mosso's original manuscripts come to light. *Brain*, *137*(Pt 2), 621–633. doi:10.1093/brain/awt091 PMID:23687118

Sandrone, S., Bacigaluppi, M., Galloni, M. R., & Martino, G. (2012). Angelo Mosso (1846–1910). *Journal of Neurology*, *259*(11), 2513–2514. doi:10.1007/s00415-012-6632-1 PMID:23010944

Stippich, C., Hofmann, R., Kapfer, D., Hempel, E., Heiland, S., Jansen, O., & Sartor, K. (1999). Somatotopic mapping of the human primary somatosensory cortex by fully automated tactile stimulation using functional magnetic resonance imaging. *Neuroscience Letters*, *277*(1), 25–28. doi:10.1016/S0304-3940(99)00835-6 PMID:10643889

KEY TERMS AND DEFINITIONS

Alt-Pas-F: This refers to a condition of alternating passive stepping at 0.5 Hz with foot loading (0-200 N).

BOLD: Blood-oxygen-level dependent refers to the change from diamagnetic oxyhemoglobin to paramagnetic deoxyhemoglobin that occurs with brain activation, resulting in decreased signal intensity on MRI.

EPI: Echo planar imaging is one of the early magnetic resonance imaging sequences (also known as Intascan) that is used in applications such as diffusion, perfusion, and functional magnetic resonance imaging.

fMRI: Functional magnetic resonance imaging is a type of specialized MRI scan used to measure the hemodynamic response (change in blood flow) related to neural activity in the brain or the spinal cord of humans or animals.

Rehabilitation: Treatments designed to facilitate the process of recovery from injury, illness, or disease to as normal a state as possible.

ROI: A region of interest (often abbreviated ROI) is a selected subset of samples within a dataset identified for a particular purpose.

SPECT: Single-photon emission computed tomography (SPECT, or less commonly, SPET) is a nuclear medicine tomographic imaging technique that uses gamma rays.

Chapter 13
The Present Visual Equipment System and Its Application in fMRI

Jiayue Guo
Okayama University, Japan

Meng Wang
Okayama University, Japan

Yang Feng
Okayama University, Japan

Jinglong Wu
Okayama University, Japan

ABSTRACT

The visual system is the part of the central nervous system that gives organisms the ability to process visual details and enables the formation of several non-image photo response functions. It detects and explains information from visible by the light to build a representation of the surrounding environment. One reason why the visual system is so important is that it enables us to perceive information at a distance. We need not be in immediate contact with a stimulus to process it. We must experiment with visual equipment to understand how we process visual information. This article summarizes current visual system equipment and how this equipment can be used to determine how the visual system functions.

INTRODUCTION

The presentation of high-quality visual stimuli to a subject undergoing functional fMRI is very important but has been difficult to achieve. Currently, brain functional activation studies, either for basic research or pre-operative brain mapping, are becoming increasingly common (Fox, Lancaster, Parsons, Xiong, & Zamarripa,

DOI: 10.4018/978-1-5225-0925-7.ch013

1997). Visual stimuli are very important and are the most commonly used stimuli for brain functional activation. For conventional positron emission tomography (PET), computed tomography (CT), single-photon emission tomography (SPECT), and other modalities, the presentation of visual stimuli poses some logistical problems because conventional video monitors can be used, and the scanner typically does not encroach on the subject's field of view. MRI scanners and three-dimensional PET scanners bores are longer, so restrict the patient's view.

There are significant conditional logistical problems involved in MRI. Every device placed within the MR scanning suite must be free of radiofrequency (RF) emissions so as not to degrade the quality of the MRI data that are acquired. Thus, devices must be properly functional in the elevated magnetic field and non-magnetic so they are not drawn into the magnet bore. Moreover, devices placed within the bore must be small enough to accommodate the patient but also non-metallic so as not to distort the magnetic or RF fields and the resultant image. However, the viewing surface should be placed as close to the subject as possible to maximize the viewing angle. Finally, the stimulus presentation system should be compatible with a wide range of input devices (computers, videos, etc.) (Roby, Gao, & Fox, 2000).

FMRI equipment creates images that are both projected onto a mirror inside by refraction and projected directly to the eye through the optical fiber. In addition, some types of visual equipment primarily focus on the central visual field and use high-speed visual stimulation systems (Richlan et al., 2013). However, more attention has recently been placed on peripheral vision, and consequently, peripheral vision visual equipment has been developed (Wu et al., 2013; Yan, Jin, He, & Wu, 2011).

MAIN FOCUS OF THE CHAPTER

1. A Versatile, Low-Cost Method for Presenting Visual Stimuli during MRI Was Developed in 2000

This method consists of passing light through a pattern of holes onto a screen (Hajnal et al., 1994). Pattern-flash systems activate the visual system, whereas complex visual stimuli (e.g., words, objects, moving patterns) can be used to induce activation in a wider range of brain areas.

The most common way to present complex stimuli is through the video projection of a computer-generated image. Systems designed for presenting relaxation videos are commercially available (e.g., MSI, MR Resources, and Magnetic Resonance Technology) and have been adapted for fMRI brain activation research (Cohen, Noll, & Schneider, 1993; Glover, Lemieux, Drangova, & Pauly, 1996; Lewin et al., 1996). In some commercial systems, the screen is normally placed at the subject's feet, and the images are viewed through mirrors. Out-of-bore screen placement greatly reduces the available field of view. To increase the field of view, the projection screen must be moved into the scanner (Glover et al., 1996; Kruger, Kleinschmidt, & Frahm, 1996). Thus, in-bore screen placement decreases the screen size and increases the optical path length. The latter two obstacles can be overcome by using a lens with a long focal length. Placing the projection system within the scanner room can decrease the focal length and avoid projecting though an RF screen. Commercially available liquid crystal display (LCD) projectors and flat screen LCD monitors functionally tolerate high magnetic fields but emit RF interference and must be RF isolated. Because they are manufactured with steel internal structures and contain electrical components, LCD projectors and displays must be placed outside the 50 Gauss field line of the MRI magnet. This present system, termed the Research Imaging Center Visual Projection System (RIC VPS), was designed to improve on previously described systems.

This RIC VPS uses an in-bore screen and an in-room, RF-shielded LCD projector. This system uses readily available, low-cost components. It is magnet-safe and free from RF interference. Because it uses a standard LCD projector, it can be driven by a wide variety of computer and video sources. The RIC VPS has been tested in MRI and in PET. In principle, it is adaptable to any imaging modality.

This system consists of a desktop computer for computer-generated displays, a VCR for taped videos, a video projector, an appropriately long lens, a back projection screen, and mirrors to bend the light path. In our MRI scanner, an angled front surface mirror is paired with a vertical screen to allow the subject to be face up and view the projected image. Because of this system's simplicity, modifications to the setup and adaptations to different scanners are simple and rapid. The MRI configuration of the complete system is illustrated in Figure 1.

Figure 1. The components of the Research Imaging Center Visual Projection System

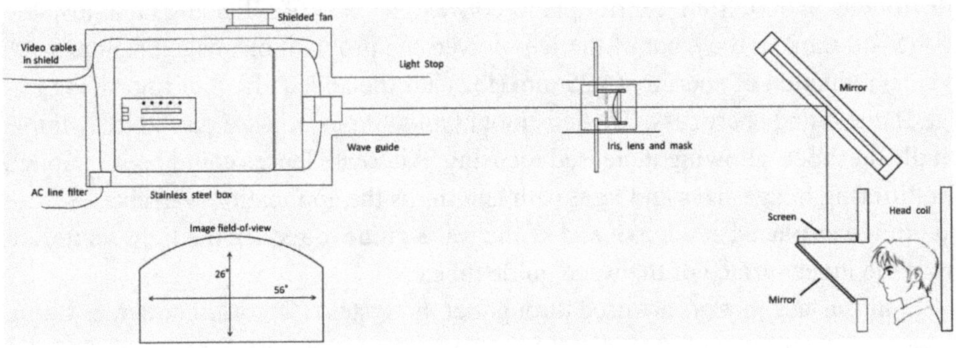

This system uses two LED video projectors, the NEC MultiSync MT and the Sharp HV-H30UA. No modifications were made to the projectors except to remove the standard lens. The Elscint 1.9 T magnet is passively self-shielded; therefore, the projector can be placed near the magnet shielding but outside of the 50 Gauss field line, as recommended by the magnet supplier (Elscint). The adaptability of a multiple digital input projector (NEC MultiSync MT) eliminates the necessity of converting to the NTSC video standard and the associated bandwidth loss and blurred pixels.

This system uses LCD projectors and computers to produce RF interference and must be shielded or removed from the scanner room. A copper screen RF shield was initially placed around the projector to reduce the electromagnetic noise produced by the LCD display with the wiring to the computer run outside the scanner suite. However, the video image quality was degraded by projecting through the screen wire. The current RF shield uses a solid stainless steel case for the projector with copper screen-covered vents and a fan and an aluminum wave guide tube (10 cm diameter, 30 cm long) to allow an obstruction-free light path. One additional requirement for the projector is that the normally supplied lens can be easily removed. The six cables to the projector (Belden, RG59) were run from the console room, through the MRI suite's RF panel, inside the solid and braided copper shielding, and into the shielded projector case. The projector case was grounded to the MRI room shield. The AC line current is required to run the projector and case-cooling fan, which passes into the case through an AC line filter (Corcom, PS0S0DHXB and 10EHT1).

An initial lens (Buhl Optical, 36"/914 mm, f6) was evaluated but yielded unsatisfactory results because of depth of field, focusing, and image flatness problems. The image was also too bright to be viewed comfortably. An 800/63 mm achromatic lens (Melles Griot, 01LAO357) was evaluated and found to solve the image distortion problems because of its simple design and smaller aperture. The current lens used is a 800/50 mm plano-convex lens (Melles Griot, 01LPX343) that displays no perceptual chromatic or spherical aberrations and is very inexpensive (Buhl 36"/f6 lens $3600, Melles Griot plano-convex lens $33.60). Placing an adjustable iris (5–40 mm) in the front of the lens solved the problem of image brightness. A typical reduction of aperture to 25 mm (f32) has the added effect of improving image flatness and sharpness. The lens mount and 40 mm iris are placed in a simple cradle on slides, allowing increased focusing. Alternate lenses could be substituted for differing image sizes and light path lengths as the application warrants. A 5 cm aperture was placed at the exit end of the wave-guide to reduce the light scattering from the inner surface of the wave guide tube.

Front surface mirrors are used throughout the system (Opton). The screens were made from both frosted acrylic and from back-projection screen material (DaLite) that was cut and mounted on an acrylic sheet. The screen and mirror assembly was placed on the top of the head coil above the subject's eyes. The optical path length from the projector to the screen is approximately 4 m, with adjustments to vary the image size. The subject views the back-projection screen from a distance of approximately 19–20 cm, which is comfortable for most people and can be viewed by most subjects without corrective lenses.

This visual presentation system passed the following performance tests:

1. RF interference introduced into the scanner room,
2. Visual field of view, and
3. Image quality.

2. A New High-Speed Visual Stimulation Method Was Used in 2013

The present visual stimulation system should be used in brain electrophysiological studies requiring reliable high-speed visual stimulation.

1. The general projector setup. This present visual stimulation system consists of two projectors (placed behind a semi-transparent screen) that are switched on to visualize the projection areas.
2. Presentation before the invisible boundary was crossed. Only the lower part of the display (containing the degraded sentence on the right-hand side of the invisible boundary) was visible to the participant.
3. Presentation after the invisible boundary was crossed. Only the upper part of the display (containing the un-degraded sentence) was visible to the participant. The red circle indicates the position of the eye of the participant.

A forehead and chin rest stabilized the participant's head 52 cm in front of the monitor. For presentation of the stimuli, they used a PC with a Pentium 4 processor (2.8 GH processor speed), 2 GB RAM, a Nvidia GeForce 6200 graphics card, and a Windows XP operating system. Two presentation setups were compared: the novel projector setup, which was realized with two projectors, and a monitor setup, which was realized with one of the fastest CRT monitors available.

First, a state-of-the-art setup was used to estimate the latencies of gaze-contingent display changes for refresh rates of 150 and 200 Hz with the Vision Master Pro 454 monitor (Iiyama, Japan). For the 150 Hz refresh rate, the display resolution was 1024 × 768 pixels, and for the 200 Hz refresh rate, the display resolution was 640 × 480 pixels.

The projector setup is a new approach to present gaze-contingent displays. Two projectors (with resolutions of 1024 × 768 pixels) that were mounted on top of one another behind a semi-transparent screen were either switched on or off by an electronic circuit. The switching circuit allows very fast display changes despite the low refresh rate of the projectors' LCD units (60 Hz; display change latency of approximately 45 ms as measured by the electronic circuit described in the Display Change Latency Measurement section). An invisible boundary paradigm with one display change was used, which was realized by switching from one projector to the other in the present experiment. To be independent from the refresh rate of the projectors, the same display was presented by both projectors, with the lower part of projector 1 and the upper part of projector 2 converging at the center of a semi-transparent screen (Figure 2c). Projector 1 presented the degraded sentence in the lower part of the display, which was visible to the participant, before the boundary was crossed (Figure 2c). Then, the boundary was crossed, projector 1 was switched off and the un-degraded sentence was presented at the very same position by projector 2 (see Figure 2c). Importantly, only the area where the two projectors converged was visible to the participant sitting in front of the screen. The display change occurred by switching projector 1 off and projector 2 on at the moment the boundary was crossed. This on-and-off switching is independent of the actual refresh rate of the projectors, resulting in faster display change latencies.

The display change content was controlled by the display PC (Figure 3). After the eye tracker indicated that the eye had crossed the invisible boundary, the display change was initiated by a TTL trigger (latency between boundary cross and TTL trigger: between 1 and 2 ms). This trigger was read out by the electronic circuit and resulted in an immediate switching of the two projectors. The fast switching was

Figure 2. The general projector setup

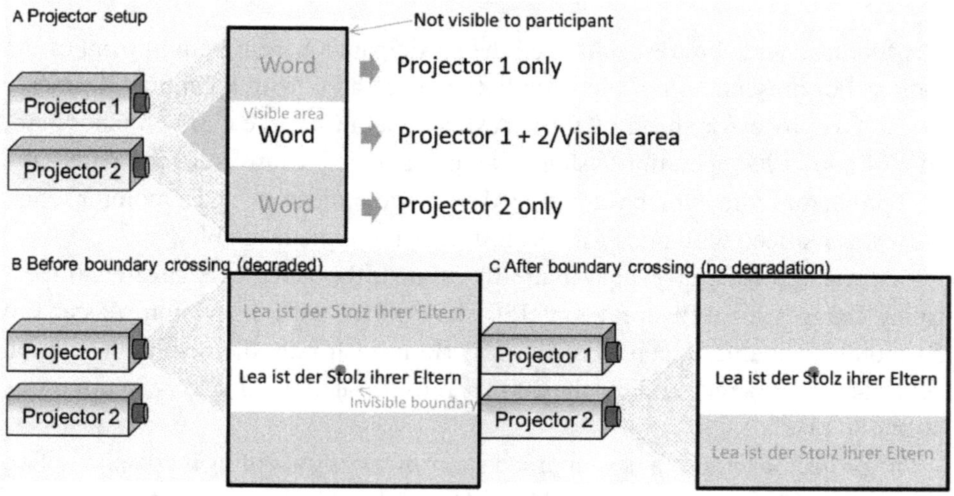

Figure 3. Schematic depiction of the switching circuit

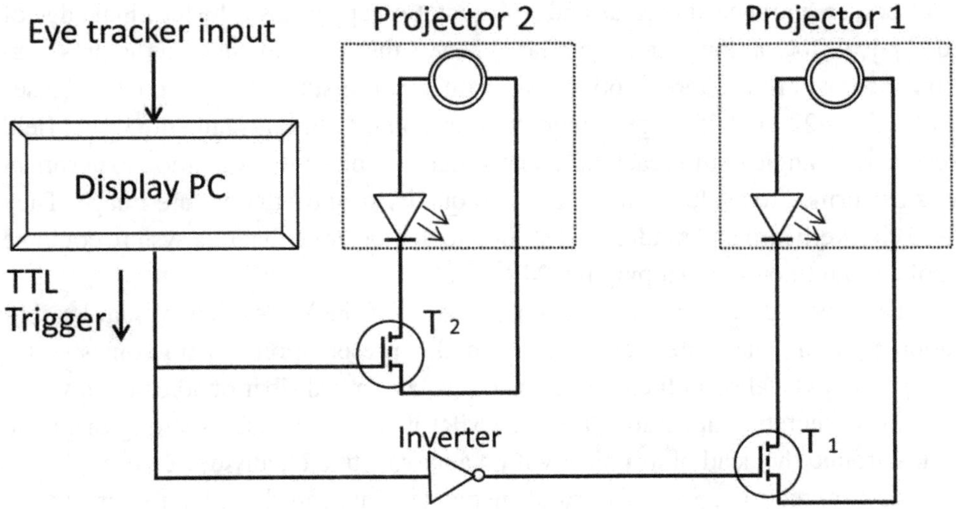

possible because both projectors (SP-F10M, Samsung Electronics Co., Ltd., South Korea) used lighting based on LEDs, which were either switched on or off by transistors. As a consequence, the transistors either connected or disconnected the projectors' LEDs from their original power sources.

Figure 3 shows a schematic depiction of the switching circuit. T1 and T2 mark the power transistors that were used to switch the projectors either on or off. After the eye tracker indicated that the eye had crossed the invisible boundary, the display change was initiated by a TTL trigger. This trigger was read out by the electronic circuit, which either connected or disconnected the projectors' LEDs from their original power sources. Note that this illustration is simplified and that the actual circuit included six transistors—one for each LED of the two projectors.

This present video projection system offers a completely novel method for experiments in fMRI. This present video projection system provides a solution for high-speed visual stimulation as required by many psychological and neuroscientific experiments.

3. Possible Peripheral Vision Visual Equipment Was Also Developed in 2011

A novel wide-view visual presentation system with a horizontal and vertical eccentricity angle of 60° for retinotopic mapping by functional MRI (fMRI) was developed and validated in 2011.

This wide-view stimuli presentation system consists of a 52-mm diameter optical fiber, an entrance apparatus and a presentation apparatus. The terminal edge of the optical fiber at the entrance is flat, whereas the terminal edge on the presentation apparatus is a sphere of 60 mm in diameter. The subjects wore contact lenses with +20, +22, or +25 magnification to focus on the stimulus, and the visual field eccentricity angle could reach 60°. The signal-to-noise ratio valuation experiment was performed to evaluate the clarity and quality of the MRI picture image. They used checkerboard and random dot stimuli to demonstrate that this system could be applied to retinotopic mapping by fMRI.

The above description provides an overview of the Wide-View Visual Presentation System. The wide-view visual stimulus presentation system consists of a computer, a visual stimuli entrance apparatus, an optical fiber bundle, and a visual stimuli presentation apparatus. Because MRI involves the use of strong magnetic fields around the head of a subject within a narrow tunnel, any device used during MRI is required to be free of ferromagnetic elements and should not interact with the magnetic field. Therefore, nonmagnetic materials were used to build the device and optical fiber bundle to present the visual stimulus patterns. The computer was used to control the presentation of stimuli by the operator in the operation room.

The visual stimuli presentation apparatus includes a section of the optical fiber bundle and a holder. Inside the scanner, a plastic optical bundle holder rests on the head coil and supports the optical bundle. The holder is composed of nonferrous materials (PVC) and is easy to set up and remove. Thus, it also allows easy adjustment of the optic bundle position to accommodate various head sizes, eye positions, and inter-pupillary distances. The visual field of the stimulus was 120° horizontal × 120° vertical. Monocular (right eye) presentations were performed with the optical-fiber screen (with a curved surface having a 30-mm curvature radius) placed in the center of the bore, 30 mm from the subjects' eyes. Because the screen was so close to the eyes, the subjects wore contact lenses (Menicon soft MA; Menicon, Japan) with +20, +22, or +25 magnification to retain their length of focus. Enlargement was taken into account when the sizes of the stimuli were calculated. The refraction of light in the three diopter lenses increased the stimulus size by approximately 8.9% (+20) to 11.3% (+25) of the stimuli.

The visual stimuli entrance apparatus consisted of an entrance display, a section of the optical fiber bundle, a supporting stand for the fiber bundle and a display box . The visual stimuli were created on a display with a resolution of 800 × 600 pixels.

The optical fiber bundle was composed of 8700 optical fibers (0.5 mm in diameter, CK-20, Eska; Mitsubishi, Japan) for a total outer bundle diameter of 52 mm, and the length was approximately 5500 mm. The center of the optical fibers was arranged so that the stimuli could be presented in the same way as they were presented at the entrance. The edge side in the entrance part of the optical fiber bundle was a planar surface, whereas the edge side of the presentation part was a sphere of 60 mm in diameter. To make the presentation part into a sphere of 60 mm in diameter, the presentation part was bonded by using soap bubbles that were 60 mm in diameter while performing a positional match at each spatial position. To prevent light from mixing into the plasmotomy and the outside of the optical fiber with the visual stimulus, the optical fiber bundle was covered with a plastic sleeve.

The fMRI experiment was performed using a 1.5 Tesla (T) Philips clinical scanner (Intera Achieva; Best, The Netherlands) for safety and the signal-to-noise ratio tests. The following parameters were used: TR/TE = 2000/50 ms; FA = 90°; matrix size = 64 × 64; and voxel size = 3 × 3 × 3 mm. Before acquiring the functional images, T2-weighted anatomical images were obtained in the same planes as the functional images using the spin echo sequence. A T1-weighted high-resolution image (1 × 1 × 1 mm) was also acquired after each functional experiment. The signal-to-noise (SNR) was calculated using the following formula [1]:

$$SNR = \frac{\left(2 - \frac{\grave{A}}{2}\right)^{\frac{1}{2}}}{N_{air}} \times S_p \tag{1}$$

Sp is the mean of the signals in the phantom; N_{air} is the standard deviation of outside noise. The average SNR was calculated from ten MRI images for the two conditions and is shown in Figure 5. The SNR results with and without the wide-view visual presentation system were 110.85 and 117.22, respectively. The image digressive rate with the device was 6.37%. They found no artifacts created by radiofrequency noise in the phantom's phase encoding.

4. A New Wide-View Visual Stimuli System in MRI Was Developed in 2013

This wide-view visual stimulus presentation system consists of a presentation apparatus, a projection apparatus and an operation computer. Computer-generated stimuli were projected onto a translucent hemispheric screen inside the MRI bore. The operator used a computer located in the observation room to control the presentation of the stimuli.

The presentation apparatus was attached to the MRI head coil via the mirror stand placed on the head coil. The subjects were able to directly view the stimuli when lying in the MRI scanner. The visual stimulus presentation apparatus included a hemispheric screen and a screen fixture with a mirror fixture. The visual stimulus presentation apparatus inside the MRI core in Figure 4a and Figure 4b shows a frontal view of the presentation apparatus.

Figure 5. Front view showing the design and size of the screen fixture. A screw was used to easily adjust and fix the screen.

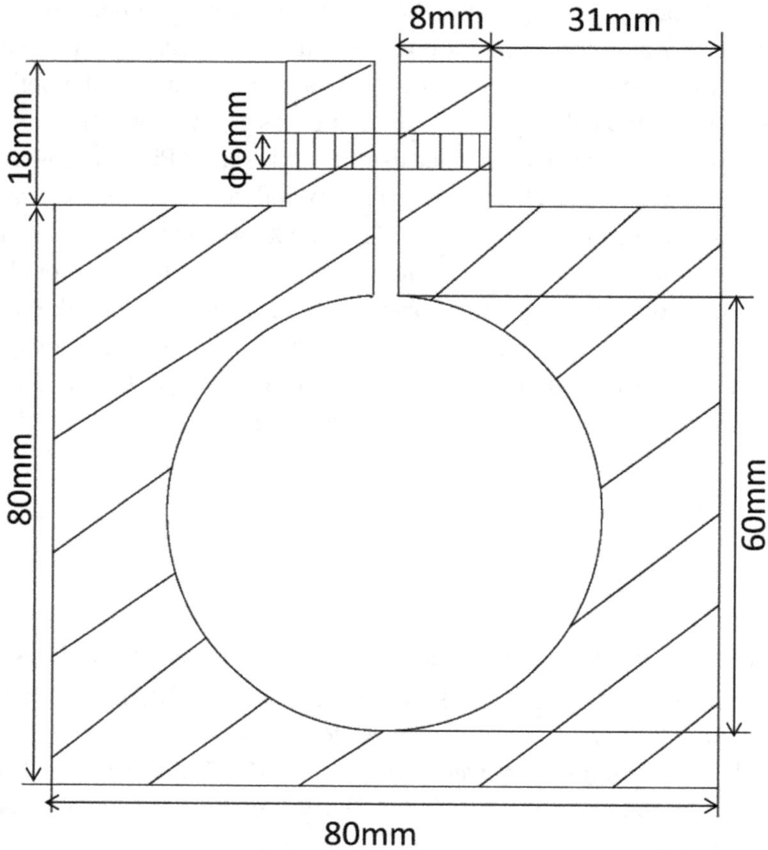

Figure 4. The composition and mechanism of the presentation apparatus

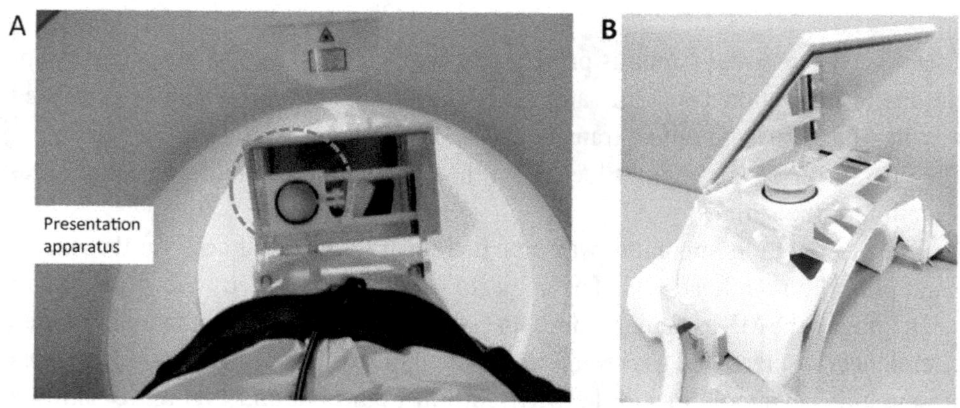

The screen fixture was made using a transparent poly plant with a thickness of 10 mm. The position of the screen fixture could be regulated to match variations in the subjects' head sizes. Figure 5 shows the square outside and round inside design of the parts. The round interior had a diameter of approximately 60 mm, which was regulated by a screw. To keep the screen steady, a layer of 4 mm thick ethylene-vinyl acetate was pasted on the surface of the inner diameter.

The mirror fixture was used to fix the mirror and to support the screen fixture. The design and size of the mirror fixture is shown in Figure 6. A female screw and

Figure 6. Front view showing the design and size of the mirror fixture. (a) The design of the support part was used on both sides of the mirror fixture. A female screw and a male screw were used on this part to adjust the mirror angle. The two holes at the bottom of the component were used to fix the component during the machining process. (b) The bars linking the two support parts.

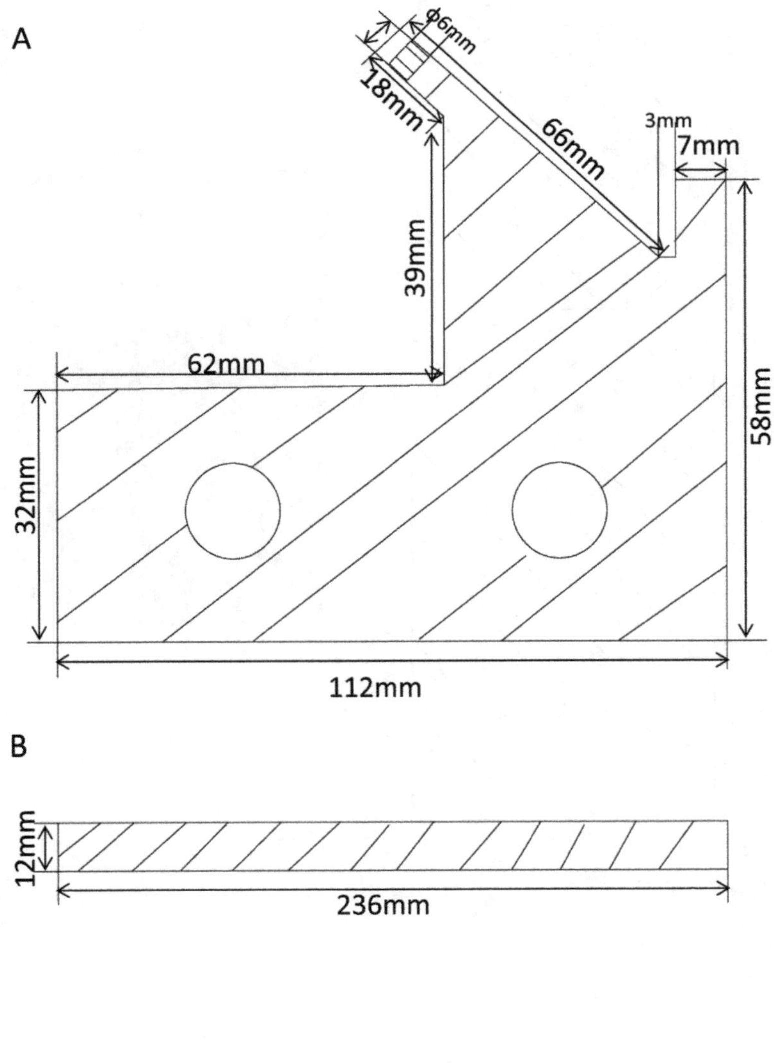

a male screw located on the mirror fixture were used to adjust the mirror angle from 40° to 50°. The completed part was pasted together using a-cyanoacrylate adhesive super glue. A 3D view of the assembled mirror fixture is shown in Figure 6c.

As shown Figure 7a, the hemispheric screen was made from a transparent poly (methyl methacrylate) column measuring 52 mm in diameter and 75 mm in length. On one of the column's extremities, a hemisphere measuring 52 mm in diameter with a curvature of 30 mm was made. Because of the size limitations of the head coil, the upper and lower edges of the hemisphere were cut by 2 mm to a final size of 48 mm. The inner surface of the hemisphere was coated with a thin layer of photographer's dulling spray to make a translucent screen (Figure 7b).

Figure 7. (a) The design and size of the hemispheric screen. (b) The hemispheric screen (the white surface is the screen).

A

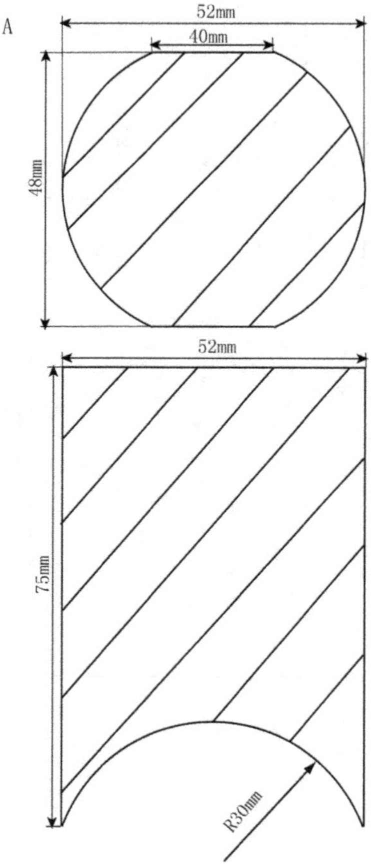

B

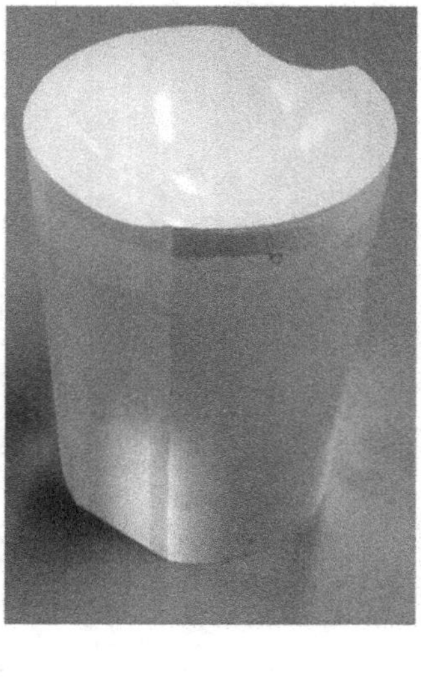

1. The visual stimulus presentation apparatus in the bore of the MRI scanner. The dashed line outlines the presentation apparatus.
2. The front view shows the components of the presentation apparatus, which include a hemispheric screen, screen fixture, mirror fixture and mirror. The mirror fixture was fixed onto the head coils of the MRI machine. The mirror angle could be adjusted from 40° to 50° by adjusting the two screws. To match variations in subject head size, the distance between the screen and the bottom of the mirror could be adjusted from 0 to 42 mm. When the distance between the screen and the subject's eyes was 30 mm, the screen field view was 120°. Subjects wore contact lenses (Menicon soft MA, Menicon, Japan) with +20, +22, or +25 magnification to retain their focal length.

Monocular (left or right eye) presentations were performed using the hemispheric screen for this present wide-view visual stimuli system. The subject's eye was fixed on the central axis, 3 mm distant from the screen. Because of the screen's close proximity to the subjects' eyes, the subjects wore +20, +22, or +25 contact lenses (Menicon soft MA, Menicon, Japan) to retain their length of visual focus (Figure 4). Because of the size limitations of the head coil, 2 mm of the upper and lower edges of the screen were removed; thus, the final hemispheric screen size was 52 × 48 mm. The eye was located at the spherical center of the hemispheric screen. In this condition, the horizontal visual field was 120°, and the vertical visual field was 116° (Figure 4). The distance between the eye and the center of the screen could not be directly measured. A tool and method were developed for determining the position of the hemispheric screen relative to the eye. A probe bar was used to position the surface of the hemispheric screen 30 mm from the eye and to make the axis of the hemispheric screen and the axis of the eye overlap.

A Mitsubishi LVP-HC6800 projector (Mitsubishi Electric, Tokyo, Japan) was configured to operate at a 1600 × 1200 pixel resolution and a 60 Hz refresh rate for projection. The standard lens was replaced, and a 70–300 mm focal length camera zoom lens (Nikon, Tokyo, Japan) was used to achieve small, high-resolution images on a screen located inside the bore. The reconstituted projector presented 18 × 13.5 cm images at a distance of 4 m. The projector was placed approximately 3 m away from the MRI scanner and approximately 4 m away from the hemispheric screen.

The spherical coordinate system is arguably the most natural choice of coordinate systems for the study of vision. A function f, described by Equation (2), was used to generate "distorted" 2D images of geometrical shapes specified by spherical coordinates (Yu & Rosa, 2010).

The function f: $(\lambda, \phi) \rightarrow (x, y)$ is

$$x = g(ecc(\lambda, \phi)) \times \cos(ang(\lambda, \phi))$$

$$y = g(ecc(\lambda, \phi)) \times \sin(ang(\lambda, \phi)) \quad (2)$$

in which λ is the longitude of the point on the hemisphere, ϕ is the latitude of the point on the hemisphere, $ecc(\lambda, \phi)$ is the eccentricity, $ang(\lambda, \phi)$ is the polar angle in the polar coordinate system, and $g(ecc(\lambda, \phi))$ is the eccentricity of the corresponding point on the projector's image plane. The intensity of the distorted image was regulated based on the actual measurement intensity.

The light is projected through the bore, reflected by an adjustable mirror (40°–50°), and ultimately focused onto the hemispheric screen. To maximize the precision of the method and avoid geometric distortions, the central axis of the light beam was aligned with the central axis of the hemispheric screen. A 52 × 48 mm size image with a 460 × 425 pixel resolution was presented on the hemispheric screen. Approximately 154,000 pixels were presented on the screen with a round shaped hemispheric screen. The luminance at the internal surface of the hemisphere on six level eccentricities (5°, 15°, 25°, 35°, 45° and 55°) in eight directions was measured. The luminance values were averaged. As the eccentricities increased, the mean luminance values of white were 143.3, 139.2, 146.2, 145.3, 137.2 and 138.5 cd/m^2, and the mean luminance values of black were 3.1, 3.1, 3.2, 2.8, 3.3 and 3.4 cd/m^2.

This wide-view visual presentation system was tested with the stimulus during the MRI scan (spin echo, TR/TE = 3000/15 ms, 256 ×256 matrix, 15 continuous 5 mm slices without gap) for safety and signal-to-noise ratio tests. Artifacts created by the radio frequency noise from the image of the phantom were not detected. The SNR was calculated using the following formula [3]:

$$SNR = \frac{\left(2 - \frac{\grave{A}}{2}\right)^{\frac{1}{2}}}{N_{air}} \times S_p \quad (3)$$

in which Sp is the mean of the signals in the phantom; N_{air} is the standard deviation of the outside noise. The average SNR was calculated from the MRI images for two conditions. The SNR was 187.50 without the device and 189.58 when the device was active. The digressive image rate with the device was 1.11%. They did not detect any artifacts created by the radio frequency noise from the image of the phantom from this present wide-view visual stimuli system in MRI.

CONCLUSION

The above systems were present in the MRI equipment that is currently and commonly used for presenting visual stimuli. The current trends are well developed for the systematic presentation of high-resolution, wide-view images in MRI.

ACKNOWLEDGMENT

This study was supported in part by the JAPAN SOCIETY FOR THE PROMOTION OF SCIENCE (JSPS) KAKENHI, grant numbers: 25249026 and 25303013; a Grant-in-Aid for Strategic Research Promotion from Okayama University

REFERENCES

Cohen, J. D., Noll, D. C., & Schneider, W. (1993). Functional magnetic resonance imaging: Overview and methods for psychological research. *Behavior Research Methods, Instruments, & Computers*, *25*(2), 101–113. doi:10.3758/BF03204483

Fox, P. T., Lancaster, J. L., Parsons, L. M., Xiong, J. H., & Zamarripa, F. (1997). Functional volumes modeling: theory and preliminary assessment. *Hum Brain Mapp, 5*(4), 306-311. doi: 10.1002/(SICI)1097-0193(1997)5:4<306::AID-HBM17>3.0.CO;2-B

Glover, G. H., Lemieux, S. K., Drangova, M., & Pauly, J. M. (1996). Decomposition of inflow and blood oxygen level-dependent (BOLD) effects with dual-echo spiral gradient-recalled echo (GRE) fMRI. *Magnetic Resonance in Medicine*, *35*(3), 299–308. doi:10.1002/mrm.1910350306 PMID:8699940

Hajnal, J. V., Myers, R., Oatridge, A., Schwieso, J. E., Young, I. R., & Bydder, G. M. (1994). Artifacts due to stimulus correlated motion in functional imaging of the brain. *Magnetic Resonance in Medicine*, *31*(3), 283–291. doi:10.1002/mrm.1910310307 PMID:8057799

Kruger, G., Kleinschmidt, A., & Frahm, J. (1996). Dynamic MRI sensitized to cerebral blood oxygenation and flow during sustained activation of human visual cortex. *Magnetic Resonance in Medicine*, *35*(6), 797–800. doi:10.1002/mrm.1910350602 PMID:8744004

Lewin, J. S., Friedman, L., Wu, D., Miller, D. A., Thompson, L. A., Klein, S. K., & Duerk, J. L. et al. (1996). Cortical localization of human sustained attention: Detection with functional MR using a visual vigilance paradigm. *Journal of Computer Assisted Tomography*, *20*(5), 695–701. doi:10.1097/00004728-199609000-00002 PMID:8797896

Richlan, F., Gagl, B., Schuster, S., Hawelka, S., Humenberger, J., & Hutzler, F. (2013). A new high-speed visual stimulation method for gaze-contingent eye movement and brain activity studies. *Frontiers in Systems Neuroscience*, *7*, 24. doi:10.3389/fnsys.2013.00024 PMID:23847475

Roby, J. W., Gao, J. H., & Fox, P. T. (2000). A versatile, low-cost method for presenting visual stimuli during MRI. *Journal of Magnetic Resonance Imaging*, *11*(2), 223–227. doi:10.1002/(SICI)1522-2586(200002)11:2<223::AID-JMRI22>3.0.CO;2-G PMID:10713958

Wu, J., Wang, B., Yang, J., Hikino, Y., Takahashi, S., Yan, T., & Kanazawa, S. et al. (2013). Development of a method to present wide-view visual stimuli in MRI for peripheral visual studies. *Journal of Neuroscience Methods*, *214*(2), 126–136. doi:10.1016/j.jneumeth.2013.01.021 PMID:23376498

Yan, T., Jin, F., He, J., & Wu, J. (2011). Development of a wide-view visual presentation system for visual retinotopic mapping during functional MRI. *Journal of Magnetic Resonance Imaging*, *33*(2), 441–447. doi:10.1002/jmri.22404 PMID:21274987

Yu, H. H., & Rosa, M. G. P. (2010). A simple method for creating wide-field visual stimulus for electrophysiology: Mapping and analyzing receptive fields using a hemispheric display. *Journal of Vision*, *10*(14). doi:10.1167/10.14.15

KEY TERMS AND DEFINITIONS

fMRI: Functional magnetic resonance imaging is a technique for measuring and mapping brain activity that is noninvasive and safe.

Projection System: Relates to a method of and means for clearly showing luminous pictures, more particularly television images upon fluorescent screens and cinematographic pictures upon a projection screen, in illuminated rooms.

Visual Cortex: The visual cortex of the brain is the part of the cerebral cortex responsible for processing visual information. The visual cortex is made up of Brodmann area 17 (the primary visual cortex), and Brodmann areas 18 and 19, the extrastriate cortical areas.

Visual Presentation: Visual presentation aims for communicating and sharing information in a dataset visually to others (e.g., experts for detailed analysis). The visual presentation must emphasize the relevant information among the rest of the data. This is of particular importance since presentations are often realized on print media, which allow for no or only little interaction.

APPENDIX

List of Suppliers

- MRI system (Elscint, Ltd., Haifa, Israel)
- Head gradient coil (Advanced NMR, Wilmington, MA)
- Projection screen material (DaLite, Inc., Warsaw, IN)
- Lenses (Melles Griot, Irvine, CA; Buhl Optical Co., Pittsburgh, PA)
- Front surface mirror (Opton, Inc., Newport News, VA)
- Video projectors (NEC Technologies Inc., Box boro, MA; Sharp Electronics Corp., Mahwah, NJ)
- Cables (Belden Wire & Cable, Richmond, IN)
- Projection systems (Resonance Technology Co., Van Nuys, CA; MSI, Tampa, FL)
- Prism glasses (MR Resources, Gardner, MA)
- Fiber optic glasses (Avotec Inc., Jensen Beach, FL)
- Virtual retinal display (Microvision, Seattle, WA)
- AC line filters (Corcom, Libertyville, IL)
- Ophthalmic lens (Lombart, Norfolk, VA)

Chapter 14
Humanoid Robots:
Future Avatars for Humans through BCI

Si Zhang
Beijing Institute of Technology, China

Jinglong Wu
Beijing Institute of Technology, China

Qiang Huang
Beijing Institute of Technology, China

ABSTRACT

This paper provides a review of humanoid robots and mind control humanoid robots. Information was obtained mainly from journals and conference proceedings on robotics and mind control technology. We primarily focus on providing an overview of commercially available robots and prototype research-stage humanoid robots in addition to mind control humanoid robot systems. First, a history and overview of the humanoid robot is presented. Then, typical mind control humanoid robot systems are described, including the relevant brain-computer interface and the whole control framework. Finally, the remaining research challenges in the field of humanoid robot safety are summarized.

DOI: 10.4018/978-1-5225-0925-7.ch014

INTRODUCTION

A humanoid robot is a robot with human appearance and behavior. These qualities provide this kind of robot with a more human-friendly appearance that is more acceptable to individuals. Human robots are used as a research tool to promote the development of scientific areas such as biomechanics, biomechanical controls, sensors, and mechanisms, computer science, and artificial intelligence. A human shape and appearance also make it possible for humanoid robots to adapt to surroundings similar to those of humans (including a normal environment and some dangerous or dirty environments) and to utilize tools designed for humans (Sakamoto 2005; Behnke, 2008). These advantages make humanoid robots the best choice for serve humans in daily life or for improving the lives of the elderly or physically disabled people.

Brain Computer Interfaces (BCIs) are communication systems that allow external devices, including computers and robots, to be controlled by brain activity. Humanoid robot surrogates controlled using BCI can help users, especially the elderly and physical disabled, to regain autonomy. The user can meld his/her own mind and movements with a robot surrogate or avatar. The development of robotics and BCI currently make the idea of avatars a possibility. Compared to other types of robots, humanoid robots, with their human size and appearance, are more suitable for use as special avatars for individuals.

This paper presents a review of the recent literature in the field of humanoid robots. The review is divided into three inter-related sections:

1. An overview of humanoid robots,
2. Mind control humanoid robots, and
3. Safety for humanoid robots.

More specifically, the first section presents a history and overview of humanoid robots. The second section describes the mind actuated humanoid robot system, which is a new trend in the application of humanoid robots. Finally, the last section addresses key research into the safety of humanoid robots, including a discussion of safety issues for both robots and humans.

BACKGROUND

Researchers have made substantial progress in the field of humanoid robots since the first such robot, WABOT-1 (Kato,1973), was developed in 1973. The field of humanoid robots can be divided into two broad classes, fully actuated and passive robots, according to the mode of control.

Inspired by the work of McGeer (1990), passive walking humanoid robots forgo full actuation and allow gravity and natural dynamics to play a large part in the generation of their motions. They may be completely passive or partially actuated. Research into this type of humanoid robot is mainly focused on the generation of human-like and highly efficient motions (Manoj, 2006; Steve, 2005) and not on serving in human surroundings. The widely used humanoid robots that were developed for undertaking these types (human environment) of tasks are fully actuated robots, which consist of position control and force/torque control robots.

Position Control Humanoid Robots

Position control robots are driven by motors that connect joints with reducers. The control parameters in these robots are joint angle and angular velocity.

ASIMO, which was developed by Honda in 1997, is a representative of joint position controlled biped robots. ASIMO (Cleland, 2002) initially possessed the ability to walk and manipulate objects under certain circumstances, such as serving tea, carting and walking on rough terrain (Hirose, 2007). Later, these robots were constructed with decision-making and real-time planning capabilities that functioned under uncertain circumstances. It can also run at a speed of 9 km/h.

Waseda University, a pioneer in biped robots, has developed multiple generations of biped robots. In 2006, the new generation biped robot WABIAN-2R achieved human-like walking with knee stretching via the addition of degree of freedoms (DOFs) at its hip and passive toe joints (Ogura, 2006). These changes allowed the robot to achieve quick turning using a slipping motion that involved both feet.

HRP-2 (Hirukawa, 2007) and HRP-3, which were developed by AIST in 1998, can complete a variety of dexterous movements, and they possess the ability to walk, move across obstacles, lift objects from the ground and carry weights similar to those that can be carried by humans. To increase performance, HRP-4 was constructed with a decreased weight. The HRP-4C is designed to walk quickly and to achieve facial expressions. HRP3 L-JSK, which was developed by AIST and the University of Tokyo in 2012, can recognize disturbance rejection while standing and walk at a speed of 5 km/h (Ito, 2011; Urata, 2012).

The KHR series robot was developed by KAIST, Korea. The robot HUBO (KHR-3), which was developed in 2008, can achieve walking with its knee stretched at a speed of 1.4 km/h and running at a speed of 3.6 km/h (Kim, 2008). The latest version, DHR-HUBO, was the winner of the DARPA Robotics Challenge (DRC) finals in 2015. Inspired by the Fukushima-Daiichi nuclear accident, DRC is motivating the development of robotic technologies that can be used in hazardous environments. The DRC finals required the robot to attempt a circuit of consecutive physical tasks. The robot DHR-HUBO was designed to be an adaptable multifunctional device that possesses the ability to transform from a standing position that is used for bipedal walking to a kneeling pose that allows it to roll on 4 wheels by bending and using wheels that were incorporated into its knees.

The BHR series of robots can walk straight and sideways, go around objects, climb stairs, and perform "Taiji" and martial arts. These humanoid robots have been under development since 2000 at the Beijing Institute of Technology (Huang, 2002; Yu 2014). BHR-5 is a newly built bipedal robot that has abilities including vision, hearing, and force and equilibrium sensing capabilities that are focused on performing manipulations while it moves quickly. It can, for example, play table tennis. The BHR-6 is currently under development and is aimed at achieving multimode locomotion.

Force Control Humanoid Robot

There are three driven modes for force control robots, namely electric, hydraulic and pneumatic. Hydraulic and pneumatic components drive joints directly, while motors usually drive joints through a series of springs to achieve force control.

Developed by Boston Dynamics, PETMAN is an amazing robot that is famous for its life-like appearance and powerful strength. It was designed to test chemical protection clothing, and it can accomplish natural agile movements, move across obstacles, and do push-ups. The newly built robot Atlas is a high mobility humanoid robot that was designed to work in extremely environments. In extremely challenging terrain, Atlas can move through congested spaces using its hands and feet. It also received a good score at the DRC in 2015.

CHIMP, a disaster response robot with a four-limbed design that was built by Carnegie Mellon University, finished third at the DRC. It rolls across terrain on rubberized tracks like a tank. This reduces the risk of toppling over. Under rough conditions, it can drop to all fours to increase stability.

With the aim of increasing stability control when disturbed, the M2 V2 robot was developed by IHMC. It is powered by a force controllable series of elastic actuators (SEAs). These actuators provide the robot with high fidelity and low impedance, which allows it to perform controlling techniques that exploit the natural dynamics of the robot (Pratt, 2008; 2012).

To make humanoid robots that can perform more natural and human-like activities, some actuators of humanoid robots have been developed to simulate real muscle. Robot Lucy, which was developed by the University of Brussels in 2007, was built with pneumatic artificial muscles that simultaneously control the torque and stiffness of the joints. Kenshiro, which was developed by Tokyo University, more accurately simulates humans. It has the same joint arrangements and muscle structures as humans, but with complex musculoskeletal construction (64 joint DOFs except hands DOFs with 11 on spine) that makes it difficult to control (Asano, 2012; Nakanishi, 2012).

MIND CONTROL HUMANOID ROBOTS

The humanoid robot Pepper was developed in 2014 with the aim of living with humans. This robot currently greets and interacts with customers in Softbank Mobile stores. It recognizes human facial expressions, voices, and tones and key words that can help it to analyze emotions. It can also react to motions with expressions, motions and voice, and it can dance and tell jokes. The robot Pepper confirms the significance of fusing multiple sources of information. However, like traditional service robots, Pepper interacts with humans using a pre-programed control system without understanding what the humans are thinking about. Because the ultimate goal of service robots is to be companions for humans, robot Pepper is only the beginning. Humanoid robots that can understand human intentions and do tasks guided by the user's mind as an avatar will be a new trend in the future.

The idea of moving robots or prosthetic devices using human brain activity instead of manual control has fascinated researchers for the past 50 years. With gradual improvements in neuroscience and brain science, a great deal of progress has been made in research into BCIs, which make mind-controlled robot systems possible.

Brain Computer Interfaces

BCIs, which are sometimes called brain-machine interfaces (BMIs), form a direct pathway for communication between the brain and an external device that provides the human with the ability to control the machine or robot, and this would be particularly useful for the elderly and the disabled. The history of BCIs starts with discovery of electrical activity in the human brain in 1929 (Berger, 1938). Research into BCIs began in 1973 at the University of California Los Angeles (UCLA) (Vidal, 1973). Research into brain-controlled robot systems has focused mainly on three aspects: brain-actuated wheelchairs, brain-actuated prostheses and mind-controlled robot systems. As demand has grown for assisted rehabilitation and improvements in BCI performance, research into noninvasive BCIs has extended into the field of auxiliary motion. The typical symbol of this phase was the emergence of the brain-actuated wheelchair. A brain-actuated wheelchair system that was designed by Ecole Polytechnique Fe de rale de Lausanne (EPFL) was able to navigate the wheelchair using brain activity, demonstrating the feasibility of continuously controlling a complex robotic device using an asynchronous and non-invasive BCI (Millan, 2009). Many studies have examined brain-actuated prostheses, which provide a degree of real convenience to the disabled (Taylor, 2002; Hochberg, 2006; Vora, 2004; Pfurtscheller, 2003; Farwell, 1988). On the other hand, many studies have suggested using BCI to control a humanoid robot directly using brain signals transmitted non-invasively via electroencephalography (EEG). A formalized schematic of BCI-based robot systems, which consist of three elements (the user, the robot, and the BCI) is shown in Figure 1.

The techniques used to measure brain signals for BCI can be divided into two classes: invasive and non-invasive. Invasive methods, such as implanted electrodes and electrocorticography (ECoG), are more risky because they require neurosurgery, whereas non-invasive methods do not. Non-invasive methods include electroencephalography (EEG), magnetoencephalography (MEG), functional nearinfrared spectroscopy signals (fNIRS), functional magnetic resonance imaging (fMRI), positron emission tomography (PET), and event-related optical signal (EROS). Because of its small size, high temporal resolution and low cost, electroencephalography (EEG) is by far the most widely used technique for recording human brain activity in BCI applications.

Figure 1. General design of BCI-based humanoid robots

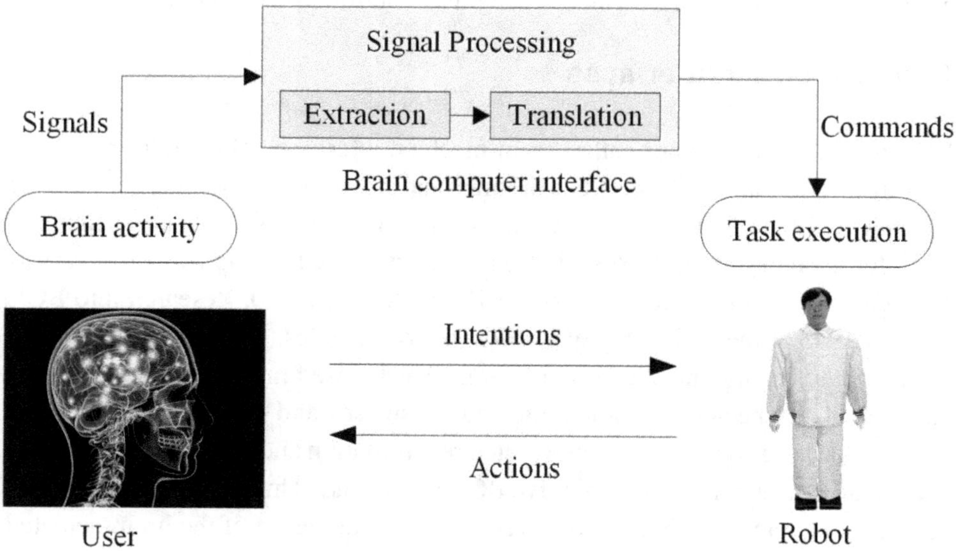

Studies have described BCI techniques that are used to control robots directly using brain signals that were obtained non-invasively via electroencephalography (EEG). Some of the popular methods of non-invasively obtaining brain signals from the scalp to control humanoid robots have included P300, motor imagery (MI), and steady state visual-evoked potentials (SSVEP).

P300 BCI-Based Humanoids

An event-related potential (ERP) is a brain response that is caused by certain events, such as light flashes or unexpected/novel stimuli. It is visible in the time domain. An ERP signal changes along several characteristic components (as positive and negative peaks) after stimulus onset. P300, which is also known as P3, is a positive peak that occurs approximately 300 ms after stimulus onset. It is most commonly elicited in an "oddball" paradigm when a subject detects an occasional target stimulus in a regular train of standard stimuli. The P300 wave only occurs if the subject is actively engaged in the task of detecting the targets. Its amplitude varies according to the improbability of the targets (Picton, 1992).

The P300 BCI presents the user with a screen on which stimuli (flashes) appear at different locations. The user must pay attention to the locations of the stimuli to count them. The target event can then be detected because it is followed by a higher amplitude P300. The typical technique for reading P300 waves is to use a P300 speller. In the speller, the BCI uses the presence or absence of P300 responses to determine which letter the user was paying attention to while watching letters on an on-screen keyboard randomly light up.

Bell C.J. et al., at the University of Washington, used a brain–computer interface (BCI) to command a Fujitsu HOAP2 humanoid robot to pick up a target box between a red box and a green box by giving it the ability to detect P300 signals. The robot then brought the box to a predefined location using a machine learning technique. This research is a remarkable example of brain-actuated humanoid robot navigation control (Bell, 2008).

HOAP-2 is a humanoid robot with 25 DOFs, including a camera on its head with which it can obtain visual feedback. The robot is programmed to be able to autonomously walk, navigate and pick up or place an object based on visual information. The robot locates the target object using its vision and then sends to the BCI for the choice of the user. In this system, then environment is already familiar to the humanoid robot, in which it has been trained to execute five complex humanoid motions.

Motor Imagery BCI-Based Humanoids

Motor imagery (MI) can be defined as a dynamic state during which an individual mentally simulates a given action. During this phenomenal experience, the subject feels herself/himself performing the action. The actions that are most commonly simulated using BCI systems are left/right hand, left/right leg and tong movements (Pfurtscheller, 1997; Henrik, 2003; Wolpaw, 2005). These activities generate sensorimotor rhythms (SMRs), which produce EEG signals with good signal-to-noise ratio (NR) that can easily be distinguished from each other when the electrodes are optimally positioned on the scalp. It has been shown that there are optimal electrode positions and frequency components for each person (Benjamin, 2007). Hence, it is necessary to train the user to utilize this method.

When the user imagines a left hand (or foot) motion, the amplitude of mu-rhythm activity in the sensory-motor area of the brain increases in the left hemisphere and decreases in the right hemisphere, while the converse occurs when the user imagines a right hand (or foot) motion.

MI BCI-Based NAO

Chae et al. (2011, 2012) designed a BCI that transmits five low level motion commands (including "stop", "turn the body", "turn the head to the left or right", and "walk around") to a humanoid robot NAO by combining three motor imagery (MI) states (e.g. "left hand", "right hand", and "foot") with a posture-dependent control architecture. To adapt to an unknown environment, a monocular camera is set on the head of the robot. This approach suggests another brain-actuated humanoid navigation system that also allows for flexible robotic motion control in unknown environments.

The framework of the whole system is shown in Figure 2. It consists of three components, including the BCI system, the interface system and the humanoid control system. The BCI system is used to classify the user's mental state. The interface system is used to display data, including the visual field of the robot's camera and the mental states that were classified by the BCI system.

Three main procedures are followed during the extent of the real-time control process, including offline non-feedback training, the online feedback test and the real-time control of the humanoid. During the offline session, the feedback system gives a training cue. The subject tries to imagine the intended motor task while the BCI records the EEG. After the training session, the BCI system extracts features. During the online feedback test, the trained BCI system extracts the subject's mental state from the ongoing EGG signals. The feedback system then identifies men-

Figure 2. System architecture for mind control NAO
Source: Adapted from Chae, 2012

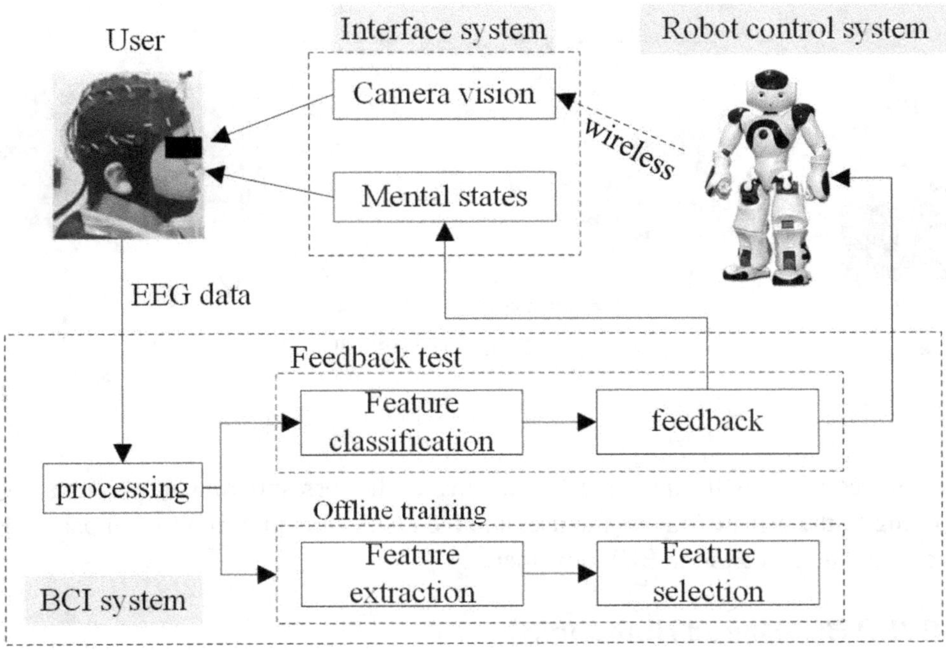

tal states from the EEG signals using fade-in rules. In the control session, the subject navigates the humanoid robot.

MI BCI-Based ASIMO

The Honda Research Institute Japan Co. uses EEG and near-infrared spectroscopy (NIRS) in combination with newly developed information extraction technology to control the humanoid ASIMO using only human thought. EEG (via electrical potentials from the scalp that reflect MI states) is used to measure changes in brain waves, and NIRS measures changes in cerebral blood flow. After being provided with body part options, the user is asked to imagine moving the corresponding body part without making any physical movements. BCI is used to measure and extract information from the complex information that is sent to two different types of sensors.

The flowchart of the full experimental process is shown in Figure 3. First, EGG and NIRS sensors are placed on the user's scalp. Then, one of the four predetermined body part options (including "left hand", "right hand", "tongue", and "feet") is provided to user. The user is asked to imagine moving that body part. During the procedure, changes in brain waves and cerebral blood flow are measured

Figure 3. Overview of mind control HRP-2 framework
Source: Adapted from Petit (2015)

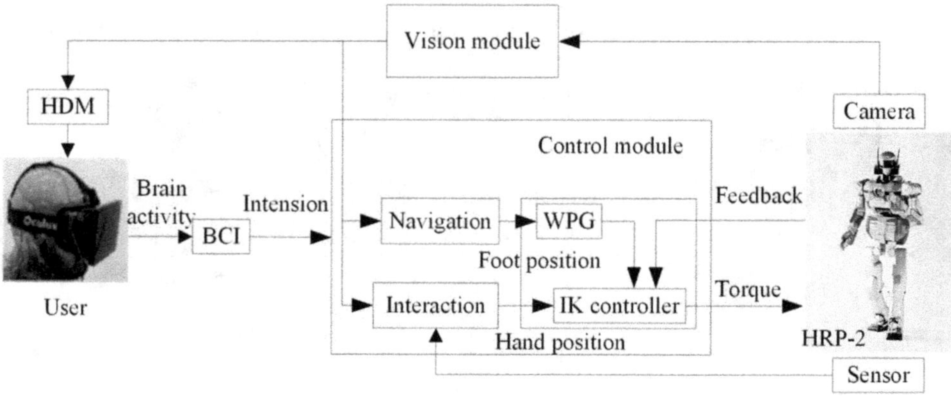

simultaneously. Finally, the robot ASIMO makes the corresponding movements according to the instructions by the use, and the results are analyzed to compare the user-imagined data to the BCI movements.

SSVEP BCI-Based Humanoid

The SSVEP is a periodic neural response that is located in the subject's central visual field. SSVEP is induced by flickering visual stimuli. It occurs in the frequency domain. Whether a certain frequency makes a high contribution or not can be determined by detecting the presence or absence of an SSVEP response while a subject is gazing at different signals with different frequencies. SSVEPs have been used in a number of BCIs that rely on voluntary control, such as wheelchair BCIs (Müller, 2008; 2010).

SSVEP-based BCIs operate by exposing the user to oscillating visual stimuli (different frequencies). The user chooses a command by concentrating on one of the stimuli (one frequency). Then, the BCI measures the electrical activity that corresponds to the frequency of the oscillation.

SSVEP BCI-Based PR2

The PR2 robot, which was developed by Willow Garage, is a wheeled robot with two arms and grippers. This semi-humanoid robot has a head with 2 DOFs and two arms with 7-8 DOFs each. It combines the ability to navigate human environments with the ability to manipulate objects. Matthew B. et al. from the University of Washington used a hierarchical EEG-based BCI to train and control the PR2 humanoid robot and to maneuver the robot's arm to pour milk over a bowl of cereal. The results showed that the humanoid robot could be instructed to perform complex tasks by using brain signals (Bryan, 2011).

The complete hierarchical architecture consists of a control interface that receives noisy input from the brain that is based on SSVEP, a robot PR2, and a hierarchical and adaptive menu. The stimuli that are used to generate the SSVEPs are LEDs, which are mounted to a screen next to the main menu. The control interface is composed of current menu options and a video feed from the robot's field of vision. The user can maneuver the robot by choosing options from the main menu.

The hierarchical and adaptive menu allows the user to control the robot directly and to teach the robot new skills. There are 5 options, including "Train", "Train Sequence", "Navigate", "Playback", and "Playback Sequence", in the main menu from which the user can choose. "Train" allows the user to teach PR2 a new arm trajectory. After choosing "stop", the user can choose to save or discard the learned trajectory. "Playback" is used to check the learned skill. "Training sequence" is used to create a command sequence, which can consist of a trained trajectory and primitives (such as rotating the wrist). The option "Navigate" is used to drive the robot. The basic primary motion of the PR2 robot is controlled using pre-programmed library functions that are provided by ROS (Quigley, 2009).

SSVEP BCI-Based HPR-2

With the aim of embodying the user's conscience into a physical robot, researchers from CNRS-AIST have proposed a method that allows the user to control the whole body of a humanoid robot by using SSVEP and a Head-Mounted Display (HMD). SSVEP allows the user to identify which option are in the user's interest, and HMD is used to display the feedback from the robot HRP2 embedded camera, which can improve the user's feeling of embodiment. A task-based controller is used to achieve instant tasks. Later, these make the user a part of the environment, which makes it possible for human-humanoid interactions to occur. In their more recent publications, they had improved the framework, which can now be used for both navigation and interaction (Petit, 2015; Gergondet, 2015).

The whole control system includes the user interface, vision modules, control module and HRP2 robot. The framework is shown in Figure 2. The user interface is integrated on the screen of the HDM, and its display changes according to the current state.

The vision modules can localize the robot in the surroundings and localize relevant objects by processing the images obtained from the camera, which is mounted on the head of HRP-2.

The Control module receives the user intention and the target object pose from the other modules and then generates the motor commands necessary to move the robot to realize the desired tasks. The module covers three aspects: Navigation, Interaction and Task execution. The navigation module is used to drive the robot according to the user's intention, which is obtained from the BCI, while the target object pose is obtained from the vision module. The output to the navigation module is the desired velocity, CoM, V_m, which is used to compute the desired foot position using a walking pattern generator. The interaction module is used to realize various actions, and the desired hand positions are also determined in this module.

The task executor is used to achieve the operations that are requested by the navigation and interaction modules. The torque metric, q, for the robot's joint is obtained using an inverse kinematic (IK) controller according the desired hand and foot position.

Hybrid BCI-Based Humanoid

A typical hybrid BCI is composed of more than one BCI and another system. The aim of these systems is to achieve specific goals better than a conventional system (Henshaw, 2014).

Choi and Jo (2013) combined P300/SSVEP/MI with image processing to control the humanoid robot NAO during navigation and task exploration. The MI-based BCI is used to navigate and explore, the P300-based BCI is used to select the object of interest, and the communication between the user and the robot is based on SSVEP. This research demonstrated that a three BCI hybrid can be combined in a serial manner. In Ma, 2013, an electrooculogram (EOG)/event-related potential (ERP)-based BCI was proposed to control the robot NAO.

KEY RESEARCHES

Mind control humanoid technology is only the beginning, and there is a long way to go before the humanoid robot can be an avatar for humans. During this process, many key technologies will need to be improved. Here, we discuss the safety of humanoid robots.

There is no such thing as absolute safety. When discussing humanoid robots, safety is a prime concern that must be addressed when the robot undertakes tasks in human surroundings. The safety of the humanoid robot mainly concerns the safety of the robot itself and the safety of human-robot interactions. That is, the robot should not perform its tasks safely and also behave in a manner that is acceptable, comfortable and understandable to humans.

Disturbance Rejection

To enhance disturbance rejection capabilities, the CoM state is controlled to realize disturbance rejection (Hyon, 2009), and steps are taken in the presence of greater disturbance (Pratt J, 2006). Some optimization methods based on a multi-link model have been proposed to coordinate whole-body motions, including the linear quadratic regulator (Humpage, 2008), dynamic programming (Liu, 2009) and convex optimization (Wang, 2012). In addition, disturbances that occur during robot walking may be related to toe-off and heel-strike (Chen, 2014).

Protection Against Falling Down

Falling is an extremely unstable state for a humanoid robot. The research into disturbance rejection for humanoid robots has mainly addressed relatively small disturbances. Sometimes, falling is unavoidable, and methods to protect the whole body from substantial damage have been studied since 2002. The research into protecting against falling down has mainly focused on three aspects: falling detection, which determines whether or not the robot is falling; falling direction, which reduces damage to the environment; and falling strategies, which attempt to reduce the damage that occurs to the humanoid robot during landing. One typical optimization-based falling strategy identifies the trajectory of the falling motion to ensure that the smallest amount of landing damage is incurred (Lee, 2012; Wang, 2012). Some bio-inspired methods to control falling motions have also been proposed to solve this problem (Ruiz, 2009; Yun, 2014).

Human-Robot Interaction Safety

To work with humans in a shared workspace, human-robot interaction (HRI) safety procedures are required to ensure human safety when the robot is operating hear humans. HRI safety can be classified into two categories: physical safety and psychological safety.

Physical safety means that all unwanted contact between humans and robots is prevented. If contact is required by the task, the contact force for the human must below the limit of what would cause an injury to ensure that injury will not occur. Psychological safety means that the HRI interaction will not cause excessive stress to humans. For example, if a robot in a hypothetical system is moving an actuator with a sharp end at high speed to within several centimeters of a human, it will cause psychological stress to the human. Even if the human is not hurt, they will be in a state of discomfort, which may have negative long-term effects. HRI safety concerns itself mainly with software and hardware components.

CONCLUSION

As a platform for mind control technology, humanoid robots with a human appearance are more suitable to becoming robot surrogates. In this paper, a history and overview of humanoid robots is provided. New trends in the field of humanoid research and mind control humanoid robots is described and summarized. It is clear that mind control systems require progress to be made that will require collaboration among numerous disciplines, including artificial technology, robotics, neuroscience, electronics, and brain science. With the development of related technologies, mind-controlled humanoid robots will revolutionize every aspect of our lives. Finally, a key technology that will allow humanoid robots to be safely used is proposed.

ACKNOWLEDGMENT

This work was supported by the National Natural Science Foundation of China (Grants 61473043).

REFERENCES

Asano, Y., Mizoguchi, H., Kozuki, T., Motegi, Y., Osada, M., & Urata, J. (2012). Lower thigh design of detailed musculoskeletal humanoid "Kenshiro". *Intelligent Robots and Systems, IEEE/RSJ International Conference on*, (pp. 4367-4372).

Behnke, S. (2008). Humanoid robots - from fiction to reality?. *KI,* (4), 5-9.

Bell, C. J., Shenoy, P., Chalodhorn, R., & Rao, R. P. (2008). Control of a humanoid robot by a noninvasive brain-computer interface in humans. *Journal of Neural Engineering*, *5*(2), 214–220. doi:10.1088/1741-2560/5/2/012 PMID:18483450

Benjamin, B., Guido, D., Matthias, K., Klaus-Robert, M., & Gabriel, C. (2007). The non-invasive berlin brain–computer interface: Fast acquisition of effective performance in untrained subjects. *NeuroImage*, *37*(2), 539–550. doi:10.1016/j.neuroimage.2007.01.051 PMID:17475513

Berger, H. (1938). Über das elektrenkephalogramm des menschen. *European Archives of Psychiatry and Clinical Neuroscience*, *108*(3), 407–431.

Bryan, M., Green, J., Chung, M., & Chang, L. (2011). An adaptive brain-computer interface for humanoid robot control.*IEEE-RAS International Conference on Humanoid Robots*, (pp. 199-204). doi:10.1109/Humanoids.2011.6100901

Chae, Y., Jeong, J., & Jo, S. (2011). Noninvasive Brain-Computer Interface-based control of humanoid navigation. *Intelligent Robots and Systems, IEEE/RSJ International Conference on*, (pp. 685-691).

Chae, Y., Jeong, J., & Jo, S. (2012). Toward brain-actuated humanoid robots: Asynchronous direct-control using an Eeg-Based BCI. *IEEE Transactions on Robotics*, *28*(5), 1131–1144. doi:10.1109/TRO.2012.2201310

Chen, X., Zhou, Y., Huang, Q., & Yu, Z. (2014). Bipedal walking with toe-off, heel-strike and compliance with external disturbances. *Humanoid Robots, IEEE-RAS International Conference on.*

Choi, B., & Jo, S. (2013). A low-cost eeg system-based hybrid brain-computer interface for humanoid robot navigation and recognition. *PLoS ONE*, *8*(9), e74583–e74583. doi:10.1371/journal.pone.0074583 PMID:24023953

Cleland, E. (2002). The intelligent ASIMO: System overview and integration.*IEEE–RSJ International Conference on Intelligent Robots and Systems*, *3*, 2478 - 2483.

Farwell, L. A., & Donchin, E. (1988). Talking off the top of your head: Toward a mental prosthesis utilizing event-related brain potentials. *Electroencephalography and Clinical Neurophysiology*, *70*(6), 510–523. doi:10.1016/0013-4694(88)90149-6 PMID:2461285

Gergondet, P., & Kheddar, A. (2015). Ssvep stimuli design for object-centric bci. *Brain-Computer Interfaces*, 2.

Henrik, H. (2003). Imagery of voluntary movement of fingers, toes, and tongue activates corresponding body-part-specific motor representations. *Journal of Neurophysiology*, *90*(5), 3304–3316. doi:10.1152/jn.01113.2002 PMID:14615433

Henshaw, J., Liu, W., & Romano, D. (2014). Problem solving using hybrid brain-computer interface methods: A review. *Cognitive Infocommunications, IEEE Conference on*, 215-219.

Hirose, M., & Ogawa, K. (2007). Honda humanoid robots development. *Philosophical Transactions of the Royal Society A Mathematical Physical & Engineering Sciences*, *365*(365), 11–19. doi:10.1098/rsta.2006.1917 PMID:17148047

Hirukawa, H. (2007). Walking biped humanoids that perform manual labour. *Philosophical Transactions of the Royal Society A Mathematical Physical & Engineering Sciences, 365*(365), 65–77. doi:10.1098/rsta.2006.1916 PMID:17148050

Hochberg, L. R., Serruya, M. D., Friehs, G. M., Mukand, J. A., Saleh, M., Caplan, A. H., & Donoghue, J. P. et al. (2006). Neuronal ensemble control of prosthetic devices by a human with tetraplegia. *Nature, 442*(7099), 164–171. doi:10.1038/nature04970 PMID:16838014

Huang, Q., Li, K., & Wang, T. (2002). Control and mechanical design of humanoid robot BHR-01. In *Proceeding of The Third IARP International Workshop on Humanoid and Human Friendly Robotics*.

Humpage, W. D., & Stott, B. (2008). Multiple balance strategies from one optimization criterion. *Humanoid Robots, IEEE-RAS International Conference on, 112*, 57-64.

Hyon, S., Osu, R., & Otaka, Y. (2009). Integration of multi-level postural balancing on humanoid robots.*Proceedings of the 2009 IEEE international conference on Robotics and Automation*, (pp. 1549 - 1556). doi:10.1109/ROBOT.2009.5152434

Ito, Y., Urata, J., Nakanishi, Y., Okada, K., & Inaba, M. (2011). Design and development of shock absorbable tendon driven ankles for high-powered humanoids. In *Advanced Robotics and its Social Impacts, 2011 IEEE Workshop on*, (pp. 58-61).

Kato, I. (1973). Development of WABOT 1. *Biomechanism, 2*, 173–214.

Kim, M. S., Kim, M. S., Park, S., & Oh, J. H. (2008). Realization of stretch-legged walking of the humanoid robot. In *8th IEEE-RAS International Conference on Humanoid Robots*. Humanoids 2008, (pp. 118 - 124).

Lee, S. H., & Goswami, A. (2012). Fall on backpack: Damage minimization of humanoid robots by falling on targeted body segments. *Journal of Computational & Nonlinear Dynamics, 8*(2), 233–246. doi:10.1115/1.4006783

Liu, C., & Atkeson, C. G. (2009). Standing Balance Control Using a Trajectory Library. *Intelligent Robots and Systems, IEEE/RSJ International Conference on*, (pp. 3031-3036).

Ma, J., Zhang, Y., Nam, Y., & Cichocki, A. (2013). EOG/ERP hybrid human-machine interface for robot control. *Intelligent Robots and Systems, IEEE/RSJ International Conference on, 40*, 859-864.

Manoj, S., & Andy, R. (2006). Computer optimization of a minimal biped model discovers walking and running. *Nature, 439*(7072), 72–75. doi:10.1038/nature04113 PMID:16155564

Mcgeer, T. (1990). Passive dynamic walking. *The International Journal of Robotics Research*, *9*(2), 62–82. doi:10.1177/027836499000900206

Millan, J. D. R., Galán, F., Vanhooydonck, D., Lew, E., Philips, J., & Nuttin, M. (2009, September). Asynchronous non-invasive brain-actuated control of an intelligent wheelchair. In *Engineering in Medicine and Biology Society, Annual International Conference of the IEEE*, (pp. 3361-3364).

Müller, S. M. T., Cardoso, W., Bastos-Filho, T. F., & Sarcinelli-Filho, M. (2010). Brain-computer interface based on visual evoked potentials to command autonomous robotic wheelchair. *Journal of Medical & Biological Engineering*, *30*(6), 407–415. doi:10.5405/jmbe.765

Müller-Putz, G. R., & Gert, P. (2008). Control of an electrical prosthesis with an ssvep-based bci. *Biomedical Engineering IEEE Transactions on*, *55*(1), 361–364. doi:10.1109/TBME.2007.897815 PMID:18232384

Nakanishi, Y., Asano, Y., Kozuki, T., Mizoguchi, H., Motegi, Y., & Osada, M. (2012). Design concept of detail musculoskeletal humanoid "Kenshiro" - Toward a real human body musculoskeletal simulator. *Humanoid Robots, 2012 12th IEEE-RAS International Conference on*, (pp. 1-6).

Ogura, Y., Shimomura, K., Kondo, H., & Morishima, A. (2006). Human-like walking with knee stretched, heel-contact and toe-off motion by a humanoid robot. *Intelligent Robots and Systems, 2006 IEEE/RSJ International Conference on*, (pp. 3976-3981).

Petit, D., Gergondet, P., Cherubini, A., & Kheddar, A. (2015). An integrated framework for humanoid embodiment with a BCI.*IEEE International Conference on Robotics & Automation*, (pp. 2882-2887). doi:10.1109/ICRA.2015.7139592

Pfurtscheller, G., Müller, G. R., Pfurtscheller, J., Gerner, H. J., & Rupp, R. (2003). 'thought'—control of functional electrical stimulation to restore hand grasp in a patient with tetraplegia. *Neuroscience Letters*, *351*(1), 33–36. doi:10.1016/S0304-3940(03)00947-9 PMID:14550907

Pfurtscheller, G., Neuper, C., Flotzinger, D., & Pregenzer, M. (1997). Eeg-based discrimination between imagination of right and left hand movement. *Electroencephalography and Clinical Neurophysiology*, *103*(6), 642–651. doi:10.1016/S0013-4694(97)00080-1 PMID:9546492

Picton, T. W. (1992). The p300 wave of the human event-related potential. *Journal of Clinical Neurophysiology Official Publication of the American Electroencephalographic Society*, *9*(4), 456–479. doi:10.1097/00004691-199210000-00002 PMID:1464675

Pratt, J., Carff, J., Drakunov, S., & Goswami, A. (2007). Capture Point: A Step toward Humanoid Push Recovery. *Humanoid Robots, IEEE-RAS International Conference on*, (pp. 200-207).

Pratt, J., Koolen, T., De Boer, T., Rebula, J., Cotton, S., Carff, J., & Neuhaus, P. et al. (2012). Capturability-based analysis and control of legged locomotion, part 2: Application to m2v2, *a lower-body humanoid. The International Journal of Robotics Research, 31*(10), 1117–1133. doi:10.1177/0278364912452762

Pratt, J., & Krupp, B. (2008). Design of a bipedal walking robot.*SPIE Defense and Security Symposium* (Vol. 6962). International Society for Optics and Photonics.

Quigley, M., Conley, K., Gerkey, B., Faust, J., Foote, T., Leibs, J., & Ng, A. Y. et al. (2009). ROS: an open-source Robot Operating System.*In IEEE International Conference on Robotics & Automation workshop on open source software.*

Ruiz-Del-Solar, J., Palma-Amestoy, R., Marchant, R., Parra-Tsunekawa, I., & Zegers, P. (2009). Learning to fall: Designing low damage fall sequences for humanoid soccer robots. *Robotics and Autonomous Systems, 57*(8), 796–807. doi:10.1016/j.robot.2009.03.011

Sakamoto, D., Kanda, T., Ono, T., Kamashima, M., Imai, M., & Ishiguro, H. (2005). Cooperative embodied communication emerged by interactive humanoid robots. *International Journal of Human-Computer Studies, 62*(2), 247–265. doi:10.1016/j.ijhcs.2004.11.001

Steve, C., Andy, R., Russ, T., & Martijn, W. (2005). Efficient bipedal robots based on passive-dynamic walkers. *Science, 307*(5712), 1082–1085. doi:10.1126/science.1107799 PMID:15718465

Taylor, D. M., Tillery, S. I. H., & Schwartz, A. B. (2002). Direct cortical control of 3d neuroprosthetic devices. *Science, 296*(5574), 1829–1832. doi:10.1126/science.1070291 PMID:12052948

Urata, J., Nshiwaki, K., Nakanishi, Y., Okada, K., Kagami, S., & Inaba, M. (2012). Online walking pattern generation for push recovery and minimum delay to commanded change of direction and speed. In *Intelligent Robots and Systems, 2012 IEEE/RSJ International Conference on,* (pp. 3411-3416).

Vermeulen, J., Lefeber, D., Verrelst, B., & Vanderborght, B. (2006). Trajectory planning for the walking biped "lucy". *The International Journal of Robotics Research, 25*(9), 867–887. doi:10.1177/0278364906069343

Vidal, J. J. (1973). Toward direct brain-computer communication. *Annual Review of Biophysics and Bioengineering*, *2*(4), 157–180. doi:10.1146/annurev.bb.02.060173.001105 PMID:4583653

Vora, J. Y., Allison, B. Z., & Moore, M. M. (2004). A P3 brain computer interface for robot arm control. *Society for Neuroscience Abstract 30*, Program No 421.19.

Wang, J. (2012). Humanoid push recovery with robust convex synthesis. *IEEE/RSJ International Conference on Intelligent Robots and Systems*, *57*, 4354-4359. doi:10.1109/IROS.2012.6386211

Wang, J., Whitman, E. C., & Stilman, M. (2012, June). Whole-body trajectory optimization for humanoid falling. In *American Control Conference*, (pp. 4837-4842).

Wolpaw, J. R., & Mcfarland, D. J. (2005). Control of a two-dimensional movement signal by a noninvasive brain-computer interface in humans. *Proceedings of the National Academy of Sciences of the United States of America*, *101*(51), 17849–17854. doi:10.1073/pnas.0403504101 PMID:15585584

Yu, Z., Huang, Q., Ma, G., Chen, X., Zhang, W., & Li, J. (2014). Design and development of the humanoid robot bhr-5. *Advances in Mechanical Engineering*, *11*, 1–11.

Yun, S. K., & Goswami, A. (2014). Tripod fall: Concept and experiments of a novel approach to humanoid robot fall damage reduction. *Robotics and Automation, IEEE International Conference on*, (pp. 2799-2805).

ADDITIONAL READING

Favot, V., Buschmann, T., Schwienbacher, M., Ewald, A., & Ulbrich, H. (2012). The sensor-controller network of the humanoid robot LOLA. *In Humanoid Robots, IEEE-RAS International Conference on*, 805-810.

Huang, D., Lin, P., Fei, D. Y., Chen, X., & Bai, O. (2009). Decoding human motor activity from EEG single trials for a discrete two-dimensional cursor control. *Journal of Neural Engineering*, *6*(4), 046005. doi:10.1088/1741-2560/6/4/046005 PMID:19556679

Moro, F. L., Tsagarakis, N. G., & Caldwell, D. G. (2011). A human-like walking for the compliant humanoid COMAN based on CoM trajectory reconstruction from kinematic Motion Primitives. *In Humanoid Robots, IEEE-RAS International Conference on*, 364-370.

Ott, C., Baumgärtner, C., Mayr, J., Fuchs, M., Burge, R., Lee, D., . . . Hirzinger, G. (2010). Development of a biped robot with torque controlled joints. *In Humanoid Robots (Humanoids), IEEE-RAS International Conference on*, 167-173.

Pfeiffer, F., Löffler, K., & Gienger, M. (2002). The concept of jogging johnnie. *In Robotics and Automation, 2002. Proceedings. ICRA'02. IEEE International Conference on*, Vol. 3, 3129-3135.

Pollard, N. S., Hodgins, J. K., Riley, M. J., & Atkeson, C. G. (2002). Adapting human motion for the control of a humanoid robot. *In Robotics and Automation, IEEE International Conference on*, 2, 1390-1397.

Tajima, R., Honda, D., & Suga, K. (2009). Fast running experiments involving a humanoid robot. *Robotics and Automation, IEEE International Conference on*, 1571 - 1576.

Taylor, D. M., Tillery, S. I. H., & Schwartz, A. B. (2003). Information conveyed through brain-control: Cursor versus robot. *Neural Systems and Rehabilitation Engineering. IEEE Transactions on*, *11*(2), 195–199.

Wolpaw, J. R., & McFarland, D. J. (1994). Multichannel EEG-based brain-computer communication. *Electroencephalography and Clinical Neurophysiology*, *90*(6), 444–449. doi:10.1016/0013-4694(94)90135-X PMID:7515787

KEY TERMS AND DEFINITIONS

Brain-Computer Interface: A communication pathway between the brain and an external device.

Force Control Humanoid: A humanoid robot that is driven by force or torque.

Humanoid Robot: A robot with human appearance and behaviors.

MI BCI-Based humanoid: A humanoid robot that is controlled using a motor imaging method.

Mind Control Robot: A robot that is controlled by brain activities.

P300 BCI-Based Humanoid: A humanoid robot that is controlled by a P300 signal.

Position Control Humanoid: A humanoid robot that is directly driven by joint angle and angular velocity.

SSVEP BCI-Based Humanoid: A humanoid robot that is controlled by an SSVEP signal.

Compilation of References

Ackerley, R., Backlund-Wasling, H., Liljencrantz, J., Olausson, H., Johnson, R. D., & Wessberg, J. (2014). Human C-tactile afferents are tuned to the temperature of a skin-stroking caress. *The Journal of Neuroscience, 34*(8), 2879–2883. doi:10.1523/JNEUROSCI.2847-13.2014 PMID:24553929

Adamic, L., & Adar, E. (2005). How to search a social network. *Social Networks, 27*(3), 187–203. doi:10.1016/j.socnet.2005.01.007

Akbaraly, T. N., Portet, F., Fustinoni, S., Dartigues, J.-F., Artero, S., Rouaud, O., & Berr, C. et al. (2009). Leisure activities and the risk of dementia in the elderly: Results from the Three-City Study. *Neurology, 73*(11), 854–861. doi:10.1212/WNL.0b013e3181b7849b PMID:19752452

Akpinar, B., & Kucukguclu, O. (2012). The validity and reliability of the Turkish version of the quality of life scale for patients with Alzheimer's disease (QOL-AD). *Journal of the Neurological Sciences, 29*(3), 554–565.

Akyar, I., & Akdemir, N. (2009). Alzheimer hastalarına bakım verenlerin yaşadıkları güçlükler[strains of caregivers of Alzheimer patients]. *Sağlık Bilimleri Fakültesi Hemşirelik Dergisi, 16*(3), 32–49.

Albert, M. L., Feldman, R. G., & Willis, A. L. (1974). The 'subcortical dementia' of progressive supranuclear palsy. *Journal of Neurology, Neurosurgery, and Psychiatry, 37*(2), 121–130. doi:10.1136/jnnp.37.2.121 PMID:4819905

Alberts, B. (2012). The breakthroughs of 2012. *Science, 388*(6114), 1511. doi:10.1126/science.1234108 PMID:23258851

Algoe, S. B., Haidt, J., & Gable, S. L. (2008). Beyond reciprocity: Gratitude and relationships in everyday life. *Emotion (Washington, D.C.), 8*(3), 425–429. doi:10.1037/1528-3542.8.3.425 PMID:18540759

Allievi, A. G., Mellendez-Calderon, A., Arichi, T., Edwards, A. D., & Burdet, E. (2012). An fMRI compatible wrist robotic interface to study brain development in neonates. *Annals of Biomedical Engineering, 41*(6), 1181–1192. doi:10.1007/s10439-013-0782-x PMID:23475437

Alzheimer Association. (2007). *Activity-Based Care*. Chicago: Alzheimer's Association. Retrieved June 2015, http://www.alz.org/professionals_and_researchers_activity_based_care.asp

Alzheimer's Association. (2011). 2011 Alzheimer's disease facts and figures. *Alzheimer's & Dementia: The Journal of the Alzheimer's Association, 7*, 208.

American Psychiatric Association. (2000). *Diagnostic criteria from dsM-iV-tr.* American Psychiatric Pub.

Anatoli, G., & Michael, E. H. (2002). A model of hippocampal circuitry mediating goal-driven navigation in a familiar environment. *Neurocomputing, 44*, 423–427.

Andreoli, P. J. H. (2003). *Monitoring evaluatie en kennisverzameling: pilotproject: senioren actief in groenkamers*. Amsterdam: Woonzorg Nederland.

Anguera, J. A., Boccanfuso, J., Rintoul, J. L., Al-Hashimi, O., Faraji, F., Janowich, J., & Gazzaley, A. et al. (2013). Video game training enhances cognitive control in older adults. *Nature, 501*(7465), 97–101. doi:10.1038/nature12486 PMID:24005416

Artikis, A., Bamidis, P. D., Billis, A., Bratsas, C., Frantzidis, C., Karkaletsis, V., … Spyropoulos, C. S. (2012). *Supporting tele-health and AI-based clinical decision making with sensor data fusion and semantic interpretation: The USEFIL case study*. Retrieved July 24, 2015, from http://airtlab.dii.univpm.it/netmed2012/sites/netmed2012.dii.univpm.it/files/papers/netmed2012.pdf#page=32

Artola, A., & Singer, W. (1987). Long-term potentiation and NMDA receptors in rat visual cortex. *Nature, 330*(6149), 649–652. doi:10.1038/330649a0 PMID:2446147

Asano, Y., Mizoguchi, H., Kozuki, T., Motegi, Y., Osada, M., & Urata, J. (2012). Lower thigh design of detailed musculoskeletal humanoid "Kenshiro". *Intelligent Robots and Systems, IEEE/RSJ International Conference on*, (pp. 4367-4372).

Ashton, K. (2009). That "Internet of Things" Thing. *RFiD Journal, 4986*. Retrieved from http://www.itrco.jp/libraries/RFIDjournal-That Internet of Things Thing.pdf\npapers3://publication/uuid/8191C095-0D90-4A17-86B0-550F2F2A6745

Au, J., Sheehan, E., Tsai, N., Duncan, G. J., Buschkuehl, M., & Jaeggi, S. M. (2015). Improving fluid intelligence with training on working memory: A meta-analysis. *Psychonomic Bulletin & Review, 22*(2), 366–377. doi:10.3758/s13423-014-0699-x PMID:25102926

Aukner, C., Eide, H. D., & Iversen, P. O. (2013). Nutritional status among older residents with dementia in open versus special care units in municipal nursing homes: An observational study. *BMC Geriatrics, 13*(1), 26–32. doi:10.1186/1471-2318-13-26 PMID:23496975

Avenanti, A., Minio-Paluello, I., Bufalari, I., & Aglioti, S. M. (2006). Stimulus-driven modulation of motor-evoked potentials during observation of others' pain. *NeuroImage, 32*(1), 316–324. doi:10.1016/j.neuroimage.2006.03.010 PMID:16675270

Babiloni, C., Binetti, G., Cassetta, E., Cerboneschi, D., Dal Forno, G., Del Percio, C., & Rossini, P. M. et al. (2004). Mapping distributed sources of cortical rhythms in mild Alzheimer's disease. A multicentric EEG study. *NeuroImage*, *22*(1), 57–67. doi:10.1016/j.neuroimage.2003.09.028 PMID:15109997

Babiloni, C., Carducci, F., Lizio, R., Vecchio, F., Baglieri, A., Bernardini, S., & Frisoni, G. B. et al. (2013). Resting state cortical electroencephalographic rhythms are related to gray matter volume in subjects with mild cognitive impairment and Alzheimer's disease. *Human Brain Mapping*, *34*(6), 1427–1446. doi:10.1002/hbm.22005 PMID:22331654

Bäckman, L. (1996). Utilizing compensatory task conditions for episodic memory in Alzheimer's disease. *Acta Neurologica Scandinavica*, *94*(S165), 109–113. doi:10.1111/j.1600-0404.1996.tb05880.x PMID:8740997

Baddeley, A. (2010). Exploring the central executive. *Quarterly Journal of Experimental Psychology A*, *1*(1), 5-28.

Bahar-Fuchs, A., Clare, L., & Woods, B. (2013). Cognitive training and cognitive rehabilitation for mild to moderate Alzheimer's disease and vascular dementia. *Cochrane Database of Systematic Reviews*, 6. PMID:23740535

Bakker, M., Verstappen, C. C. P., Bloem, B. R., & Toni, I. (2007). Recent advances in functional neuroimaging of gait. *Journal of Neural Transmission*, *114*(10), 1323–1331. doi:10.1007/s00702-007-0783-8 PMID:17622483

Bamidis, P. D., Vivas, A. B., Styliadis, C., Frantzidis, C., Klados, M., Schlee, W., & Papageorgiou, S. G. et al. (2014). A review of physical and cognitive interventions in aging. *Neuroscience and Biobehavioral Reviews*, *44*, 206–220. doi:10.1016/j.neubiorev.2014.03.019 PMID:24705268

Barber, R., Gholkar, A., Scheltens, P., Ballard, C., McKeith, I. G., & O'Brien, J. T. (1999). Medial temporal lobe atrophy on MRI in dementia with Lewy bodies. *Neurology*, *52*(6), 1153–1153. doi:10.1212/WNL.52.6.1153 PMID:10214736

Barghout-Stein, L. (1999). *On differences between peripheral and foveal pattern masking*. Berkeley, CA: University of California.

Barker, M. G., & Lawson, J. S. (1968). Nominal aphasia in dementia. *The British Journal of Psychiatry*, *114*(516), 1351–1356. doi:10.1192/bjp.114.516.1351 PMID:5702274

Baron-Cohen, S., Ring, H., Wheelwright, S., Bullmore, E. T., Brammer, M. J., Simmons, A., & Williams, S. C. R. (1999). Social intelligence in the normal and autistic brain: An fMRI study. *The European Journal of Neuroscience*, *11*(6), 1891–1898. doi:10.1046/j.1460-9568.1999.00621.x PMID:10336657

Baron-Cohen, S., Tager-Flusberg, H., & Cohen, D. J. (2000). *Understanding the minds: perspectives from developmental cognitive neuroscience*. Oxford University Press.

Bastos-Leite, A., Van Waesberghe, J., Oen, A., Van Der Flier, W., Scheltens, P., & Barkhof, F. (2006). Hippocampal sulcus width and cavities: Comparison between patients with Alzheimer disease and nondemented elderly subjects. *American Journal of Neuroradiology*, *27*, 2141–2145. PMID:17110684

Bayles, K. A. (1982). Language function in senile dementia. *Brain and Language*, *16*(2), 265–280. doi:10.1016/0093-934X(82)90086-4 PMID:7116128

Bayles, K. A., & Tomoeda, C. K. (1983). Confrontation naming impairment in dementia. *Brain and Language*, *19*(1), 98–114. doi:10.1016/0093-934X(83)90057-3 PMID:6222782

Beatty, E. L., Jobidon, M. E., Bouak, F., Nakashima, A., Smith, I., Lam, Q., & Vartanian, O. et al. (2015). Transfer of training from one working memory task to another: Behavioural and neural evidence. *Frontiers in Systems Neuroscience*, *9*, 86. doi:10.3389/fnsys.2015.00086 PMID:26082694

Bechara, A., Damasio, H., Tranel, D., & Damasio, A. R. (1997). Deciding advantageously before knowing the advantageous strategy. *Science*, *275*(5304), 1293–1295. doi:10.1126/science.275.5304.1293 PMID:9036851

Bechtel, R. B., & Churchman, A. (2003). *Handbook of Environmental Psychology*. John Wiley & Sons.

Beck, A. M., Holst, M., & Rasmussen, H. H. (2008). Efficacy of the Mini Nutritional Assessment to predict the risk of developing malnutrition or adverse health outcomes for old people. *e-SPEN, the European e-Journal of Clinical Nutrition and Metabolism*, *3*(3), e102-e107.

Beerens, H. C., Zwakhalen, S. M. G., Verbeek, H., Ruwaard, D., & Hamers, J. P. H. (2013). Factors associated with quality of life of people with dementia in long-term care facilities: A systematic review. *International Journal of Nursing Studies*, *50*(9), 1259–1270. doi:10.1016/j.ijnurstu.2013.02.005 PMID:23465959

Behnke, S. (2008). Humanoid robots - from fiction to reality?. *KI*, (4), 5-9.

Bellack, A. S., Gold, J. M., & Buchanan, R. W. (1999). Cognitive rehabilitation for schizophrenia: Problems, prospects, and strategies. *Schizophrenia Bulletin*, *25*(2), 257–274. doi:10.1093/oxfordjournals.schbul.a033377 PMID:10416730

Bell, C. J., Shenoy, P., Chalodhorn, R., & Rao, R. P. (2008). Control of a humanoid robot by a noninvasive brain-computer interface in humans. *Journal of Neural Engineering*, *5*(2), 214–220. doi:10.1088/1741-2560/5/2/012 PMID:18483450

Belleville, S., Gilbert, B., Fontaine, F., Gagnon, L., Ménard, É., & Gauthier, S. (2006). Improvement of episodic memory in persons with mild cognitive impairment and healthy older adults: Evidence from a cognitive intervention program. *Dementia and Geriatric Cognitive Disorders*, *22*(5-6), 486–499. doi:10.1159/000096316 PMID:17050952

Bellotti, F., Kapralos, B., Lee, K., Moreno-Ger, P., & Berta, R. (2013). Assessment in and of Serious Games: An Overview. *Advances in Human-Computer Interaction*, *2013*, 1–11. doi:10.1155/2013/136864

Benedek, K., Janaky, M., Braunitzer, G., Rokszin, A., Keri, S., & Benedek, G. (2010). Parallel development of contour integration and visual contrast sensitivity at low spatial frequencies. *Neuroscience Letters*, *472*(3), 175–178. doi:10.1016/j.neulet.2010.02.001 PMID:20138967

Benjamin, B., Guido, D., Matthias, K., Klaus-Robert, M., & Gabriel, C. (2007). The non-invasive berlin brain–computer interface: Fast acquisition of effective performance in untrained subjects. *NeuroImage*, *37*(2), 539–550. doi:10.1016/j.neuroimage.2007.01.051 PMID:17475513

Bennys, K., Rondouin, G., Vergnes, C., & Touchon, J. (2001). Diagnostic value of quantitative EEG in Alzheimer's disease. *Neurophysiologie Clinique. Clinical Neurophysiology*, *31*(3), 153–160. doi:10.1016/S0987-7053(01)00254-4 PMID:11488226

Berger, H. (1938). Über das elektrenkephalogramm des menschen. *European Archives of Psychiatry and Clinical Neuroscience*, *108*(3), 407–431.

Berwanger, D., Wittmann, M., von Steinbuchel, N., & von Suchodoletz, W. (2004). Measurement of temporal-order judgment in children. *Acta Neurobiologiae Experimentalis*, *64*(3), 387–394. PMID:15283480

Besle, J., Sánchez-Panchuelo, R., Bowtell, R., Francis, S., & Schluppeck, D. (2013). Single-subject fMRI mapping at 7 T of the representation of fingertips in S1: A comparison of event-related and phase-encoding designs. *Neurophysiol*, *109*(9), 2293–2305. doi:10.1152/jn.00499.2012 PMID:23427300

Besle, J., Sánchez-Panchuelo, R., Bowtell, R., Francis, S., & Schluppeck, D. (2014). Event-related fMRI at 7T reveals overlapping cortical representations for adjacent fingertips in S1 of individual subjects. *Human Brain Mapping*, *35*(5), 2027–2043. doi:10.1002/hbm.22310 PMID:24014446

Beyer, P. L. (2012). Intake: Digestion, absorption, transport, and excretion of nutrients. In L. K. Mahan, S. Escott-Stump, & J. L. Raymond (Eds.), *Krause's food & the nutrition care process* (pp. 1–18). Elsevier Health Sciences.

Bialystok, E. (2007). Cognitive effects of bilingualism: How linguistic experience leads to cognitive change. *International Journal of Bilingual Education and Bilingualism*, *10*(3), 210–223. doi:10.2167/beb441.0

Bialystok, E. (2010). Global-local and trail-making tasks by monolingual and bilingual children: Beyond inhibition. *Developmental Psychology*, *46*(1), 93–105. doi:10.1037/a0015466 PMID:20053009

Bialystok, E., Barac, R., Blaye, A., & Poulin-Dubois, D. (2010). Word mapping and executive functioning in young monolingual and bilingual children. *Journal of Cognition and Development*, *11*(4), 485–508. doi:10.1080/15248372.2010.516420 PMID:21197133

Bialystok, E., Craik, F. I. M., Cheryl, G., Wilkin, C., Ryouhei, I., & Atsuko, G. et al.. (2005). Effect of bilingualism on cognitive control in the simon task: Evidence from meg. *NeuroImage*, *24*(1), 40–49. doi:10.1016/j.neuroimage.2004.09.044 PMID:15588595

Bialystok, E., Majumder, S., & Martin, M. M. (2003). Developing phonological awareness: Is there a bilingual advantage. *Applied Psycholinguistics*, *24*(1), 27–44. doi:10.1017/S014271640300002X

Billis, A. S., Papageorgiou, E. I., Frantzidis, C., Konstantinidis, E. I., & Bamidis, P. D. (2013). Towards a hierarchically-structured decision support tool for improving seniors' independent living. In *Proceedings of the 6th International Conference on PErvasive Technologies Related to Assistive Environments - PETRA '13* (pp. 1–4). New York: ACM Press. http://doi.org/doi:10.1145/2504335.2504362

Billis, A. S., Papageorgiou, E. I., Frantzidis, C. A., Tsatali, M. S., Tsolaki, A. C., & Bamidis, P. D. (2015). A Decision-Support Framework for Promoting Independent Living and Ageing Well. *IEEE Journal of Biomedical and Health Informatics*, *19*(1), 199–209. doi:10.1109/JBHI.2014.2336757 PMID:25073180

Binder, L. I., Guillozet-Bongaarts, A. L., Garcia-Sierra, F., & Berry, R. W. (2005). Tau, tangles, and Alzheimer's disease. *Biochimica et Biophysica Acta (BBA)- Molecular Basis of Disease*, *1739*(2-3), 216–223. doi:10.1016/j.bbadis.2004.08.014

Bird, J., Levy, R., & Jacoby, R. J. (1986). Computed tomography in the elderly: Changes over time in a normal population. *The British Journal of Psychiatry*, *148*(1), 80–85. doi:10.1192/bjp.148.1.80 PMID:3485462

Bissell, K. (2010). *Designing for those with dementia using the principle of wayfinding* (Senior Thesis). Retrieved June 2015, http://muir.wrlc.org/bitstream/handle/10994/77/Final%20Thesis%20by%20Kelly%20Bissell.pdf?sequence=1

Björnsdotter, M., Morrison, I., & Olausson, H. (2010). Feeling good: On the role of C fiber mediated touch in interoception. *Experimental Brain Research*, *207*(3-4), 149–155. doi:10.1007/s00221-010-2408-y PMID:20963582

Bliss, T., & Collingridge, G. L. (1993). A synaptic model of memory: long-term potentiation in the hippocampus. *Nature, 361*(6407), 31-39.

Bliss, T., & Gardner-Medwin, A. R. (1973). Long-lasting potentiation of synaptic transmission in the dentate area of the unanaesthetized rabbit following stimulation of the perforant path. *The Journal of Physiology, 232*(2), 357-374.

Bliss, T., & Lømo, T. (1973). Long-lasting potentiation of synaptic transmission in the dentate area of the anaesthetized rabbit following stimulation of the perforant path. *The Journal of Physiology, 232*(2), 331-356.

Blumenfeld, H. K., & Marian, V. (2011). Bilingualism influences inhibitory control in auditory comprehension. *Cognition, 118*(2), 245–257. doi:10.1016/j.cognition.2010.10.012 PMID:21159332

Bodega, A., Geyer, S., Grefkes, C., Zilles, K., & Roland, P. E. (2001). Hierarchical processing of tactile shape in the human brain. *Neuron, 31*(2), 317–328. doi:10.1016/S0896-6273(01)00362-2 PMID:11502261

Bogg, T., & Lasecki, L. (2014). Reliable gains? Evidence for substantially underpowered designs in studies of working memory training transfer to fluid intelligence. *Frontiers in Psychology*, *5*, 1589. doi:10.3389/fpsyg.2014.01589 PMID:25657629

Boise, L., Morgan, D. L., Kaye, J., & Camicioli, R. (1999). Delays in the diagnosis of dementia: Perspectives of family caregivers. *American Journal of Alzheimer's Disease and Other Dementias*, *14*(1), 20–26. doi:10.1177/153331759901400101

Bolognini, N., Rossetti, A., Fusaro, M., Vallar, G., & Miniussi, C. (2014). Sharing social touch in the primary somatosensory cortex. *Current Biology*, *24*(13), 1513–1517. doi:10.1016/j.cub.2014.05.025 PMID:24954046

Bomalaski, M. N. (2011). Horticultural therapy for persons with severe dementia. *Journal of Investigative Medicine*, *59*(1), 208–209.

Borson, S., Frank, L., Bayley, P. J., Boustani, M., Dean, M., Lin, P.-J., & Ashford, J. W. et al. (2013). Improving dementia care: The role of screening and detection of cognitive impairment. *Alzheimer's & Dementia : The Journal of the Alzheimer's Association*, *9*(2), 151–159. doi:10.1016/j.jalz.2012.08.008 PMID:23375564

Bosch, L., & Sebastián-Gallés, N. (2000). Evidence of early language discrimination abilities in infants from bilingual environments. *Infancy*, *2*(1), 29–49. doi:10.1207/S15327078IN0201_3

Botvinick, M. M., & Barch, T. S. (2001). Conflict Monitoring and Cognitive Control. *Psychological Review*, *108*(3), 624–652. doi:10.1037/0033-295X.108.3.624 PMID:11488380

Boyke, J., Driemeyer, J., Gaser, C., Buchel, C., & May, A. (2008). Training-Induced Brain Structure Changes in the Elderly. *The Journal of Neuroscience*, *28*(28), 7031–7035. doi:10.1523/JNEUROSCI.0742-08.2008 PMID:18614670

Bradford, A., Kunik, M. E., Schulz, P., Williams, S. P., & Singh, H. (2009). Missed and Delayed Diagnosis of Dementia in Primary Care. *Alzheimer Disease and Associated Disorders*, *23*(4), 306–314. doi:10.1097/WAD.0b013e3181a6bebc PMID:19568149

Brannon, E. M., Suanda, S., & Libertus, K. (2007). Temporal discrimination increases in precision over development and parallels the development of numerosity discrimination. *Developmental Science*, *10*(6), 770–777. doi:10.1111/j.1467-7687.2007.00635.x PMID:17973794

Brawley, E. (2001). Environmental design for Alzheimer's disease: A quality of life issue. *Aging & Mental Health*, *5*(sup1), 79–83. doi:10.1080/713650005 PMID:11513503

Brawley, E. (2002). Therapeutic Gardens for Individuals with Alzheimer's Disease. *Alzheimer's Care Quarterly*, *3*(1), 7–11.

Breazeal, C., & Brooks, R. (2005). Robot emotion: A functional perspective. In J. Fellous (Ed.), *Who needs emotions* (pp. 271–310). Oxford, UK: Oxford University Press. doi:10.1093/acprof:oso/9780195166194.003.0010

Brewer, M. (2014). Handbook of Research Methods in Social and Personality Psychology. Retrieved from http://books.google.com/books?id=NRWTAgAAQBAJ&pgis=1

Brossard, L., & Decarie, T. (1968). Comparative reinforcing effects of eight stimulations on the smiling responses of infants. *Journal of Child Psychology and Psychiatry, and Allied Disciplines*, *9*(1), 51–59. doi:10.1111/j.1469-7610.1968.tb02207.x PMID:5729746

Browne, C. (1992). The role of nature for the promotion of wellbeing of the elderly. In D. Relf (Ed.), *The role of horticulture in human wellbeing and social development: A national symposium* (pp. 75–79). Portland, OR: Timber Press.

Bruce, H. (2014). *Gardening activities can help enrich the quality of life for those with Alzheimer's, and their caregivers*. Retrieved June 2015, http://horttherapywithhankbruce.weebly.com/alzheimers-with-a-green-thumb.html

Bryan, M., Green, J., Chung, M., & Chang, L. (2011). An adaptive brain-computer interface for humanoid robot control.*IEEE-RAS International Conference on Humanoid Robots*, (pp. 199-204). doi:10.1109/Humanoids.2011.6100901

Buhusi, C. V., & Meck, W. H. (2005). What makes us tick? Functional and neural mechanisms of interval timing. *Nature Reviews. Neuroscience*, *6*(10), 755–765. doi:10.1038/nrn1764 PMID:16163383

Buonomano, D. V., & Karmarkar, U. R. (2002). How do we tell time? *The Neuroscientist*, *8*(1), 42–51. doi:10.1177/107385840200800109 PMID:11843098

Burke, S. N., & Barnes, C. A. (2006). Neural plasticity in the ageing brain. *Nature Reviews. Neuroscience*, *7*(1), 30–40. doi:10.1038/nrn1809 PMID:16371948

Bushara, K. O., Grafman, J., & Hallett, M. (2001). Neural correlates of auditory-visual stimulus onset asynchrony detection. *The Journal of Neuroscience*, *21*, 300–304. PMID:11150347

Busse, A. L., Gil, G., Santarém, J. M., & Filho, W. J. (2009). Physical activity and cognition in the elderly: A review. *Dementia Neuropsychologia, 3*(3), 204–208. Retrieved from http://search.ebscohost.com/login.aspx?direct=true&db=psyh&AN=2010-10986-005&site=ehost-live

Byun, S., & Park, C. (2011). *Serious Game for Cognitive Testing of Elderly HCI International 2011 – Posters' Extended Abstracts* (C. Stephanidis, Ed.). Berlin: Springer Berlin Heidelberg. doi:10.1007/978-3-642-22098-2

Cahn-Weiner, D. A., Malloy, P. F., Rebok, G. W., & Ott, B. R. (2003). Results of a randomized placebo-controlled study of memory training for mildly impaired Alzheimer's disease patients. *Applied Neuropsychology*, *10*(4), 215–223. doi:10.1207/s15324826an1004_3 PMID:14690802

Calvert, G. A. (2001). Crossmodal processing in the human brain: Insights from functional neuroimaging studies. *Cerebral Cortex*, *11*(12), 1110–1123. doi:10.1093/cercor/11.12.1110 PMID:11709482

Camicioli, R., Howieson, D., Oken, B., Sexton, G., & Kaye, J. (1998). Motor slowing precedes cognitive impairment in the oldest old. *Neurology, 50*(5), 1496–1498. doi:10.1212/WNL.50.5.1496 PMID:9596020

Canu, E., McLaren, D. G., Fitzgerald, M. E., Bendlin, B. B., Zoccatelli, G., Alessandrini, F., & Frisoni, G. B. et al. (2010). Microstructural diffusion changes are independent of macrostructural volume loss in moderate to severe Alzheimer's disease. *Journal of Alzheimer's Disease, 19*(3), 963–976. doi:10.3233/JAD-2010-1295 PMID:20157252

Cao, H., Xu, X., Zhao, Y., Long, D., & Zhang, M. (2011). Altered brain activation and connectivity in early parkinson disease tactile perception. *AJNR. American Journal of Neuroradiology, 32*(10), 1969–1974. doi:10.3174/ajnr.A2672 PMID:21998100

Caporale, N., & Dan, Y. (2008). Spike timing-dependent plasticity: A Hebbian learning rule. *Annual Review of Neuroscience, 31*(1), 25–46. doi:10.1146/annurev.neuro.31.060407.125639 PMID:18275283

Capraiello, P. A., & Reis, H. T. (2010). Perceived partner responsiveness minimizes defensive reactions to failure. *Social Psychological & Personality Science, 2*(4), 365–372. doi:10.1177/1948550610391914

Carr, C. E. (1993). Processing of temporal information in the brain. *Annual Review of Neuroscience, 16*(1), 223–243. doi:10.1146/annurev.ne.16.030193.001255 PMID:8460892

Carruthers, P. (2007). The illusion of conscious will. *Synthese, 159*(2), 197–213. doi:10.1007/s11229-007-9204-7

Cassady, J. C., & Johnson, R. E. (2002). Cognitive Test Anxiety and Academic Performance. *Contemporary Educational Psychology, 27*(2), 270–295. doi:10.1006/ceps.2001.1094

Cave, A., & Brown, J. (1992). *Planning and Design Guide for Community Based Day Care Centres*. Alzheimer's Disease Society.

Cedervall, Y., & Aberg, A. C. (2010). Physical activity and implications on well-being in mild Alzheimer's disease: A qualitative case study on two men with dementia and their spouses. *Physiotherapy Theory and Practice, 26*(4), 226–239. doi:10.3109/09593980903423012 PMID:20397857

Chae, Y., Jeong, J., & Jo, S. (2011). Noninvasive Brain-Computer Interface-based control of humanoid navigation. *Intelligent Robots and Systems, IEEE/RSJ International Conference on*, (pp. 685-691).

Chae, Y., Jeong, J., & Jo, S. (2012). Toward brain-actuated humanoid robots: Asynchronous direct-control using an Eeg-Based BCI. *IEEE Transactions on Robotics, 28*(5), 1131–1144. doi:10.1109/TRO.2012.2201310

Chakravartya, M. M., Broadbenta, S., Rosa-Neto, P., Lambert, C. M., & Collins, L. (2009). Design, construction, and validation of an MRI-compatible vibrotactile stimulator intended for clinical use. *Journal of Neuroscience Methods, 184*(1), 129–135. doi:10.1016/j.jneumeth.2009.07.018 PMID:19631690

Chan, I. W. P., Chu, L. W., Lee, P. W., Li, S. W., & Yu, K. K. (2011). Effects of cognitive function and depressive mood on the quality of life in Chinese Alzheimer's disease patients in Hong Kong. *Geriatrics & Gerontology International*, *11*(1), 69–76. doi:10.1111/j.1447-0594.2010.00643.x PMID:20738410

Chan, J. S., Wu, Q., Liang, D., & Yan, J. H. (2015). Visuospatial working memory training facilitates visually-aided explicit sequence learning. *Acta Psychologica*, *161*, 145–153. doi:10.1016/j.actpsy.2015.09.008 PMID:26398484

Chantal, S., Labelle, M., Bouchard, R. W., Braun, C. M., & Boulanger, Y. (2002). Correlation of regional proton magnetic resonance spectroscopic metabolic changes with cognitive deficits in mild Alzheimer disease. *Archives of Neurology*, *59*(6), 955–962. doi:10.1001/archneur.59.6.955 PMID:12056931

Chapman, P. F., Kairiss, E. W., Keenan, C. L., & Brown, T. H. (1990). Long-Term synaptic potentiation in the amygdala. *Synapse (New York, N.Y.)*, *6*(3), 271–278. doi:10.1002/syn.890060306 PMID:2237784

Chen, X., Zhou, Y., Huang, Q., & Yu, Z. (2014). Bipedal walking with toe-off, heel-strike and compliance with external disturbances. *Humanoid Robots, IEEE-RAS International Conference on*.

Cheng, C. P., Chan, S. S., Mak, A. D., Chan, W. C., Cheng, S. T., Shi, L., & Lam, L. C. et al. (2015). Would transcranial direct current stimulation (tDCS) enhance the effects of working memory training in older adults with mild neurocognitive disorder due to Alzheimer's disease: Study protocol for a randomized controlled trial. *Trials*, *16*(1), 479. doi:10.1186/s13063-015-0999-0 PMID:26499250

Cheng, Y., Lin, C. P., Liu, H. L., Hsu, Y. Y., Lim, K. E., Hung, D., & Decety, J. (2007). Expertise modulates the perception of pain in others. *Current Biology*, *17*(19), 1708–1713. doi:10.1016/j.cub.2007.09.020 PMID:17900903

Chen, L. M., Dillenburger, B. C., Wang, F., & Tang, C. H. (2012). Differential fMRI activation to noxious heat and tactile stimuli in parasylvian areas of new world monkeys. *Pain*, *153*(1), 158–169. doi:10.1016/j.pain.2011.10.006 PMID:22115923

Chen, Z., Fan, L., Huan, L., Liu, Y., Ma, W. Y., & Liu, W. Y. (2002). User Intention Modelling in Web Applications Using Data Mining. *Internet and Web Information Systems Journal Kluwer Academic Publishers*, *5*, 181–192.

Chertkow, H., Whitehead, V., Phillips, N., Wolfson, C., Atherton, J., & Bergman, H. (2010). Multilingualism (but not always bilingualism) delays the onset of Alzheimer disease: Evidence from a bilingual community. *Alzheimer Disease and Associated Disorders*, *24*(2), 118–125. doi:10.1097/WAD.0b013e3181ca1221 PMID:20505429

Chiriac, S., Röll, N., Parada, J., & Rosales, B. (2012). Towards combining validation concepts for short and long-term ambient health monitoring. *2012 6th International Conference on Pervasive Computing Technologies for Healthcare and Workshops, PervasiveHealth 2012*. http://doi.org/ doi:<ALIGNMENT.qj></ALIGNMENT>10.4108/icst.pervasivehealth.2012.248676

Choi, B., & Jo, S. (2013). A low-cost eeg system-based hybrid brain-computer interface for humanoid robot navigation and recognition. *PLoS ONE*, *8*(9), e74583–e74583. doi:10.1371/journal.pone.0074583 PMID:24023953

Chong, W. K. O., & Hermreck, C. (2011). *ICSDC 2011: Integrating Sustainability Practices in the Construction Industry*. American Society of Civil Engineers.

Christensen, L. O. D., Johannsen, P., Sinkjaer, T., Petersen, N., Pyndt, H. S., & Nielsen, J. B. (2000). Cerebral activation during bicycle movements in man. *Experimental Brain Research*, *135*, 66–72. doi:10.1007/s002210000493 PMID:11104128

Ciccarelli, O., Toosy, A. T., Marsden, J. F., Wheeler-Kingshott, C. M., Sahyoun, C., Matthews, P. M., & Thompson, A. J. et al. (2005). Identifying brain regions for integrative sensorimotor processing with ankle movements. *Experimental Brain Research*, *166*(1), 31–42. doi:10.1007/s00221-005-2335-5 PMID:16034570

Cienkowski, K. M., & Carney, A. E. (2002). Auditory-visual speech perception and aging. *Ear and Hearing*, *23*(5), 439–449. doi:10.1097/00003446-200210000-00006 PMID:12411777

Ciesielska-Wrobel, I. L., Langenhove, L. V., & Grabowska, K. (2014). Fingertip skin models for analysis of the haptic perception of textiles. *Journal of Biomedical Science and Engineering*, 7(01), 1–6. doi:10.4236/jbise.2014.71001

Clayton, S. D. (2012). *The Oxford Handbook of Environmental and Conservation Psychology (Oxford Library of Psychology)*. Oxford University Press. doi:10.1093/oxfordhb/9780199733026.001.0001

Cleland, E. (2002). The intelligent ASIMO: System overview and integration.*IEEE–RSJ International Conference on Intelligent Robots and Systems*, *3*, 2478 - 2483.

Clugnet, M.-C., & LeDoux, J. E. (1990). Synaptic plasticity in fear conditioning circuits: Induction of LTP in the lateral nucleus of the amygdala by stimulation of the medial geniculate body. *The Journal of Neuroscience*, *10*(8), 2818–2824. PMID:2388089

Cohen, J. D., Noll, D. C., & Schneider, W. (1993). Functional magnetic resonance imaging: Overview and methods for psychological research. *Behavior Research Methods, Instruments, & Computers*, *25*(2), 101–113. doi:10.3758/BF03204483

Cohen-Mansfield, J., & Werner, P. (1998). Visits to an outdoor garden: impact on behaviour and mood of nursing home residents who pace. In B. J. Vellas & L. J. Fitten (Eds.), *Research and practice in Alzheimer's disease* (pp. 419–436). New York: Springer Publishing Company.

Cohen, U., & Weisman, G. D. (1991). *Holding on to Home Designing Environments for people with Dementia*. Baltimore, MD: The John Hopkins University press.

Colcombe, S., & Kramer, A. F. (2003). Fitness effects on the cognitive function of older adults: A Meta-Analytic study. *Psychological Science*, *14*(2), 125–130. doi:10.1111/1467-9280.t01-1-01430 PMID:12661673

Cole, J., Bushnell, M. C., McGlone, F., Elam, M., Lamarre, Y., Vallbo, A., & Olausson, H. (2006). Unmyelinated tactile afferents underpin detection of low-force monofilaments. *Muscle & Nerve, 34*(1), 105–107. doi:10.1002/mus.20534 PMID:16518853

Collerton, J., Collerton, D., Arai, Y., Barrass, K., Eccles, M., Jagger, C., & Kirkwood, T. et al. (2007). A comparison of computerized and pencil-and-paper tasks in assessing cognitive function in community-dwelling older people in the Newcastle 85+ Pilot Study. *Journal of the American Geriatrics Society, 55*(10), 1630–1635. doi:10.1111/j.1532-5415.2007.01379.x PMID:17697099

Collier, V. P. (1995). Acquiring a second language for school. *Directions in Language & Education, 1*, 14.

Collinger, J. L., Wodlinger, B., Downey, J. E., Wang, W., Tyler-Kabara, E. C., Weber, D. J., & Schwartz, A. B. et al. (2013). High-performance neuroprosthetic control by an individual with tetraplegia. *Lancet, 381*(9866), 557–564. doi:10.1016/S0140-6736(12)61816-9 PMID:23253623

Connell, B. R., Sanford, J. A., & Lewis, D. (2007). Therapeutic effects of an outdoor activity program on nursing home residents with dementia. In S. Rodiek & B. Schwarz (Eds.), *Outdoor Environments for People with Dementia*. Haworth Press. doi:10.1300/J081v21n03_10

Conte, A., Modugno, N., Lena, F., Dispenza, S., Gandolfi, B., Iezzi, E., & Berardelli, A. et al. (2010). Subthalamic nucleus stimulation and somatosensory temporal discrimination in Parkinson's disease. *Brain, 133*(9), 2656–2663. doi:10.1093/brain/awq191 PMID:20802206

Corneil, B. D., Van Wanrooij, M., Munoz, D. P., & Van Opstal, A. J. (2002). Auditory-visual interactions subserving goal-directed saccades in a complex scene. *Journal of Neurophysiology, 88*, 438–454. PMID:12091566

Corpas, E., Harman, S. M., & Blackman, M. R. (1993). Human growth hormone and human aging. *Endocrine Reviews, 14*(1), 20–39. doi:10.1210/edrv-14-1-20 PMID:8491152

Corsellis, J. A. N. (1963). Encephalitides. *British Journal of Psychiatry the Journal of Mental Science,* (459), 324.

Costa, T.L., Nogueira, R.M., Pereira, A.G., and Santos, N.A. (2013). Differential effects of aging on spatial contrast sensitivity to linear and polar sine-wave gratings. *Brazilian Journal of Medical and Biological Research, 46*, 855-860.

Costa, A., Hernández, M., & Sebastián-Gallés, N. (2008). Bilingualism aids conflict resolution: Evidence from the ant task. *Cognition, 106*(1), 59–86. doi:10.1016/j.cognition.2006.12.013 PMID:17275801

Costa, A., & Santesteban, M. (2004). Lexical access in bilingual speech production: Evidence from language switching in highly proficient bilinguals and l2 learners. *Journal of Memory and Language, 50*(4), 491–511. doi:10.1016/j.jml.2004.02.002

Costa, M., Priplata, A. A., Lipsitz, L. A., Wu, Z., Huang, N. E., Goldberger, A. L., & Peng, C. K. (2007). Noise and poise: Enhancement of postural complexity in the elderly with a stochastic-resonance-based therapy. *Europhysics Letters*, *77*(6), 68008. doi:10.1209/0295-5075/77/68008 PMID:17710211

Coull, J. T., Cheng, R. K., & Meck, W. H. (2011). Neuroanatomical and neurochemical substrates of timing. *Neuropsychopharmacology*, *36*(1), 3–25. doi:10.1038/npp.2010.113 PMID:20668434

Coull, J. T., & Nobre, A. C. (1998). Where and when to pay attention: The neural systems for directing attention to spatial locations and to time intervals as revealed by both PET and fMRI. *The Journal of Neuroscience*, *18*(18), 7426–7435. PMID:9736662

Coull, J., & Nobre, A. (2008). Dissociating explicit timing from temporal expectation with fMRI. *Current Opinion in Neurobiology*, *18*(2), 137–144. doi:10.1016/j.conb.2008.07.011 PMID:18692573

Covey, E., & Casseday, J. H. (1999). Timing in the auditory system of the bat. *Annual Review of Physiology*, *61*(1), 457–476. doi:10.1146/annurev.physiol.61.1.457 PMID:10099697

Craig, A. D. (2008). *In handbook of emotions* (3rd ed.). New York, NY: Guilford Press.

Crews, L., & Masliah, E. (2010). Molecular mechanisms of neurodegeneration in Alzheimer's disease. *Human Molecular Genetics*. PMID:20413653

Cuervo, M., Ansorena, D., García, A., Astiasaran, I., & Martinez, J. A. (2008). Food consumption analysis in spanish elderly based upon the mini nutritional assessment test. *Annals of Nutrition & Metabolism*, *52*(4), 299–307. doi:10.1159/000151483 PMID:18714147

Cuervo, M., Ansorena, D., Martínez-González, M. A., García, A., Astiasarán, I., & Martínez, J. A. (2009). Impact of global and subjective mini nutritional assessment (MNA) questions on the evaluation of the nutritional status: The role of gender and age. *Archives of Gerontology and Geriatrics*, *49*(1), 69–73. doi:10.1016/j.archger.2008.05.003 PMID:18573549

Czaplicka, A., Holyst, J. A., & Sloot, P. M. A. (2013). Noise enhances information transfer in hierarchical networks. *Scientific Reports*, *3*, 1223. doi:10.1038/srep01223 PMID:23390574

Damasio, A. R. (2000). Eighth C.U. Ariëns Kappers Lecture. The fabric of the mind: A neurobiological perspective. *Progress in Brain Research*, *126*, 457–467. doi:10.1016/S0079-6123(00)26029-9 PMID:11105662

Damasio, A. R. (Ed.). (1994). *Descartes' error: emotion, reason, and the human brain*. New York, NY: Vintage Press.

Damasio, A. R. (Ed.). (1994). *Descartes' Error: Emotion, Reason, and the Human Brain*. New York: Vintage Press.

Danysz, W., & Parsons, C. G. (2012). Alzheimer's disease, β-amyloid, glutamate, NMDA receptors and memantine–searching for the connections. *British Journal of Pharmacology*, *167*(2), 324–352. doi:10.1111/j.1476-5381.2012.02057.x PMID:22646481

Davis, R. N., Massman, P. J., & Doody, R. S. (2001). Cognitive intervention in Alzheimer disease: A randomized placebo-controlled study. *Alzheimer Disease and Associated Disorders*, *15*(1), 1–9. doi:10.1097/00002093-200101000-00001 PMID:11236819

Daydamony, E. M., Gayar, M. E., & Chadi, F. (2008). A computerized system for SEMG signals analysis and classifieation.*25th National Radio Science Conference* (pp. 1-7). Tanta: IEEE. doi:10.1109/NRSC.2008.4542388

de Portugal, A. J., de Portugal, F., Rivera, B. L., Chimpén, R. V., González, S. M. F., & Sánchez, R. A. Waist/hip ratio and vascular risk factors in obese and not obese individuals. Anales de Medicina Interna, 14(1), 3-8.

de Sousa, O. L. V., & do Amaral, T. F. (2014). LB014-MON: Quality of life and nutritional status in moderate Alzheimer's disease patients. *Clinical Nutrition (Edinburgh, Lothian)*, *33*(1), S256. doi:10.1016/S0261-5614(14)50672-3

De Vreese, L. P., Neri, M., Fioravanti, M., Belloi, L., & Zanetti, O. (2001). Memory rehabilitation in Alzheimer's disease: A review of progress. *International Journal of Geriatric Psychiatry*, *16*(8), 794–809. doi:10.1002/gps.428 PMID:11536347

Delbeuck, X., Collette, F., & Van der Linden, M. (2007). Is Alzheimer's disease a disconnection syndrome? Evidence from a crossmodal audio-visual illusory experiment. *Neuropsychologia*, *45*(14), 3315–3323. doi:10.1016/j.neuropsychologia.2007.05.001 PMID:17765932

Detweiler, M. B., Murphy, P. F., Kim, K. Y., Myers, L. C., & Ashiai, A. (2009). Scheduled medications and falls in dementia patients utilizing a wander garden. *American Journal of Alzheimer's Disease and Other Dementias*, *24*(4), 322–332. doi:10.1177/1533317509334036 PMID:19366885

Detweiler, M. B., Murphy, P. F., Myers, L. C., & Kim, K. Y. (2008). Does a wander garden influence inappropriate behaviors in dementia residents? *American Journal of Alzheimer's Disease and Other Dementias*, *23*(1), 31–45. doi:10.1177/1533317507309799 PMID:18276956

Diederich, A., & Colonius, H. (2004). Bimodal and trimodal multisensory enhancement: Effects of stimulus onset and intensity on reaction time. *Perception & Psychophysics*, *66*(8), 1388–1404. doi:10.3758/BF03195006 PMID:15813202

Diehl, R. L., Lotto, A. J., & Holt, L. L. (2004). Speech perception. *Annual Review of Psychology*, *55*(1), 149–179. doi:10.1146/annurev.psych.55.090902.142028 PMID:14744213

Dietz, V., & Duysens, J. (2000). Significance of load receptor input during locomotion: A review. *Gait & Posture*, *11*(2), 102–110. doi:10.1016/S0966-6362(99)00052-1 PMID:10899663

Dietz, V., Gollhofer, A., Kleiber, M., & Trippel, M. (1992). Regulation of bipedal stance: Dependency on "load" receptors. *Experimental Brain Research*, *89*(1), 229–231. doi:10.1007/BF00229020 PMID:1601101

Dietz, V., Grillner, S., Trepp, A., Hubli, M., & Bolliger, M. (2009). Changes in spinal reflex and locomotor activity after a complete spinal cord injury: A common mechanism? *Brain*, *132*(8), 2196–2205. doi:10.1093/brain/awp124 PMID:19460795

Dietz, V., Muller, R., & Colombo, G. (2002). Locomotor activity in spinal man: Significance of afferent input from joint and load receptors. *Brain, 125*(12), 2626–2634. doi:10.1093/brain/awf273 PMID:12429590

Ding, Q. P., Tong, R. K., & Li, G. (2006). Development of an EOG (electro-oculography) based human-computer interface. In *Engineering in Medicine and Biology Society 27th Annual International Conference* (pp. 6829-6831). Shanghai: IEEE.

Dixon, C. J. M. (2002). A Return to the garden: Design Criteria for Therapeutic Exterior Environments for People with Alzheimer Disease. (Master's Thesis). University of Manitoba, Winnipeg, Manitoba, Canada.

Dobkin, B. H., Firestine, A., West, M., Saremi, K., & Woods, R. (2004). Ankle dorsiflexion as an fMRI paradigm to assay motor control for walking during rehabilitation. *NeuroImage, 23*(1), 370–381. doi:10.1016/j.neuroimage.2004.06.008 PMID:15325385

Dresel, C., Parzinger, A., Rimpau, C., Zimmer, C., Ceballos-Baumann, A. O., & Haslinger, B. (2008). A new device for tactile stimulation during fMRI. *NeuroImage, 39*(3), 1094–1103. doi:10.1016/j.neuroimage.2007.09.033 PMID:17997331

Droit-Volet, S., Clement, A., & Wearden, J. (2001). Temporal generalization in 3- to 8-year-old children. *Journal of Experimental Child Psychology, 80*(3), 271–288. doi:10.1006/jecp.2001.2629 PMID:11583526

Droit-Volet, S., & Wearden, J. H. (2001). Temporal bisection in children. *Journal of Experimental Child Psychology, 80*(2), 142–159. doi:10.1006/jecp.2001.2631 PMID:11529672

Droogsma, E., Van Asselt, D. Z. B., Scholzel-Dorenbos, C. J. M., Van Steijn, J. H. M., Van Walderveen, P. E., & Van Der Hooft, C. S. (2013). Nutritional status of community-dwelling elderly with newly diagnosed Alzheimer's disease: Prevalence of malnutrition and the relation of various factors to nutritional status. *The Journal of Nutrition, Health & Aging, 17*(7), 606–610. doi:10.1007/s12603-013-0032-9 PMID:23933871

Dubois, B., Feldman, H. H., Jacova, C., Dekosky, S. T., Barberger-Gateau, P., Cummings, J., & Scheltens, P. et al. (2007). Research criteria for the diagnosis of Alzheimer's disease: Revising the NINCDS-ADRDA criteria. *Lancet Neurology, 6*(8), 734–746. doi:10.1016/S1474-4422(07)70178-3 PMID:17616482

Duchowski, A. (2007). *Eye tracking methodology: Theory and practice*. Springer.

Dvorak, R. V., & Poehlman, E. T. (1998). Appendicular skeletal muscle mass, physical activity, and cognitive status in patients with Alzheimer's disease. *Neurology, 51*(5), 1386–1390. doi:10.1212/WNL.51.5.1386 PMID:9818865

Dykes, R. W., Miquee, A., Xerri, C., Zennou-Azogui, Y., Rainville, C., Dumoulin, A., & Marineau, D. (2007). A delivery device for presentation of tactile stimuli during functional magnetic resonance imaging. *Journal of Neuroscience Methods, 159*(2), 308–317. doi:10.1016/j.jneumeth.2006.07.020 PMID:16945420 *dynanets.org*. (2015). Retrieved July 25, 2015, from http://dynanets.org/

Edwards, C. A., McDonnell, C., & Merl, H. (2013). An evaluation of a therapeutic garden's influence on the quality of life of aged care residents with dementia. *Dementia (London), 12*(4), 494–510. doi:10.1177/1471301211435188 PMID:24336957

Ekman, P., & Friesen, W. V. (1971). Constants across cultures in the face and emotion. *Journal of Personality and Social Psychology, 17*(2), 124–129. doi:10.1037/h0030377 PMID:5542557

Elia, M., Jones, B., & Russell, C. (2008). Malnutrition in various care settings in the UK: The 2007 nutrition screening week survey. *Clinical Medicine*, *8*(4), 364–365. doi:10.7861/clinmedicine.8-4-364 PMID:18724599

Elings, M. (2006). People-plant interaction: the physiological, psychological and sociological effects of plants on people. In Farming for Health. Green-Care Farming Across Europe and the United States of America. Springer. doi:10.1007/1-4020-4541-7_4

ERIN Research Inc. (2010). *Landscape architecture and public welfare*. Council of Landscape Architectural Registration Boards. Retrieved June 2015, https://www.clarb.org/CLARBDocuments/PublicWelfareFINAL.pdf

Erol, A., Bebis, G., Nicolescu, M., Boyle, R. D., & Twombly, X. (2007). Vision-based hand pose estimation: A review. *Computer Vision and Image Understanding, 108*(1-2), 52–73. doi:10.1016/j.cviu.2006.10.012

Esiri, M., Matthews, F., Brayne, C., Ince, P., Matthews, F., & Xuereb, J. (2001). Pathological correlates of late-onset dementia in a multicenter, community-based population in England and Wales. *Lancet*, *357*(9251), 169–175. doi:10.1016/S0140-6736(00)03589-3 PMID:11213093

Farwell, L. A., & Donchin, E. (1988). Talking off the top of your head: Toward a mental prosthesis utilizing event-related brain potentials. *Electroencephalography and Clinical Neurophysiology, 70*(6), 510–523. doi:10.1016/0013-4694(88)90149-6 PMID:2461285

Faxen-Irving, G., Andren-Olsson, B., Geijerstam, A. A., Basun, H., & Cederholm, T. (2002). Original Communications-The effect of nutritional intervention in elderly subjects residing in group-living for the demented. *European Journal of Clinical Nutrition, 56*(3), 221–227. doi:10.1038/sj.ejcn.1601304 PMID:11960297

Fellgiebel, A., Dellani, P. R., Greverus, D., Scheurich, A., Stoeter, P., & Müller, M. J. (2006). Predicting conversion to dementia in mild cognitive impairment by volumetric and diffusivity measurements of the hippocampus. *Psychiatry Research: Neuroimaging, 146*(3), 283–287. doi:10.1016/j.pscychresns.2006.01.006 PMID:16530394

Fernández, A., Turrero, A., Zuluaga, P., Gil, P., Maestú, F., Campo, P., & Ortiz, T. (2006). Magnetoencephalographic parietal delta dipole density in mild cognitive impairment: Preliminary results of a method to estimate the risk of developing Alzheimer disease. *Archives of Neurology, 63*(3), 427–430. doi:10.1001/archneur.63.3.427 PMID:16533970

Ferri, C. P., Prince, M., Brayne, C., Brodaty, H., Fratiglioni, L., Ganguli, M., & Scazufca, M. et al. (2005). Global prevalence of dementia: A Delphi consensus study. *Lancet*, *366*(9503), 2112–2117. doi:10.1016/S0140-6736(05)67889-0 PMID:16360788

Fiorio, M., Marotta, A., Ottaviani, S., Pozzer, L., & Tinazzi, M. (2014). Aristotle's illusion in parkinson's disease: Evidence for normal interdigit tactile perception. *PLoS ONE*, *9*(2), e88686. doi:10.1371/journal.pone.0088686 PMID:24523929

Fleischer, C., & Hommel, G. A. (2008). A human-exoskeleton interface utilizing electromyography. *IEEE Transactions on Robotics*, *24*(4), 872–882. doi:10.1109/TRO.2008.926860

Flicker, L. (1999). Book: Dementia Reconsidered: the Person Comes First. *BMJ (Clinical Research Ed.)*, *318*(7187), 880–880. doi:10.1136/bmj.318.7187.880a PMID:10092286

Folstein, M. F., Folstein, S. E., & Mchugh, P. R. (1975). "Mini-mental state". A practical method for grading the cognitive state of patients for the clinician. *Journal of Psychiatric Research*, *12*(1), 189–198. doi:10.1016/0022-3956(75)90026-6 PMID:1202204

Fontaine, K. R., & Barofsky, I. (2001). Obesity and health-related quality of life. *Obesity Reviews*, *2*(3), 173–182. doi:10.1046/j.1467-789x.2001.00032.x PMID:12120102

Fox, P. T., Lancaster, J. L., Parsons, L. M., Xiong, J. H., & Zamarripa, F. (1997). Functional volumes modeling: theory and preliminary assessment. *Hum Brain Mapp*, *5*(4), 306-311. doi: 10.1002/(SICI)1097-0193(1997)5:4<306::AID-HBM17>3.0.CO;2-B 10.1002/(SICI)1097-0193(1997)5:4<306::AID-HBM17>3.0.CO;2-B

Fox, N. C., & Freeborough, P. A. (1997). Brain atrophy progression measured from registered serial MRI: Validation and application to alzheimer's disease. *Journal of Magnetic Resonance Imaging*, *7*(6), 1069–1075. doi:10.1002/jmri.1880070620 PMID:9400851

Francis, D. D., Caldji, C., Champagne, F., Plotsky, P. M., & Meaney, M. J. (1999). The role of corticotropin-releasing factor--norepinephrine systems in mediating the effects of early experience on the development of behavioral and endocrine responses to stress. *Biological Psychiatry*, *46*(9), 1153–1166. doi:10.1016/S0006-3223(99)00237-1 PMID:10560022

Frank, S. M., & Greenlee, M. W. (2014). An MRI-compatible caloric stimulation device for the investigation of human vestibular cortex. *Journal of Neuroscience Methods*, *235*, 208–218. doi:10.1016/j.jneumeth.2014.07.008 PMID:25064191

Frantzidis, C. A., Vivas, A. B., Tsolaki, A., Klados, M. A., Tsolaki, M., & Bamidis, P. D. (2014). Functional disorganization of small-world brain networks in mild Alzheimer's Disease and amnestic Mild Cognitive Impairment: An EEG study using Relative Wavelet Entropy (RWE). *Frontiers in Aging Neuroscience*, *6*, 224. doi:10.3389/fnagi.2014.00224 PMID:25206333

Fratiglioni, L., Wang, H. X., Ericsson, K., Maytan, M., & Winblad, B. (2000). Influence of social network on occurrence of dementia: A community-based longitudinal study. *Lancet*, *355*(9212), 1315–1319. doi:10.1016/S0140-6736(00)02113-9 PMID:10776744

French, C., & Llorente, A. M. (2008). *Language: Development, Bilingualism, and Abnormal States. Principles of Neuropsychological Assessment with Hispanics*. Springer New York.

Frisancho, A. R. (1999). *Anthropometric standards for the assesment of growth and nutritional status*. The University of Michigan Press.

Frisoni, G. B., Fox, N. C., Jack, C. R., Scheltens, P., & Thompson, P. M. (2010). The clinical use of structural MRI in Alzheimer disease. *Nature Reviews. Nephrology*, *6*(2), 67–77. doi:10.1038/nrneurol.2009.215 PMID:20139996

Frith, C. (2002). Attention to action and awareness of other minds. *Consciousness and Cognition*, *11*(4), 481–487. doi:10.1016/S1053-8100(02)00022-3 PMID:12470618

Fukuyama, H., Ouchi, Y., Matsuzaki, S., Nagahama, Y., Yamauchi, H., Ogawa, M., & Shibasaki, H. et al. (1997). Brain functional activity during gait in normal subjects: A SPECT study. *Neuroscience Letters*, *228*(3), 183–186. doi:10.1016/S0304-3940(97)00381-9 PMID:9218638

Gallagher, M. L. (2012). Intake: The nutrients and their metabolism. In L. K. Mahan, S. Escott-Stump, & J. L. Raymond (Eds.), *Krause's food & the nutrition care process* (pp. 32–128). Elsevier Health Sciences.

Gallasch, E., Fend, M., Rafolt, D., Nardone, R., Kunz, A. B., Kronbichler, M., & Golaszewski, S. et al. (2010). Cuff-type pneumatic stimulator for studying somatosensory evoked responses with fMRI. *NeuroImage*, *50*(3), 1067–1073. doi:10.1016/j.neuroimage.2010.01.014 PMID:20079447

Gallasch, E., Golaszewski, S. M., Fend, M., Siedentopf, C. M., Koppelstaetter, F., Eisner, W., & Felber, S. R. et al. (2006). Contact force- and amplitude-controllable vibrating probe for somatosensory mapping of plantar afferences with fMRI. *Journal of Magnetic Resonance Imaging*, *24*(5), 1177–1182. doi:10.1002/jmri.20742 PMID:17031838

Gallese, V. (2003). The manifold nature of interpersonal relations: The quest for a common mechanism. *Philosophical Transactions of the Royal Society of London. Series B, Biological Sciences*, *358*(1431), 517–528. doi:10.1098/rstb.2002.1234 PMID:12689377

Garcés, P., Angel Pineda-Pardo, J., Canuet, L., Aurtenetxe, S., López, M. E., Marcos, A., & Maestú, F. et al. (2014). The Default Mode Network is functionally and structurally disrupted in amnestic mild cognitive impairment - a bimodal MEG-DTI study. *NeuroImage. Clinical*, *6*, 214–221. doi:10.1016/j.nicl.2014.09.004 PMID:25379433

Garcia, C. (2014). *The Benefits of Memory Gardens at Nursing Homes*. Retrieved June 2015, http://studio-sprout.com/files/The-Benefits-of-Memory-Gardens-at-Nursing-Homes.pdf

Garry, P. J., & Vellas, B. J. (1996). Aging and nutrition. In E. E. Ziegler & L. J. Filer Jr., (Eds.), *Present knowledgein nutrition* (pp. 414–419). Washington, DC: ILSI Press.

Gascon, G. G., & Gilles, F. (1973). Limbic dementia. *Journal of Neurology, Neurosurgery, and Psychiatry*, *36*(3), 421–430. doi:10.1136/jnnp.36.3.421 PMID:4714104

Gaugler, J. E., Kane, R. L., Kane, R. A., & Newcomer, R. (2005). Unmet care needs and key outcomes in dementia. *Journal of the American Geriatrics Society*, *53*(12), 2098–2105. doi:10.1111/j.1532-5415.2005.00495.x PMID:16398893

Gazzaley, A., & Nobre, A. C. (2012). Top-down modulation: Bridging selective attention and working memory. *Trends in Cognitive Sciences*, *16*(2), 129–135. doi:10.1016/j.tics.2011.11.014 PMID:22209601

Gazzaniga, M. S., Ivry, R. B., & Mangun, G. R. (Eds.). (2013). *Cognitive neuroscience: the biology of the mind* (4th ed.). W. W. Norton & Company.

Geldard, F. A. (1960). Some neglected possibilities of communication. *Science*, *131*(3413), 1583–1588. doi:10.1126/science.131.3413.1583 PMID:13827173

Gergondet, P., & Kheddar, A. (2015). Ssvep stimuli design for object-centric bci. *Brain-Computer Interfaces*, 2.

Gewirth, L. R., Shindler, A. G., & Hier, D. B. (1984). Altered patterns of word associations in dementia and aphasia. *Brain and Language*, *21*(21), 307–317. doi:10.1016/0093-934X(84)90054-3 PMID:6704703

Gewirtz, J. L., & Peláez-Nogueras, M. B. (1992). Skinner's legacy to human infant behavior and development. *The American Psychologist*, *47*(11), 1411–1422. doi:10.1037/0003-066X.47.11.1411 PMID:1482005

Giacobini, E. (2000). Cholinesterase inhibitors stabilize Alzheimer's disease. *Annals of the New York Academy of Sciences*, *920*(1), 321–327. doi:10.1111/j.1749-6632.2000.tb06942.x PMID:11193171

Gibbon, J., Malapani, C., Dale, C. L., & Gallistel, C. (1997). Toward a neurobiology of temporal cognition: Advances and challenges. *Current Opinion in Neurobiology*, *7*(2), 170–184. doi:10.1016/S0959-4388(97)80005-0 PMID:9142762

Gierthmuhlen, J., Schumacher, S., Deuschl, G., Fritzer, E., Llein, C., & Baron, R. (2010). Somatosensory function in asymptomatic Parkin-mutation carriers. *European Journal of Neurology*, *17*(3), 513–517. doi:10.1111/j.1468-1331.2009.02797.x PMID:19863651

Gigliotti, C. M., Jarrott, S. E., & Yorgason, J. (2004). Harvesting health: Effects of three types of horticultural therapy activities for persons with dementia. *Dementia (London)*, *3*(2), 161–180. doi:10.1177/1471301204042335

Gillette-Guyonnet, S., Lauque, S., & Ousset, P. J. (2005). Nutrition and Alzheimer's disease. *Psychologie & Neuropsychiatrie du Vieillissement*, *3*, S35–S41. PMID:15899603

Gillette-Guyonnet, S., Nourhashémi, F., Andrieu, S., de Glisezinski, I., Ousset, P. J., Rivière, D., & Vellas, B. (2000). Weight loss in Alzheimer disease. *The American Journal of Clinical Nutrition*, *71*(2), 637s–642s. PMID:10681272

Gillioz, A. S., Villars, H., Voisin, T., Cortes, F., Gillette-Guyonnet, S., Andrieu, S., & Vellas, B. (2009). Spared and impaired abilities in community-dwelling patients entering the severe stage of Alzheimer's disease. *Dementia and Geriatric Cognitive Disorders*, *28*(5), 412–417. doi:10.1159/000255635 PMID:19907179

Glover, G. H., Lemieux, S. K., Drangova, M., & Pauly, J. M. (1996). Decomposition of inflow and blood oxygen level-dependent (BOLD) effects with dual-echo spiral gradient-recalled echo (GRE) fMRI. *Magnetic Resonance in Medicine*, *35*(3), 299–308. doi:10.1002/mrm.1910350306 PMID:8699940

Goes, V. F., Horst, J. A. E., Paganini, J. C. D. A., da Silva, W. C. F. N., Khalil, N. M., & Bonini, J. S. (2015). Nutritional status and food intake of Brazilian patients at various stages of Alzheimer's disease: A cross-sectional study. *Revista de Ciências Farmacêuticas Básica e Aplicada*, *35*(2), 211–215.

Goes, V. F., Mello-Carpes, P. B., Oliveira, L. O. D., Hack, J., Magro, M., & Bonini, J. S. (2014). Evaluation of dysphagia risk, nutritional status and caloric intake in elderly patients with Alzheimer's. *Revista Latino-Americana de Enfermagem*, *22*(2), 317–324. doi:10.1590/0104-1169.3252.2418 PMID:26107841

Golaszewski, S. M., Siedentopf, C. M., Baldauf, E., Koppelstaetter, F., Eisner, W., Unterrainer, J., & Felber, S. R. et al. (2002, September). Functional magnetic resonance imaging of the human sensorimotor cortex using a novel ibrotactile stimulator. *NeuroImage*, *17*(1), 421–430. doi:10.1006/nimg.2002.1195 PMID:12482095

Golaszewsk, S. M., Siedentopf, C. M., Koppelstaetter, F., Fend, M., Ischebeck, E., & Gonzalez-Felipe, V. et al.. (2006). Human brain structures related to plantar vibrotactile stimulation: A functional magnetic resonance imaging study. *NeuroImage*, *29*(3), 923–929. doi:10.1016/j.neuroimage.2005.08.052 PMID:16253525

Gollan, T. H., Montoya, R. I., & Werner, G. A. (2002). Semantic and letter fluency in Spanish-English bilinguals. *Neuropsychology*, *16*(4), 562–576. doi:10.1037/0894-4105.16.4.562 PMID:12382994

Gollan, T. H., Salmon, D. P., Montoya, R. I., & Galasko, D. R. (2011). Degree of bilingualism predicts age of diagnosis of Alzheimer's disease in low-education but not in highly educated Hispanics. *Neuropsychologia*, *49*(14), 3826–3830. doi:10.1016/j.neuropsychologia.2011.09.041 PMID:22001315

Golle, P., & Partridge, K. (2009). Pervasive Computing (Vol. 5538). Berlin: Springer Berlin Heidelberg. http://doi.org/ doi:<ALIGNMENT.qj></ALIGNMENT>10.1007/978-3-642-01516-8_26

Gomez-Ramirez, J., & Wu, J. (2014). Network-based biomarkers in Alzheimer's disease: review and future directions. *Frontiers in Aging Neuroscience, 6*.

Gordon, E. L., Cindee, M., Vaughn, B. N., Cheong, A. M. Y., & Miller, J. C. (2008). Retention of high tactile acuity throughout the life span in blindness. *Perception & Psychophysics*, *70*(8), 1471–1488. doi:10.3758/PP.70.8.1471 PMID:19064491

Gordon, I., Voos, A. C., Bennett, R. H., Bolling, D. Z., Pelphrey, K. A., & Kaiser, M. D. (2013). Brain mechanisms for processing affective touch. *Human Brain Mapping*, *34*(4), 914–922. doi:10.1002/hbm.21480 PMID:22125232

Graham, S. J., Staines, W. R., Nelson, A., Plewes, D. B., & McIlroy, W. E. (2001). New devices to deliver somatosensory stimuli during functional MRI. *Magnetic Resonance in Medicine*, *46*(3), 436–442. doi:10.1002/mrm.1211 PMID:11550233

Gray-Donald, K., Payette, H., & Boutier, V. (1995). Randomized clinical trial of nutritional supplementation shows little effect on functional status among free-living frail elderly. *The Journal of Nutrition*, *125*(12), 2965–2971. PMID:7500174

Green, C. T., Long, D. L., Green, D., Iosif, A.-M., Dixon, J. F., Miller, M. R., & Schweitzer, J. B. et al. (2012). Will working memory training generalize to improve off-task behavior in children with attention-deficit/hyperactivity disorder? *Neurotherapeutics: The Journal of the American Society for Experimental NeuroTherapeutics*, *9*(3), 639–648. doi:10.1007/s13311-012-0124-y PMID:22752960

Greenwood, C. E., Tam, C., Chan, M., Young, K. W., Binns, M. A., & Van Reekum, R. (2005). Behavioral disturbances, not cognitive deterioration, are associated with altered food selection in seniors with Alzheimer's disease. *The Journals of Gerontology. Series A, Biological Sciences and Medical Sciences*, *60*(4), 499–505. doi:10.1093/gerona/60.4.499 PMID:15933391

Greicius, M. D., Srivastava, G., Reiss, A. L., & Menon, V. (2004). Default-mode network activity distinguishes Alzheimer's disease from healthy aging: Evidence from functional MRI. *Proceedings of the National Academy of Sciences of the United States of America*, *101*(13), 4637–4642. doi:10.1073/pnas.0308627101 PMID:15070770

Griffin, J. W., McArthur, J. C., & Polydefkis, M. (2001). Assessment of cutaneous innervation by skin biopsies. *Current Opinion in Neurology*, *14*(5), 655–659. doi:10.1097/00019052-200110000-00016 PMID:11562579

Groessl, E. J., Kaplan, R. M., Barrett-Connor, E., & Ganiats, T. G. (2004). Body mass index and quality of well-being in a community of older adults. *American Journal of Preventive Medicine*, *26*(2), 126–129. doi:10.1016/j.amepre.2003.10.007 PMID:14751323

Grove, K. (2012). *Gardens for People with Dementia*. Retrieved June 2015, http://www.kimgrove-gardendesigner.co.uk/resources/Gardens%20for%20People%20with%20Dementia%20-%20A%20Guide%20to%20Make%20Them%20Safe%20and%20Suitable%20-%202013.pdf

Grunwald, M., Weiss, T., Mueller, S., & Rall, L. (2014). EEG changes caused by spontaneous facial self-touch may represent emotion regulating processes and working memory maintenance. *Brain Research*, *1557*, 111–126. doi:10.1016/j.brainres.2014.02.002 PMID:24530432

Guérin, O., Andrieu, S., Schneider, S. M., Milano, M., Boulahssass, R., Brocker, P., & Vellas, B. (2005). Different modes of weight loss in Alzheimer disease: A prospective study of 395 patients. *The American Journal of Clinical Nutrition*, *82*(2), 435–441. PMID:16087990

Guigoz, Y. (2006). The Mini Nutritional Assessment (MNA) review of the literature-what does it tell us? *The Journal of Nutrition, Health & Aging*, *10*(6), 466–485. PMID:17183419

Gujar, S. K., Maheshwari, S., Björkman-Burtscher, I., & Sundgren, P. C. (2005). Magnetic resonance spectroscopy. *Journal of Neuro-Ophthalmology*, *25*, 217–226. doi:10.1097/01.wno.0000177307.21081.81 PMID:16148633

Gurvit, H. I. (2004). Demans sendromu. [Dementia syndrome]. In S. Z. Bahar & A. E. Öge (Eds.), *Alzheimer hastalığı ve Alzheimer dışı Demanslar* [Alzheimer's disease and non-Alzheimer's dementias] (pp. 367–415). İstanbul: Nobel Tıp Kitabevleri. (in Turkish)

Gurvit, H., Emre, M., Tinaz, S., Bilgic, B., Hanagasi, H., Sahin, H., & Harmanci, H. (2008). The prevalence of dementia in an urban Turkish population. *American Journal of Alzheimer's Disease and Other Dementias*, *23*(1), 67–76. doi:10.1177/1533317507310570 PMID:18276959

Hagler, S., Austin, D., Hayes, T. L., Kaye, J., & Pavel, M. (2010). Unobtrusive and ubiquitous in-home monitoring: A methodology for continuous assessment of gait velocity in elders. *IEEE Transactions on Bio-Medical Engineering*, *57*(4), 813–820. doi:10.1109/TBME.2009.2036732 PMID:19932989

Hagler, S., Jimison, H. B., & Pavel, M. (2014). Assessing executive function using a computer game: Computational modeling of cognitive processes. *IEEE Journal of Biomedical and Health Informatics*, *18*(4), 1442–1452. doi:10.1109/JBHI.2014.2299793 PMID:25014944

Hajnal, J. V., Myers, R., Oatridge, A., Schwieso, J. E., Young, I. R., & Bydder, G. M. (1994). Artifacts due to stimulus correlated motion in functional imaging of the brain. *Magnetic Resonance in Medicine*, *31*(3), 283–291. doi:10.1002/mrm.1910310307 PMID:8057799

Hakuta, K. (1986). Cognitive development of bilingual children. *Acculturation*, *44*(1), 36–54.

Hamers, J. F., & Blanc, M. (2000). *Bilinguality and Bilingualism*. Cambridge University Press. doi:10.1017/CBO9780511605796

Hampel, H., Frank, R., Broich, K., Teipel, S. J., Katz, R. G., Hardy, J., & Hoessler, Y. C. et al. (2010). Biomarkers for Alzheimer's disease: Academic, industry and regulatory perspectives. *Nature Reviews. Drug Discovery*, *9*(7), 560–574. doi:10.1038/nrd3115 PMID:20592748

Hanakawa, T., Katsumi, Y., Fukuyama, H., Honda, M., Hayashi, T., Kimura, J., & Shibasaki, H. (1999). Mechanisms underlying gait disturbance in Parkinson's disease—a single photon emission computed tomography study. *Brain*, *122*(7), 1271–1282. doi:10.1093/brain/122.7.1271 PMID:10388793

Hao, Y., Manor, B., Liu, J., Zhang, K., Chai, Y., Lipsitz, L., & Fang, J. et al. (2013). A novel MRI-compatible tactile stimulator for cortical mapping of foot sole pressure stimuli with fMRI. *Magnetic Resonance in Medicine*, *69*(4), 1194–1199. doi:10.1002/mrm.24330 PMID:22678849

Harrington, G. S., Wright, C. T., & Downs, J. R. (2000). A new vibrotactile stimulator for functional MRI. *Human Brain Mapping*, *10*(3), 140–145. doi:10.1002/1097-0193(200007)10:3<140::AID-HBM50>3.0.CO;2-0 PMID:10912593

Harris, C. W., Dines, N. T., & Brown, K. D. (1998). *Time-Saver Standards for Landscape Architecture*. McGraw-Hill Education.

Hartig, T., & Cooper-Marcus, C. (2006). Healing Gardens: Places for nature in health care. *Lancet*, *368*, 36–37. doi:10.1016/S0140-6736(06)69920-0

Hartig, T., Evans, G. W., Jamner, L. D., Davis, D. S., & Garling, T. (2003). Tracking restoration in natural and urban field settings. *Journal of Environmental Psychology*, *23*(2), 109–123. doi:10.1016/S0272-4944(02)00109-3

Hayashi, M. J., Kantele, M., Walsh, V., Carlson, S., & Kanai, R. (2014). Dissociable neuroanatomical correlates of subsecond and suprasecond time perception. *Journal of Cognitive Neuroscience*, *26*(8), 1685–1693. doi:10.1162/jocn_a_00580 PMID:24456398

Hayes, T. L., Abendroth, F., Adami, A., Pavel, M., Zitzelberger, T. A., & Kaye, J. A. (2008). Unobtrusive assessment of activity patterns associated with mild cognitive impairment. *Alzheimer's & Dementia : The Journal of the Alzheimer's Association*, *4*(6), 395–405. doi:10.1016/j.jalz.2008.07.004 PMID:19012864

Hayes, T. L., Riley, T., Mattek, N., Pavel, M., & Kaye, J. A. (2014). Sleep habits in mild cognitive impairment. *Alzheimer Disease and Associated Disorders*, *28*(2), 145–150. doi:10.1097/WAD.0000000000000010 PMID:24145694

Health Council of the Netherlands and Dutch Advisory Council for Research on Spatial Planning Nature and the Environment (HCNDACRSP). (2004). *Nature and Health. The influence of nature on social, psychological and physical wellbeing*. Health Council of the Netherlands and RMNO.

Hebb, D. (1949). *The Organization of Behaviour: A Neuropsychological Theory*. Academic Press.

Hebert, L. E., Weuve, J., Scherr, P. A., & Evans, D. A. (2013). Alzheimer disease in the United States (2010–2050) estimated using the 2010 census. *Neurology*, *80*(19), 1778–1783. doi:10.1212/WNL.0b013e31828726f5 PMID:23390181

Hedden, T., & Gabrieli, J. D. E. (2004). Insights into the ageing mind: A view from cognitive neuroscience. *Nature Reviews. Neuroscience*, *5*(2), 87–96. doi:10.1038/nrn1323 PMID:14735112

Hegner, Y. L., Lee, Y., Grodd, W., & Braun, C. (2010). Comparing Tactile Pattern and Vibrotactile Frequency Discrimination: A Human fMRI Study. *Journal of Neurophysiology*, *103*(6), 3115–3122. doi:10.1152/jn.00940.2009 PMID:20457848

Helfer, K. S. (1998). Auditory and auditory-visual recognition of clear and conversational speech by older adults. *Journal of the American Academy of Audiology*, *9*, 234–242. PMID:9644622

Henrik, H. (2003). Imagery of voluntary movement of fingers, toes, and tongue activates corresponding body-part-specific motor representations. *Journal of Neurophysiology*, *90*(5), 3304–3316. doi:10.1152/jn.01113.2002 PMID:14615433

Henshaw, J., Liu, W., & Romano, D. (2014). Problem solving using hybrid brain-computer interface methods: A review. *Cognitive Infocommunications, IEEE Conference on*, 215-219.

Herrera, C., Chambon, C., Michel, B. F., Paban, V., & Alescio-Lautier, B. (2012). Positive effects of computer-based cognitive training in adults with mild cognitive impairment. *Neuropsychologia*, *50*(8), 1871–1881. doi:10.1016/j.neuropsychologia.2012.04.012 PMID:22525705

Hertenstein, M. J., Holmes, R., McCullough, M., & Keltner, D. (2009). The communication of emotion via touch. *Emotion (Washington, D.C.)*, *9*(4), 566–573. doi:10.1037/a0016108 PMID:19653781

Hertenstein, M. J., & Keltner, D. (2011). Gender and the communication of emotion via touch. *Sex Roles*, *64*(1-2), 70–80. doi:10.1007/s11199-010-9842-y PMID:21297854

Hertenstein, M. J., Keltner, D., App, B., Bulleit, B. A., & Jaskollka, A. R. (2006). Touch communicates distinct emotions. *Emotion (Washington, D.C.)*, *6*(3), 528–533. doi:10.1037/1528-3542.6.3.528 PMID:16938094

Hertenstein, M. J., Verkamp, J. M., Kerestes, A. M., & Holmes, R. M. (2006). The communicative functions of touch in humans, nonhuman primates, and rats: A review and synthesis of the empirical research. *Genetic, Social, and General Psychology Monographs*, *132*(1), 5–94. doi:10.3200/MONO.132.1.5-94 PMID:17345871

Heywood, C. A., Nicholas, J. J., & Cowey, A. (1996). Behavioural and electrophysiological chromatic and achromatic contrast sensitivity in an achromatopsic patient. *Journal of Neurology, Neurosurgery, and Psychiatry*, *60*(6), 638–643. doi:10.1136/jnnp.60.6.638 PMID:8648330

Hikosaka, K., Iwai, E., Saito, H., & Tanaka, K. (1988). Polysensory properties of neurons in the anterior bank of the caudal superior temporal sulcus of the macaque monkey. *Journal of Neurophysiology*, *60*, 1615–1637. PMID:2462027

Hirose, M., & Ogawa, K. (2007). Honda humanoid robots development. *Philosophical Transactions of the Royal Society A Mathematical Physical & Engineering Sciences*, *365*(365), 11–19. doi:10.1098/rsta.2006.1917 PMID:17148047

Hirukawa, H. (2007). Walking biped humanoids that perform manual labour. *Philosophical Transactions of the Royal Society A Mathematical Physical & Engineering Sciences*, *365*(365), 65–77. doi:10.1098/rsta.2006.1916 PMID:17148050

Hochberg, L. R., Serruya, M. D., Friehs, G. M., Mukand, J. A., Saleh, M., Caplan, A. H., & Donoghue, J. P. et al. (2006). Neuronal ensemble control of prosthetic devices by a human with tetraplegia. *Nature*, *442*(7099), 164–171. doi:10.1038/nature04970 PMID:16838014

Hofmann, M., Hock, C., Kühler, A., & Müller-Spahn, F. (1996). Interactive computer-based cognitive training in patients with Alzheimer's disease. *Journal of Psychiatric Research*, *30*(6), 493–501. doi:10.1016/S0022-3956(96)00036-2 PMID:9023793

Holland, A. L., Mcburney, D. H., Moossy, J., & Reinmuth, O. M. (1985). The dissolution of language in pick's disease with neurofibrillary tangles: A case study. *Brain and Language*, *24*(1), 36–58. doi:10.1016/0093-934X(85)90096-3 PMID:3971135

Holmes, N. P. (2007). The law of inverse effectiveness in neurons and behaviour: Multisensory integration versus normal variability. *Neuropsychologia*, *45*(14), 3340–3345. doi:10.1016/j.neuropsychologia.2007.05.025 PMID:17663007

Hore, J., Wild, B., & Diener, H. C. (1991). Cerebellar dysmetria at the elbow, wrist, and fingers. *Journal of Neurophysiology*, *65*(3), 563–571. PMID:2051195

Huang, Q., Li, K., & Wang, T. (2002). Control and mechanical design of humanoid robot BHR-01. In *Proceeding of The Third IARP International Workshop on Humanoid and Human Friendly Robotics*.

Hubacher, M., Kappos, L., Weier, K., Stocklin, M., Opwis, K., & Penner, I. K. (2015). Case-Based fMRI Analysis after Cognitive Rehabilitation in MS: A Novel Approach. *Front Neurol*, *6*, 78. doi:10.3389/fneur.2015.00078 PMID:25904893

Huettel, S. A., Song, A. W., &McCarthy, G. (2009). *Functional Magnetic Resonance Imaging* (2nd ed.). Sinauer.

Hughes, J. C., Robinson, L., & Volicer, L. (2005). Specialist palliative care in dementia. *BMJ (Clinical Research Ed.)*, *330*(7482), 57–58. doi:10.1136/bmj.330.7482.57 PMID:15637354

Humpage, W. D., & Stott, B. (2008). Multiple balance strategies from one optimization criterion. *Humanoid Robots, IEEE-RAS International Conference on*, *112*, 57-64.

Hyon, S., Osu, R., & Otaka, Y. (2009). Integration of multi-level postural balancing on humanoid robots.*Proceedings of the 2009 IEEE international conference on Robotics and Automation*, (pp. 1549 - 1556). doi:10.1109/ROBOT.2009.5152434

Iqbal, S. T., Zheng, X. S., & Bailey, B. P. (2004). Task-evoked pupillary response to mental workload in human-computer interaction. *Conference on Human factors in computing systems* (pp. 1477-1480). Association for Computing Machinery. doi:10.1145/985921.986094

Ito, Y., Urata, J., Nakanishi, Y., Okada, K., & Inaba, M. (2011). Design and development of shock absorbable tendon driven ankles for high-powered humanoids. In *Advanced Robotics and its Social Impacts, 2011 IEEE Workshop on*, (pp. 58-61).

Ito, M. (2005). Bases and implications of learning in the cerebellum—adaptive control and internal model mechanism. *Progress in Brain Research*, *148*, 95–109. doi:10.1016/S0079-6123(04)48009-1 PMID:15661184

Ivanenko, Y. P., Grasso, R., Macellari, V., & Lacquaniti, F. (2002). Control of foot trajectory in human locomotion: Role of ground contact forces in simulated reduced gravity. *Journal of Neurophysiology*, *87*, 3070–3089. PMID:12037209

Jackson, P. L., Meltzoff, A. N., & Decety, J. (2005). How do we perceive the pain of others? A window into the neural processes involved in empathy. *NeuroImage*, *24*(3), 771–779. doi:10.1016/j.neuroimage.2004.09.006 PMID:15652312

Jackson, S. (2005). The Potential on the Door step: The Importance of Gardens in the Psychological Well-being of Older People. *Journal of Therapeutic Horticulture*, *16*, 29–36.

Jaeggi, S. M., Buschkuehl, M., Jonides, J., & Perrig, W. J. (2008). Improving fluid intelligence with training on working memory. *Proceedings of the National Academy of Sciences of the United States of America*, *105*(19), 6829–6833. doi:10.1073/pnas.0801268105 PMID:18443283

Jagust, W. J., Budinger, T. F., & Reed, B. R. (1987). The diagnosis of dementia with single photon emission computed tomography. *Archives of Neurology*, *44*(3), 258–262. doi:10.1001/archneur.1987.00520150014011 PMID:3493756

Jahanshahi, M., Jones, C. R., Dirnberger, G., & Frith, C. D. (2006). The substantia nigra pars compacta and temporal processing. *The Journal of Neuroscience*, *26*(47), 12266–12273. doi:10.1523/JNEUROSCI.2540-06.2006 PMID:17122052

Jahn, K., Deutschlander, A., Stephan, T., Strupp, M., Wiesmann, M., & Brandt, T. (2004). Brain activation patterns during imagined stance and locomotion in functional magnetic resonance imaging. *NeuroImage*, *22*(4), 1722–1731. doi:10.1016/j.neuroimage.2004.05.017 PMID:15275928

Jaimes, A., & Sebe, N. (2007). Multimodal human–computer interaction: A survey. *Computer Vision and Image Understanding*, *108*(1-2), 116–134. doi:10.1016/j.cviu.2006.10.019

James, T. W., Kim, S., & Fisher, J. S. (2007). The neural basis of haptic object processing. *Canadian Journal of Experimental Psychology*, *61*(3), 219–229. doi:10.1037/cjep2007023 PMID:17974316

Janata, P., & Grafton, S. T. (2003). Swinging in the brain: Shared neural substrates for behaviors related to sequencing and music. *Nature Neuroscience*, *6*(7), 682–687. doi:10.1038/nn1081 PMID:12830159

Jared, D. (2010). Social science. The benefits of multilingualism. *Science*, *330*(6002), 332–333. doi:10.1126/science.1195067 PMID:20947754

Jean, L., Bergeron, M.-È., Thivierge, S., & Simard, M. (2010). Cognitive intervention programs for individuals with mild cognitive impairment: Systematic review of the literature. *The American Journal of Geriatric Psychiatry*, *18*(4), 281–296. doi:10.1097/JGP.0b013e3181c37ce9 PMID:20220584

Jeong, J. (2004). EEG dynamics in patients with Alzheimer's disease. *Clinical Neurophysiology: Official Journal of the International Federation of Clinical Neurophysiology*, *115*(7), 1490–1505. doi:10.1016/j.clinph.2004.01.001 PMID:15203050

Jin, M., Shepardson, N., Yang, T., Chen, G., Walsh, D., & Selkoe, D. J. (2011). Soluble amyloid β-protein dimers isolated from Alzheimer cortex directly induce Tau hyperphosphorylation and neuritic degeneration. *Proceedings of the National Academy of Sciences of the United States of America*, *108*(14), 5819–5824. doi:10.1073/pnas.1017033108 PMID:21421841

Johansson, R. S., Landstrom, U., & Lundstrom, R. (1982). Responses of mechanoreceptive afferent units in the glabrous skin of the human hand to sinusoidal skin displacements. *Brain Research*, *244*(1), 17–25. doi:10.1016/0006-8993(82)90899-X PMID:6288178

Jolles, D. D., & Crone, E. A. (2012). Training the developing brain: A neurocognitive perspective. *Frontiers in Human Neuroscience*, 6. PMID:22509161

Jolles, D. D., van Buchem, M. A., Crone, E. A., & Rombouts, S. A. R. B. (2013). Functional brain connectivity at rest changes after working memory training. *Human Brain Mapping*, *34*(2), 396–406. doi:10.1002/hbm.21444 PMID:22076823

Jung, K. K., Kim, J. W., Lee, H. K., Chung, S. B., & Eom, K. H. (2007). EMG pattern classification using spectral estimation and neural network.*SICE Annual Conference* (pp. 1108-1111). IEEE.

Juri, C., Rodriguez-Oroz, M., & Obeso, J. A. (2010). The pathophysiological basis of sensory disturbances in Parkinson's disease. *Neurological Sciences*, *289*(1-2), 60–65. doi:10.1016/j.jns.2009.08.018 PMID:19758602

Kahneman, D., & Beatty, J. (1977). Pupil diameter and load on memory. *Science*, *154*(3756), 1583–1585. doi:10.1126/science.154.3756.1583 PMID:5924930

Kamibayashi, K., Nakajima, T., Takahashi, M., Akai, M., & Nakazawa, K. (2009). Facilitation of corticospinal excitability in the tibialis anterior muscle during robot-assisted passive stepping in humans. *The European Journal of Neuroscience*, *30*(1), 100–109. doi:10.1111/j.1460-9568.2009.06795.x PMID:19523098

Kanaan, S. F., McDowd, J. M., Colgrove, Y., Burns, J. M., Gajewski, B., & Pohl, P. S. (2014). Feasibility and efficacy of intensive cognitive training in early-stage Alzheimer's disease. *American Journal of Alzheimer's Disease and Other Dementias*, *29*(2), 150–158. doi:10.1177/1533317513506775 PMID:24667905

Kantarci, K., Senjem, M. L., Avula, R., Zhang, B., Samikoglu, A. R., Weigand, S. D., & Jack, C. R. et al. (2011). Diffusion tensor imaging and cognitive function in older adults with no dementia. *Neurology*, *77*(1), 26–34. doi:10.1212/WNL.0b013e31822313dc PMID:21593440

Kaplan, R. (1993). The role of nature in the context of the workplace. *Landscape and Urban Planning*, *26*(1-4), 193–201. doi:10.1016/0169-2046(93)90016-7

Kaplan, R. (2001). The nature of the view from home: Psychological benefits. *Environment and Behavior*, *33*(4), 507–542. doi:10.1177/00139160121973115

Karbach, J., & Kray, J. (2009). How useful is executive control training? Age differences in near and far transfer of task-switching training. *Developmental Science*, *12*(6), 978–990. doi:10.1111/j.1467-7687.2009.00846.x PMID:19840052

Kato, I. (1973). Development of WABOT 1. *Biomechanism*, *2*, 173–214.

Katzouris, N., Artikis, A., & Paliouras, G. (2014). Event Recognition for Unobtrusive Assisted Living. In A. Likas, K. Blekas, & D. Kalles (Eds.), Lecture Notes in Computer Science: Vol. 8445. *Artificial Intelligence: Methods and Applications* (pp. 237–250). Cham: Springer International Publishing; doi:10.1007/978-3-319-07064-3

Kaushanskaya, M., & Marian, V. (2009). The bilingual advantage in novel word learning. *Psychonomic Bulletin & Review*, *16*(4), 705–710. doi:10.3758/PBR.16.4.705 PMID:19648456

Kennard, C. (2006). *The Alzheimer's Garden Plan*. Retrieved June 2015, http://alzheimers.about.com/od/familyandfriends/a/garden_design.htm

Khader, F. (2011). Quality of life in the nursing homes in Jordan: Perspectives of residents. *Care Management Journals*, *12*(4), 149–162. doi:10.1891/1521-0987.12.4.169 PMID:23214238

Khan, F., Risheh, N. A. A., Al-Neghaimshi, H. S., Alhomaidhi, N. A., Siddiqui, A. A., Al-Muammar, M. N., & Adewole, A. H. (2013). Assessment of nutritional status of alzheimer patients in Riyadh, Saudi Arabia. *International Journal of Health Sciences and Research*, *3*(4), 1–10.

Khanicheh, A., & Muto, A., Triantafyllou, C., Weinberg, B., Astrakas, L., Mavroidis, C., et al. (2006). fMRI-compatible rehabilitation hand device. *Journal of Neuroengineering and Rehabilitation*, *3*(24), 1–11. PMID:17022828

Kiguchi, K., & Hayashi, Y. (2012). A study of EMG and EEG during perception-assist with an upper-limb power-assist robot. *IEEE International Conference on Robotics and Automation* (vol. 162, pp. 2711-2716). IEEE. doi:10.1109/ICRA.2012.6225027

Killiany, R. J., Gomez-Isla, T., Moss, M., Kikinis, R., Sandor, T., Jolesz, F., & Albert, M. S. et al. (2000). Use of structural magnetic resonance imaging to predict who will get Alzheimer's disease. *Annals of Neurology*, *47*(4), 430–439. doi:10.1002/1531-8249(200004)47:4<430::AID-ANA5>3.0.CO;2-I PMID:10762153

Kim, M. S., Kim, M. S., Park, S., & Oh, J. H. (2008). Realization of stretch-legged walking of the humanoid robot. In *8th IEEE-RAS International Conference on Humanoid Robots*. Humanoids 2008, (pp. 118 - 124).

King, D. P., & Takahashi, J. S. (2000). Molecular genetics of circadian rhythms in mammals. *Annual Review of Neuroscience*, *23*(1), 713–742. doi:10.1146/annurev.neuro.23.1.713 PMID:10845079

Kivipelto, M., Ngandu, T., Fratiglioni, L., Viitanen, M., Kåreholt, I., Winblad, B., & Nissinen, A. (2005). Obesity and vascular risk factors at midlife and the risk of dementia and Alzheimer disease. *Archives of Neurology*, *62*(10), 1556–1560. doi:10.1001/archneur.62.10.1556 PMID:16216938

Klatzky, R. L., & Lederman, S. J. (2010). Multisensory texture perception. In Multisensory Object Perception in the Primate Brain (pp. 211-230). Springer-Verlag. doi:10.1007/978-1-4419-5615-6_12

Klein, S., Allison, D. B., Heymsfield, S. B., Kelley, D. E., Leibel, R. L., Nonas, C., & Kahn, R. (2007). Waist circumference and cardiometabolic risk: a consensus statement from shaping America's health: Association for weight management and obesity prevention; NAASO, the Obesity Society; the American Society for Nutrition; and the American Diabetes Association. *The American Journal of Clinical Nutrition*, *85*(5), 1197–1202. PMID:17490953

Klocker, A., Oddo, C. M., Camboni, D., Penta, M., & Thonnard, J. (2014). Physical factors influencing pleasant touch during passive fingertip stimulation. *PLoS ONE*, *9*(7), e101361. doi:10.1371/journal.pone.0101361 PMID:25000561

Knapp, M. L., & Hall, J. A. (Eds.). (1997). *Nonverbal communication in human interaction*. Boston, MA: Harcourt Brace College Press.

Knupfer, L., & Spiegel, R. (1986). Differences in olfactory test performance between normal aged, Alzheimer and vascular type dementia individuals. *International Journal of Geriatric Psychiatry*, *1*(1), 3–14. doi:10.1002/gps.930010103

Konczak, J., Sciutti, A., Avanzino, L., Squeri, V., Gori, M., Masia, L., & Sandini, G. et al. (2012). Parkinson's disease accelerates age-related decline in haptic perception by altering somatosensory integration. *Brain*, *135*(11), 3371–3379. doi:10.1093/brain/aws265 PMID:23169922

Konrad, P. (2005). *The abc of emg: A practical introduction to kinesiological electromyography*. Noraxon INC.

Konstantinidis, E., Billis, A., Mouzakidis, C., Zilidou, V., Antoniou, P., & Bamidis, P. (2014). Design, implementation and wide pilot deployment of FitForAll: an easy to use exergaming platform improving physical fitness and life quality of senior citizens. *IEEE Journal of Biomedical and Health Informatics*, 1–1. http://doi.org/<ALIGNMENT.qj></ALIGNMENT>10.1109/JBHI.2014.2378814

Konstantinidis, E. I., Antoniou, P. E., Bamparopoulos, G., & Bamidis, P. D. (2014). A lightweight framework for transparent cross platform communication of controller data in ambient assisted living environments. *Information Sciences*, *300*, 124–139. doi:10.1016/j.ins.2014.10.070

Konstantinidis, E. I., Bamidis, P. D., Billis, A. S., Kartsidis, P., & Papageorgiou, S. G. (2015). Physical training in-game metrics for cognitive assessment: Evidence from extended trials with the FitForAll exergame platform. *PLoS ONE*.

Konstantinidis, E., Antoniou, P., Billis, A., Bamparopoulos, G., Costas, P., & Bamidis, P. (2014). *Universal Access in Human-Computer Interaction. Aging and Assistive Environments* (C. Stephanidis & M. Antona, Eds.). Cham: Springer International Publishing. doi:10.1007/978-3-319-07446-7

Kopf, A., Bicak, M., Kottmann, R., Schnetzer, J., Kostadinov, I., Lehmann, K., & Glockner, F. O. et al. (2015). The ocean sampling day consortium. *Gigascience*, *4*(1), 27. doi:10.1186/s13742-015-0066-5 PMID:26097697

Kornhuber, H. H., & Deecke, L. (1965). Changes in the brain potential in voluntary movements and passive movements in man: Readiness potentials and reafferent potentials. *Pflügers Archiv für die Gesamte Physiologie des Menschen und der Tiere*, *284*, 1–17. doi:10.1007/BF00412364 PMID:14341490

Kotagal, V., Langa, K. M., Plassman, B. L., Fisher, G. G., Giordani, B. J., Wallace, R. B., & Foster, N. L. et al. (2015). Factors associated with cognitive evaluations in the United States. *Neurology*, *84*(1), 64–71. doi:10.1212/WNL.0000000000001096 PMID:25428689

Kovach, C. R., Noonan, P. E., Schlidt, A. M., & Wells, T. (2005). A model of consequences of need-driven, dementia-compromised behavior. *Journal of Nursing Scholarship*, *37*(2), 134–140. doi:10.1111/j.1547-5069.2005.00025_1.x PMID:15960057

Kramer, H. H., Lundblad, L., Birklein, F., Linde, M., Karlsson, T., Elam, M., & Olausson, H. (2007). Activation of the cortical pain network by soft tactile stimulation after injection of sumatriptan. *Pain*, *133*(1-3), 72–78. doi:10.1016/j.pain.2007.03.001 PMID:17449179

Kruger, G., Kleinschmidt, A., & Frahm, J. (1996). Dynamic MRI sensitized to cerebral blood oxygenation and flow during sustained activation of human visual cortex. *Magnetic Resonance in Medicine*, *35*(6), 797–800. doi:10.1002/mrm.1910350602 PMID:8744004

Kucukerdonmez, O., Koksal, E., Rakicioglu, N., & Pekcan, G. (2005). Assessment and evaluation of the nutritional status of the elderly using 2 different instruments. *Saudi Medical Journal*, *26*(10), 1611–1616. PMID:16228066

Kucukerdonmez, O., Rakıcıoglu, N., Eroglu, E., Portakal, O., & Ayaz, S. (2006). Alzheimer tipi senil demanslı hastalarda beslenme durumunun değerlendirilmesi [The determination of nutritional status of patients with Alzheimer type senil dementia]. *Beslenme ve Diyet Dergisi*, *34*(1), 11–22.

Kuo, F.E. & Taylor, A.F. (2004). A Potential Natural Treatment for Attention-Deficit/Hyperactivity Disorder: Evidence from a National Study. *American Journal of Public Health, 94*(9), 1580.

Kuzu-Kurban, N., Zencir, M., Kartal, A., & Şahiner, T. (2010). Alzheimer hastalığıolanveolmaya nyaşlıbireylerinyaşamkalitesivedepresyondüzeylerininkarşılaştırılması [Comparison of quality of life and depression levels of elderly persons with Alzheimer's disease and not]. *Yaşlı Sorunları Arastırma Dergisi*, *1*, 34–43.

Kvamme, J. M., Olsen, J. A., Florholmen, J., & Jacobsen, B. K. (2011). Risk of malnutrition and health-related quality of life in community-living elderly men and women: The Tromsø study. *Quality of Life Research: An International Journal of Quality of Life Aspects of Treatment, Care and Rehabilitation*, *20*(4), 575–582. doi:10.1007/s11136-010-9788-0 PMID:21076942

Laakso, M., Partanen, K., Riekkinen, P., Lehtovirta, M., Helkala, E.-L., Hallikainen, M., & Soininen, H. et al. (1996). Hippocampal volumes in Alzheimer's disease, Parkinson's disease with and without dementia, and in vascular dementia An MRI study. *Neurology*, *46*(3), 678–681. doi:10.1212/WNL.46.3.678 PMID:8618666

Lakatos, P., Chen, C. M., O'connell, M. N., Mills, A., & Schroeder, C. E. (2007). Neuronal oscillations and multisensory interaction in primary auditory cortex. *Neuron*, *53*(2), 279–292. doi:10.1016/j.neuron.2006.12.011 PMID:17224408

Landi, F., Liperoti, R., Fusco, D., Mastropaolo, S., Quattrociocchi, D., Proia, A., & Onder, G. (2012). Prevalence and risk factors of sarcopenia among nursing home older residents. *The Journals of Gerontology. Series A, Biological Sciences and Medical Sciences*, *67*(1), 48–55. doi:10.1093/gerona/glr035 PMID:21393423

Landscape, P. R. P. (2013). *Landscape Design for Dementia, Factsheet 35*. CareHousing Learning & Improvement Network Press. Retrieved June 2015, http://www.housinglin.org.uk/_library/Resources/Housing/Support_materials/Factsheets/HLIN_Factsheet35_Landscape.pdf

Larner, A. (2010). *Cholinesterase inhibitors: beyond Alzheimer's disease*. Academic Press.

Lauque, S., Arnaud-Battandier, F., Gillette, S., Plaze, J. M., Andrieu, S., Cantet, C., & Vellas, B. (2004). Improvement of weight and fat-free mass with oral nutritional supplementation in patients with Alzheimer's disease at risk of malnutrition: A prospective randomized study. *Journal of the American Geriatrics Society*, *52*(10), 1702–1707. doi:10.1111/j.1532-5415.2004.52464.x PMID:15450048

Lawlor-Savage, L., & Goghari, V. M. (2014). Working memory training in schizophrenia and healthy populations. *Behav Sci (Basel)*, *4*(3), 301–319. doi:10.3390/bs4030301 PMID:25379283

Lecheta, D. R., Schieferdecker, M. M., de Mello, A. P., Berkenbrock, I., Neto, J. C., & Maluf, E. P. (2015). Dietary inadequacies in the elderly with Alzhimer's disease followed at the reference health center for elderly care in Curitiba-Brazil. *Journal of Aging Clinical Practice*, *4*(2), 85–91.

Lederman, S. J. (1981). The perception of surface roughness by active and passive touch. *Bulletin of the Psychonomic Society*, *18*(5), 253–255. doi:10.3758/BF03333619

Lederman, S. J., & Klatzky, R. L. (2009). Tutorial review haptic perception: A tutorial. *Attention, Perception & Psychophysics*, *71*(7), 1439–1459. doi:10.3758/APP.71.7.1439 PMID:19801605

Lee, G. Y., Yip, C. K., Yu, E., & Man, D. (2013). Evaluation of a computer-assisted errorless learning-based memory training program for patients with early Alzheimer's disease in Hong Kong: A pilot study. *Clinical Interventions in Aging*, *8*, 623. PMID:23766638

Lee, R. D., & Nieman, D. C. (2003). Assessment of the hospitalized patient. In R. D. Lee & D. C. Nieman (Eds.), *Nutritional Assessment* (pp. 216–250). New York: McGraw Hill.

Lee, S. H., & Goswami, A. (2012). Fall on backpack: Damage minimization of humanoid robots by falling on targeted body segments. *Journal of Computational & Nonlinear Dynamics*, *8*(2), 233–246. doi:10.1115/1.4006783

Lee, Y., & Kim, S. (2008). Effects of indoor gardening on sleep, agitation, and cognition in dementia patients: A pilot study. *International Journal of Geriatric Psychiatry*, *23*(5), 485–489. doi:10.1002/gps.1920 PMID:17918774

Leung, P., Orrell, M., & Orgeta, V. (2015). Social support group interventions in people with dementia and mild cognitive impairment: A systematic review of the literature. *International Journal of Geriatric Psychiatry*, *30*(1), 1–9. doi:10.1002/gps.4166 PMID:24990344

Lew, E., Chavarriaga, R., Silvoni, S., & Millán, J. (2012). Detection of self-paced reaching movement intention from EEG signals. *Frontiers in Neuroengineering, 5*.

Lewin, J. S., Friedman, L., Wu, D., Miller, D. A., Thompson, L. A., Klein, S. K., & Duerk, J. L. et al. (1996). Cortical localization of human sustained attention: Detection with functional MR using a visual vigilance paradigm. *Journal of Computer Assisted Tomography*, *20*(5), 695–701. doi:10.1097/00004728-199609000-00002 PMID:8797896

Lewis, P. A., & Miall, R. C. (2003). Brain activation patterns during measurement of sub- and supra-second intervals. *Neuropsychologia*, *41*(12), 1583–1592. doi:10.1016/S0028-3932(03)00118-0 PMID:12887983

Li, Wu, & Liu. (2012). the effect of bilingual experiences on cognition abilities. *Advances in Psychological Science*, *20*(7), 995-1002.

Liu, C., & Atkeson, C. G. (2009). Standing Balance Control Using a Trajectory Library. *Intelligent Robots and Systems, IEEE/RSJ International Conference on*, (pp. 3031-3036).

Liu, S., Shen, Z., Mei, J., & Ji, J. (2013). Parkinson's Disease Predictive Analytics through a Pad Game Based on Personal Data. *Int. J. Inf. Technol*, *19*(2).

Liu, D., Diorio, J., Tannenbaum, B., Caldji, C., Francis, D., & Freedman, A. et al.. (1997). Maternal care, hippocampal glucocorticoid receptors, and hypothalamic-pituitary-adrenal responses to stress. *Science*, *277*(5332), 1659–1662. doi:10.1126/science.277.5332.1659 PMID:9287218

Liu, Y., Wang, K., Yu, C., He, Y., Zhou, Y., Liang, M., & Jiang, T. et al. (2008). Regional homogeneity, functional connectivity and imaging markers of Alzheimer's disease: A review of resting-state fMRI studies. *Neuropsychologia*, *46*(6), 1648–1656. doi:10.1016/j.neuropsychologia.2008.01.027 PMID:18346763

Livesey, A. C., Wall, M. B., & Smith, A. T. (2007). Time perception: Manipulation of task difficulty dissociates clock functions from other cognitive demands. *Neuropsychologia*, *45*(2), 321–331. doi:10.1016/j.neuropsychologia.2006.06.033 PMID:16934301

Logothetis, N. K. (2008). What we can do and what we cannot do with fMRI. *Nature*, *453*(7197), 869–878. doi:10.1038/nature06976 PMID:18548064

Loken, L. S., Wessberg, J., Morrison, I., McGlone, F., & Olausson, H. (2009). Coding of pleasant touch by unmyelinated afferents in humans. *Nature Neuroscience*, *12*(5), 547–548. doi:10.1038/nn.2312 PMID:19363489

Loreck, E., Chimakurthi, R., & Steinle, N. I. (2012). Nutritional assessment of the geriatric patient: A comprehensive approach toward evaluating and managing nutrition. *Clinical Geriatrics*, *20*(4), 20–26.

Lotze, M., & Cohen, L. G. (2006). Volition and imagery in neurorehabilitation. *Cognitive and Behavioral Neurology*, *19*(3), 135–140. doi:10.1097/01.wnn.0000209875.56060.06 PMID:16957491

Low, G., & Molzahn, A. E. (2007). Predictors of quality of life in old age: A cross-validation study. *Research in Nursing & Health*, *30*(2), 141–150. doi:10.1002/nur.20178 PMID:17380515

Lucas-Carrasco, R., Lamping, D. L., Banerjee, S., Rejas, J., Smith, S. C., & Gómez-Benito, J. (2010). Validation of the Spanish version of the DEMQOL system. *International Psychogeriatrics*, *22*(04), 589–597. doi:10.1017/S1041610210000207 PMID:20447322

Luft, A. R., Forrester, L., Macko, R. F., McCombe-Waller, S., Whitall, J., Villagra, F., & Hanley, D. F. (2005). Brain activation of lower extremity movement in chronically impaired stroke survivors. *NeuroImage*, *26*(1), 184–194. doi:10.1016/j.neuroimage.2005.01.027 PMID:15862218

Luft, A. R., Smith, G. V., Forrester, L., Whitall, J., Macko, R. F., Hauser, T.-K., & Hanley, D. F. et al. (2002). Comparing brain activation associated with isolated upper and lower limb movement across corresponding joints. *Human Brain Mapping*, *17*(2), 131–140. doi:10.1002/hbm.10058 PMID:12353246

Luo & Peng. (2001). Perspective on Dementia. *Contemporary Linguistics,* (2), 109-118.

Luo, H., Fang, X., Liao, Y., Elliott, A., & Zhang, X. (2010). Associations of special care units and outcomes of residents with dementia: 2004 national nursing home survey. *The Gerontologist*, *50*(4), 509–518. doi:10.1093/geront/gnq035 PMID:20462932

Luxenberg, J., Haxby, J. V., Creasey, H., Sundaram, M., & Rapoport, S. (1987). Rate of ventricular enlargement in dementia of the Alzheimer type correlates with rate of neuropsychological deterioration. *Neurology*, *37*(7), 1135–1135. doi:10.1212/WNL.37.7.1135 PMID:3496557

Lyketsos, C. G., Lopez, O., Jones, B., Fitzpatrick, A. L., Breitner, J., & DeKosky, S. (2002). Prevalence of Neuropsychiatric Symptoms in Dementia and Mild Cognitive Impairment. *Journal of the American Medical Association*, *288*(12), 1475. doi:10.1001/jama.288.12.1475 PMID:12243634

Lyons, B. E., Austin, D., Seelye, A., Petersen, J., Yeargers, J., & Riley, T., … Kaye, J. a. (2015). Pervasive Computing Technologies to Continuously Assess Alzheimerâ€™s Disease Progression and Intervention Efficacy. *Frontiers in Aging Neuroscience*, *7*(June), 1–14. doi:10.3389/fnagi.2015.00102 PMID:25653617

Ma, J., Zhang, Y., Nam, Y., & Cichocki, A. (2013). EOG/ERP hybrid human-machine interface for robot control. *Intelligent Robots and Systems, IEEE/RSJ International Conference on*, *40*, 859-864.

Macaluso, E., George, N., Dolan, R., Spence, C., & Driver, J. (2004). Spatial and temporal factors during processing of audiovisual speech: A PET study. *NeuroImage*, *21*(2), 725–732. doi:10.1016/j.neuroimage.2003.09.049 PMID:14980575

MacIntosh, B. J., Mraz, R., Baker, N., Tam, F., Staines, W. R., & Graham, S. J. (2004). Optimizing the experimental design for ankle dorsiflexion fMRI. *NeuroImage*, *22*(4), 1619–1627. doi:10.1016/j.neuroimage.2004.03.035 PMID:15275918

Maclean, P. D. (1949). Psychosomatic disease and the visceral brain; recent developments bearing on the Papez theory of emotion. *Psychosomatic Medicine*, *11*(6), 338–353. doi:10.1097/00006842-194911000-00003 PMID:15410445

Mahendra, N. (n.d.). Direct interventions for improving the performance of individuals with Alzheimer's disease. Seminars in Speech and Language, 291-303.

Mahncke, H. W., Connor, B. B., Appelman, J., Ahsanuddin, O. N., Hardy, J. L., Wood, R. A., … Merzenich, M. M. (2006). Memory enhancement in healthy older adults using a brain plasticity-based training program: a randomized, controlled study. *Proceedings of the National Academy of Sciences of the United States of America*, *103*(33), 12523–8. http://doi.org/ doi:10.1073/pnas.0605194103

Majerus, S., Cowan, N., Peters, F., Van Calster, L., Phillips, C., & Schrouff, J. (2014). Cross-Modal Decoding of Neural Patterns Associated with Working Memory: Evidence for Attention-Based Accounts of Working Memory. *Cereb Cortex*. doi:10.1093/cercor/bhu189 PMID:25146374

Majerus, S., D'Argembeau, A., Perez, T. M., Belayachi, S., Van der Linden, M., Collette, F., & Maquet, P. et al. (2010). The commonality of neural networks for verbal and visual short-term memory. *Journal of Cognitive Neuroscience*, *22*(11), 2570–2593. doi:10.1162/jocn.2009.21378 PMID:19925207

Malouin, F., Richards, C. L., Jackson, P. L., Dumas, F., & Doyon, J. (2003). Brain activations during motor imagery of locomotor-related tasks: A PET study. *Human Brain Mapping*, *19*(1), 47–62. doi:10.1002/hbm.10103 PMID:12731103

Manoj, S., & Andy, R. (2006). Computer optimization of a minimal biped model discovers walking and running. *Nature*, *439*(7072), 72–75. doi:10.1038/nature04113 PMID:16155564

Manor, B., Costa, M. D., Hu, K., Newton, E., Starobinets, O., Kang, H. G., & Lipsitz, L. A. et al. (2010). Physiological complexity and system adaptability: Evidence from postural control dynamics of older adults. *Journal of Applied Physiology (Bethesda, Md.)*, *109*(6), 1786–1791. doi:10.1152/japplphysiol.00390.2010 PMID:20947715

Marcus, C. C. (2005). *Healing Gardens in Hospitals*. Retrieved June 2015, http://www.umcg.nl/SiteCollectionDocuments/UMCG/C1_Cooper_Marcus.ppt.pdf

Marcus, C.C. (2008). Garden of the Family Life Center, Grand Rapids, Michigan. *Journal of Housing For the Elderly Publication*, 285-304.

Marshall S. P. (2000). *Method and apparatus for eye tracking and monitoring pupil dilation to evaluate cognitive activity*. US: US6090051.

Mather, J. A., Nemecek, D., & Oliver, K. (1999). The effect of a walled garden on behavior of individuals with Alzheimer's. *American Journal of Alzheimer's Disease*, *12*(6), 252–257. doi:10.1177/153331759701200603

Matthews, P., & Jezzard, P. (2004). Functional magnetic resonance imaging. *Journal of Neurology, Neurosurgery, and Psychiatry*, *75*, 6–12. PMID:14707297

Mattis, S., & Mattis, S. (1976). *Mental status examination for organic mental syndrome in the elderly patient*. Grune & Stratton Inc.

Mauk, M. D., & Buonomano, D. V. (2004). The neural basis of temporal processing. *Annual Review of Neuroscience*, *27*(1), 307–340. doi:10.1146/annurev.neuro.27.070203.144247 PMID:15217335

McCabe, C., Rolls, E. T., Bilderbeck, A., & McGlone, F. (2008). Cognitive influences on the affective representation of touch and the sight of touch in the human brain. *Social Cognitive and Affective Neuroscience*, *3*(2), 97–108. doi:10.1093/scan/nsn005 PMID:19015100

McCormick, W. C., Kukull, W. A., van Belle, G., Bowen, J. D., Teri, L., & Larson, E. B. (1994). Symptom Patterns and Comorbidity in the Early Stages of Alzheimer's Disease. *Journal of the American Geriatrics Society*, *42*(5), 517–521. doi:10.1111/j.1532-5415.1994.tb04974.x PMID:8176147

Mcgeer, T. (1990). Passive dynamic walking. *The International Journal of Robotics Research*, *9*(2), 62–82. doi:10.1177/027836499000900206

Mcgleenon, B., Dynan, K., & Passmore, A. (1999). Acetylcholinesterase inhibitors in Alzheimer's disease. *British Journal of Clinical Pharmacology*, *48*(4), 471–480. doi:10.1046/j.1365-2125.1999.00026.x PMID:10583015

McGlone, F., Olausson, H., Boyle, J. A., Jones-Gotman, M., Dancer, C., Guest, S., & Essick, G. (2012). Touching and feeling: Differences in pleasant touch processing between glabrous and hairy skin in humans. *The European Journal of Neuroscience*, *35*(11), 1782–1788. doi:10.1111/j.1460-9568.2012.08092.x PMID:22594914

McGlone, F., Vallbo, A. B., Olausson, H., Loken, L., & Wessberg, J. (2007). Discriminative touch and emotional touch. *Journal of Experimental Social Psychology*, *61*(3), 173–183. PMID:17974312

McGlone, F., Wessberg, J., & Olausson, H. (2014). Discriminative and affective touch: Sensing and feeling. *Neuron*, *82*(4), 737–755. doi:10.1016/j.neuron.2014.05.001 PMID:24853935

McKanna, J. A., Jimison, H., & Pavel, M. (2009). Divided attention in computer game play: analysis utilizing unobtrusive health monitoring. *Conference Proceedings: ... Annual International Conference of the IEEE Engineering in Medicine and Biology Society. IEEE Engineering in Medicine and Biology Society. Annual Conference, 2009.* http://doi.org/ doi:10.1109/IEMBS.2009.5334662

McKeith, I. G., Dickson, D. W., Lowe, J., Emre, M., O'Brien, J. T., Feldman, H., & Yamada, M. et al. (2005). Diagnosis and management of dementia with Lewy bodies: Third report of the DLB Consortium. *Neurology*, *65*(12), 1863–1872. doi:10.1212/01.wnl.0000187889.17253.b1 PMID:16237129

Mckhann, G., Drachman, D., Folstein, M., Katzman, R., Price, D., & Stadlan, E. (1984a). Report of the NINCDS-ADRDA work group under the auspices of Department of Health and Human Services task force on Alzheimer's disease. *Neurology*, *34*(7), 939–943. doi:10.1212/WNL.34.7.939 PMID:6610841

McNab, F., Varrone, A., Farde, L., Jucaite, A., Bystritsky, P., Forssberg, H., & Klingberg, T. (2009). Changes in cortical dopamine D1 receptor binding associated with cognitive training. *Science*, *323*(5915), 800–802. doi:10.1126/science.1166102 PMID:19197069

Meaney, M. J., Aitken, D. H., Bodnoff, S. R., Bhatnagar, S., & Sapolsky, R. M. (2013). Early postnatal handling alters glucocorticoid receptor concentrations in selected brain regions. *Behavioral Neuroscience, 127*(5), 637–641. doi:10.1037/a0034187 PMID:24128353

Meaney, M. J., Aitken, D. H., van-Berkel, C., Bhatnagar, S., & Sapolsky, R. M. (1988). Effect of neonatal handling on age-related impairments associated with the hippocampus. *Science, 239*(4841 Pt 1), 766–768. doi:10.1126/science.3340858 PMID:3340858

Meaney, M. J., Mitchell, J. B., Aitken, D., Bhatnagar, S., Bodnoff, S. R., Iny, L. J., & Sarrieau, A. (1991). The effects of neonatal handling on the development of the adrenocortical response to stress: Implications for neuropathology and cognitive deficits in later life. *Psychoneuroendocrinology, 16*(1-3), 85–103. doi:10.1016/0306-4530(91)90072-2 PMID:1961847

Meftah, E. M., Belingard, L., & Chapman, C. E. (2000). Relative effects of the spatial and temporal characteristics of scanned surfaces on human perception of tactile roughness using passive touch. *Experimental Brain Research, 132*(3), 351–361. doi:10.1007/s002210000348 PMID:10883383

Mehta, J. P., Verber, M. D., Wieser, J. A., Schmit, B. D., & Schindler-Ivens, S. M. (2009). A novel technique for examining human brain activity associated with pedaling using fMRI. *Journal of Neuroscience Methods, 179*(2), 230–239. doi:10.1016/j.jneumeth.2009.01.029 PMID:19428532

Mehta, K. M., Yaffe, K., & Covinsky, K. E. (2002). Cognitive Impairment, Depressive Symptoms, and Functional Decline in Older People. *Journal of the American Geriatrics Society, 50*(6), 1045–1050. doi:10.1046/j.1532-5415.2002.50259.x PMID:12110064

Meredith, M. A., Nemitz, J. W., & Stein, B. E. (1987). Determinants of multisensory integration in superior colliculus neurons. I. Temporal factors. *The Journal of Neuroscience, 7*, 3215–3229. PMID:3668625

Meredith, M. A., & Stein, B. E. (1983). Interactions among converging sensory inputs in the superior colliculus. *Science, 221*(4608), 389–391. doi:10.1126/science.6867718 PMID:6867718

Meredith, M. A., & Stein, B. E. (1986). Spatial Factors Determine the Activity of Multisensory Neurons in Cat Superior Colliculus. *Brain Research, 365*(2), 350–354. doi:10.1016/0006-8993(86)91648-3 PMID:3947999

Mevel, K., Chételat, G., Eustache, F., & Desgranges, B. (2011). The default mode network in healthy aging and Alzheimer's disease. *International Journal of Alzheimer's Disease, 535816.* doi:10.4061/2011/535816 PMID:21760988

Michael, E. B., & Gollan, T. H. (2009). Being and becoming bilingual. Handbook of bilingualism, 389.

Mihailidis, A. (2008). *Technology and Aging: Selected Papers from the 2007 International Conference on Technology and Aging*. Retrieved from https://books.google.com/books?hl=el&lr=&id=OSCScvzDPrwC&pgis=1

Millan, J. D. R., Galán, F., Vanhooydonck, D., Lew, E., Philips, J., & Nuttin, M. (2009, September). Asynchronous non-invasive brain-actuated control of an intelligent wheelchair. In *Engineering in Medicine and Biology Society, Annual International Conference of the IEEE*, (pp. 3361-3364).

Miller, J. (1982). Divided attention: Evidence for coactivation with redundant signals. *Cognitive Psychology*, *14*(2), 247–279. doi:10.1016/0010-0285(82)90010-X PMID:7083803

Mirela, K., Tiest, W. M. B., & Kappers, A. M. L. (2011). Discrimination thresholds for haptic perception of volume, surface area, and weight. *Attention, Perception & Psychophysics*, *73*(8), 2649–2656. doi:10.3758/s13414-011-0202-y PMID:21870206

Miyai, I., Suzuki, M., Hatakenaka, M., & Kubota, K. (2006). Effect of body weight support on cortical activation during gait in patients with stroke. *Experimental Brain Research*, *169*(1), 85–91. doi:10.1007/s00221-005-0123-x PMID:16237521

Miyai, I., Tanabe, H. C., Sase, I., Eda, H., Oda, I., Konishi, I., & Kubota, K. et al. (2001). Cortical mapping of gait in humans: A near-infrared spectroscopic topography study. *NeuroImage*, *14*(5), 1186–1192. doi:10.1006/nimg.2001.0905 PMID:11697950

Molholm, S., Ritter, W., Murray, M. M., Javitt, D. C., Schroeder, C. E., & Foxe, J. J. (2002). Multisensory auditory-visual interactions during early sensory processing in humans: A high-density electrical mapping study. *Brain Research. Cognitive Brain Research*, *14*(1), 115–128. doi:10.1016/S0926-6410(02)00066-6 PMID:12063135

Monekosso, D. N., & Remagnino, P. (2010). Behavior Analysis for Assisted Living. *IEEE Transactions on Automation Science and Engineering*, *7*(4), 879–886. doi:10.1109/TASE.2010.2049840

Mooney, P., & Nicel, P. L. (1992). The Importance of Exterior Environment for Alzheimer Residents: Effective Care and Risk Management. *Healthcare Management Forum*, *5*(2), 23–29. doi:10.1016/S0840-4704(10)61202-1 PMID:10171068

Morales, J., Padilla, F., Gomez-Ariza, C. J., & Bajo, M. T. (2015). Simultaneous interpretation selectively influences working memory and attentional networks. *Acta Psychologica*, *155*, 82–91. doi:10.1016/j.actpsy.2014.12.004 PMID:25577491

Moran, J., & Desimone, R. (1985). Selective attention gates visual processing in the extrastriate cortex. *Science*, *229*(4715), 782–784. doi:10.1126/science.4023713 PMID:4023713

Moreno, S., Bialystok, E., Wodniecka, Z., & Alain, C. (2010). Conflict resolution in sentence processing by bilinguals. *Journal of Neurolinguistics*, *23*(6), 564–579. doi:10.1016/j.jneuroling.2010.05.002 PMID:21057658

Morillon, B., Kell, C. A., & Giraud, A. L. (2009). Three stages and four neural systems in time estimation. *The Journal of Neuroscience*, *29*(47), 14803–14811. doi:10.1523/JNEUROSCI.3222-09.2009 PMID:19940175

Morimoto, C. H., & Mimica, M. R. M. (2005). Eye gaze tracking techniques for interactive applications. *Computer Vision and Image Understanding*, *98*(1), 4–24. doi:10.1016/j.cviu.2004.07.010

Morrison, I., & Downing, P. E. (2007). Organization of felt and seen pain responses in anterior cingulate cortex. *NeuroImage*, *37*(2), 642–651. doi:10.1016/j.neuroimage.2007.03.079 PMID:17588777

Morrison, I., Lloyd, D., di Pellegrino, G., & Roberts, N. (2004). Vicarious responses to pain in anterior cingulate cortex: Is empathy a multisensory issue? *Cognitive, Affective & Behavioral Neuroscience*, *4*(2), 270–278. doi:10.3758/CABN.4.2.270 PMID:15460933

Morrison, I., Loken, L. S., & Olausson, H. (2010). The skin as a social organ. *Experimental Brain Research*, *204*(3), 305–314. doi:10.1007/s00221-009-2007-y PMID:19771420

Mountcastle, V. B. (2005). *The sensory hand.* Cambridge, MA: Harvard University Press.

Müller-Putz, G. R., & Gert, P. (2008). Control of an electrical prosthesis with an ssvep-based bci. *Biomedical Engineering IEEE Transactions on*, *55*(1), 361–364. doi:10.1109/TBME.2007.897815 PMID:18232384

Müller, S. M. T., Cardoso, W., Bastos-Filho, T. F., & Sarcinelli-Filho, M. (2010). Brain-computer interface based on visual evoked potentials to command autonomous robotic wheelchair. *Journal of Medical & Biological Engineering*, *30*(6), 407–415. doi:10.5405/jmbe.765

Nakanishi, Y., Asano, Y., Kozuki, T., Mizoguchi, H., Motegi, Y., & Osada, M. (2012). Design concept of detail musculoskeletal humanoid "Kenshiro" - Toward a real human body musculoskeletal simulator. *Humanoid Robots, 2012 12th IEEE-RAS International Conference on*, (pp. 1-6).

Niall McLaughlin Architects Bedford House. (2012). *The Alzheimer's Respite Centre*. Retrieved June 2015, http://www.niallmclaughlin.com/wp-content/uploads/2014/07/AAIAwards2010-reduced.pdf

Nicholas, M., Obler, L., Albert, M., & Goodglass, H. (1985). Lexical retrieval in healthy aging. *Cortex*, *21*(4), 595–606. doi:10.1016/S0010-9452(58)80007-6 PMID:4092486

Nobili, A., Piana, I., Balossi, L., Pasina, L., Matucci, M., Tarantola, M., & Tettamanti, M. (2008). Alzheimer special care units compared with traditional nursing home for dementia care: Are there differences at admission and in clinical outcomes? *Alzheimer Disease and Associated Disorders*, *22*(4), 352–361. doi:10.1097/WAD.0b013e31818207d0 PMID:18978601

Nord, R. D. (2004). *Architecture for alzheimer disease*. Alinea Editrice Press.

Nourhashemi, F., Ousset, P. J., Guyonnet, S., Andrieu, S., Rolland, Y., Adoue, D. & Albarède, J. L. (2000). *La Revue de medecine interne/fondee... par la Societe nationale francaise de medecine interne* [Alzheimer's disease: from pathology to preventive methods?]. Academic Press. (in French)

Novak, P., & Novak, V. (2006, May4). Effect of step-synchronized vibration stimulation of soles on gait in Parkinson's disease: A pilot study. *Journal of Neuroengineering and Rehabilitation*, *3*(1), 9. doi:10.1186/1743-0003-3-9 PMID:16674823

Nystrom, L. E., Braver, T. S., Sabb, F. W., Delgado, M. R., Noll, D. C., & Cohen, J. D. (2000). Working memory for letters, shapes, and locations: fMRI evidence against stimulus-based regional organization in human prefrontal cortex. *NeuroImage*, *11*(5), 424–446. doi:10.1006/nimg.2000.0572 PMID:10806029

Obler, L. K. (1983). *Language and brain dysfunction in dementia - language functions and brain organization.* Language Functions & Brain Organization. doi:10.1016/B978-0-12-635640-3.50020-5

Ogura, Y., Shimomura, K., Kondo, H., & Morishima, A. (2006). Human-like walking with knee stretched, heel-contact and toe-off motion by a humanoid robot. *Intelligent Robots and Systems, 2006 IEEE/RSJ International Conference on*, (pp. 3976-3981).

Oishi, K., Mielke, M. M., Albert, M., Lyketsos, C. G., & Mori, S. (2012). The fornix sign: A potential sign for Alzheimer's disease based on diffusion tensor imaging. *Journal of Neuroimaging : Official Journal of the American Society of Neuroimaging*, *22*(4), 365–374. doi:10.1111/j.1552-6569.2011.00633.x PMID:21848679

Okun, M., Steinmetz, N. A., Cossell, L., Iacaruso, M. F., Ko, H., Barthó, P., & Harris, K. D. et al. (2015). Diverse coupling of neurons to populations in sensory cortex. *Nature*, *521*(7553), 511–515. doi:10.1038/nature14273 PMID:25849776

Olausson, H., Lamarre, Y., Backlund, H., Morin, C., Wallin, B. G., Starck, G., & Bushnell, M. C. et al. (2002). Unmyelinated tactile afferents signal touch and project to insular cortex. *Nature Neuroscience*, *5*(9), 900–904. doi:10.1038/nn896 PMID:12145636

Olesen, P. J., Westerberg, H., & Klingberg, T. (2004). Increased prefrontal and parietal activity after training of working memory. *Nature Neuroscience*, *7*(1), 75–79. doi:10.1038/nn1165 PMID:14699419

Olivares, D. K., Deshpande, V., Shi, Y. K., Lahiri, D. H., Greig, N. T., Rogers, J., & Huang, X. (2012). N-Methyl D-Aspartate (NMDA) receptor antagonists and memantine treatment for Alzheimer's disease, vascular dementia and Parkinson's disease. *Current Alzheimer Research*, *9*, 746–758. doi:10.2174/156720512801322564 PMID:21875407

Onoda, K., & Yamaguchi, S. (2013). Small-worldness and modularity of the resting-state functional brain network decrease with aging. *Neuroscience Letters*, *556*, 104–108. doi:10.1016/j.neulet.2013.10.023 PMID:24157850

Organization, World Health. (2012). *Dementia: a public health priority.* World Health Organization.

Ousset, P. J., Nourhashemi, F., Reynish, E., & Vellas, B. (2008). Nutritional status is associated with disease progression in very mild Alzheimer disease. *Alzheimer Disease and Associated Disorders*, *22*(1), 66–71. doi:10.1097/WAD.0b013e31815a9dbb PMID:18317249

Overduin, S. A. & Servos, P. (2008). Symmetric Sensorimotor Somatotopy. *PLoS One, 3*(1), e1505.

Overduin, S. A., & Servos, P. (2004). Distributed digit somatotopy in primary somatosensory cortex. *NeuroImage*, *23*(2), 462–472. doi:10.1016/j.neuroimage.2004.06.024 PMID:15488396

Packer, M., & Ginsburg, A. P. (2007). Contrast sensitivity and aging. *Ophthalmology, 114*(8), 1589, author reply 1589–1590. doi:10.1016/j.ophtha.2007.03.046 PMID:17678702

Páez, M. M., Tabors, P. O., & López, L. M. (2007). Dual language and literacy development of Spanish-speaking preschool children. *Journal of Applied Developmental Psychology, 28*(2), 85–102. doi:10.1016/j.appdev.2006.12.007 PMID:20396646

Palop, J. J., Jones, B., Kekonius, L., Chin, J., Yu, G.-Q., Raber, J., & Mucke, L. et al. (2003). Neuronal depletion of calcium-dependent proteins in the dentate gyrus is tightly linked to Alzheimer's disease-related cognitive deficits. *Proceedings of the National Academy of Sciences of the United States of America, 100*(16), 9572–9577. doi:10.1073/pnas.1133381100 PMID:12881482

Panagiotis, D., Bamidis, Tarnanas, I., Tsolaki, M., & Hadjileontiadis, L. (2015). *Handbook of Research on Innovations in Database Technologies and Applications: Current and Future Trends.* Retrieved July 29, 2015, from http://www.igi-global.com/book/handbook-research-innovations-diagnosis-treatment/121164

Papageorgiou, E. I., Billis, A. S., Frantzidis, C., Konstantinidis, E. I., & Bamidis, P. D. (2013). A preliminary fuzzy cognitive map - based desicion support tool for geriatric depression assessment. In *2013 IEEE International Conference on Fuzzy Systems (FUZZ-IEEE)* (pp. 1–8). IEEE. http://doi.org/ doi:10.1109/FUZZ-IEEE.2013.6622485

Paraskevopoulos, E., Kuchenbuch, A., Herholz, S. C., & Pantev, C. (2014). Multisensory integration during short-term music reading training enhances both uni- and multisensory cortical processing. *Journal of Cognitive Neuroscience, 26*(10), 2224–2238. doi:10.1162/jocn_a_00620 PMID:24669793

Pardhan, S. (2004). Contrast sensitivity loss with aging: Sampling efficiency and equivalent noise at different spatial frequencies. *Journal of the Optical Society of America. A, Optics, Image Science, and Vision, 21*(2), 169–175. doi:10.1364/JOSAA.21.000169 PMID:14763759

Paskulin, L. M. G., & Molzahn, A. (2007). Quality of life of older adults in Canada and Brazil. *Western Journal of Nursing Research, 29*(1), 10–26. doi:10.1177/0193945906292550 PMID:17228059

Peiffer, A. M., Mozolic, J. L., Hugenschmidt, C. E., & Laurienti, P. J. (2007). Age-related multisensory enhancement in a simple audiovisual detection task. *Neuroreport, 18*(10), 1077–1081. doi:10.1097/WNR.0b013e3281e72ae7 PMID:17558300

Peláez-Nogueras, M., Field, T. M., Hossain, Z., & Pickens, J. (1996). Depressed mothers' touching increases infants' positive affect and attention in still-face interactions. *Child Development, 67*(4), 1780–1792. doi:10.2307/1131731 PMID:8890507

Penfield, W., & Rasmussen, T. (Eds.). (1950). *The cerebral cortex of man*. New York: Macmillan.

Petersen, S. E., & Posner, M. I. (2012). The attention system of the human brain: 20 years after. *Annual Review of Neuroscience, 35*(1), 73–89. doi:10.1146/annurev-neuro-062111-150525 PMID:22524787

Petit, D., Gergondet, P., Cherubini, A., & Kheddar, A. (2015). An integrated framework for humanoid embodiment with a BCI.*IEEE International Conference on Robotics & Automation*, (pp. 2882-2887). doi:10.1109/ICRA.2015.7139592

Petitto, L. A. (2009). New discoveries from the bilingual brain and mind across the life span: Implications for education. *Mind Brain & Education*, *3*(4), 185–197. doi:10.1111/j.1751-228X.2009.01069.x

Pfurtscheller, G., Müller, G. R., Pfurtscheller, J., Gerner, H. J., & Rupp, R. (2003). 'thought'—control of functional electrical stimulation to restore hand grasp in a patient with tetraplegia. *Neuroscience Letters*, *351*(1), 33–36. doi:10.1016/S0304-3940(03)00947-9 PMID:14550907

Pfurtscheller, G., Neuper, C., Flotzinger, D., & Pregenzer, M. (1997). Eeg-based discrimination between imagination of right and left hand movement. *Electroencephalography and Clinical Neurophysiology*, *103*(6), 642–651. doi:10.1016/S0013-4694(97)00080-1 PMID:9546492

Phillips-Silver, J., & Trainor, L. J. (2005). Feeling the beat: Movement influences infant rhythm perception. *Science*, *308*(5727), 1430. doi:10.1126/science.1110922 PMID:15933193

Phung, H., Nguyen, C. T., Nguyen, T. D., Lee, C., Kim, U., Lee, D., & Choi, H. R. et al. (2015). Tactile display with rigid coupling based on soft actuator. *Meccanica*, *50*(11), 2825–2837. doi:10.1007/s11012-015-0270-5

Picton, T. W. (1992). The p300 wave of the human event-related potential. *Journal of Clinical Neurophysiology Official Publication of the American Electroencephalographic Society*, *9*(4), 456–479. doi:10.1097/00004691-199210000-00002 PMID:1464675

Pivi, G. A., da Silva, R. V., Juliano, Y., Novo, N. F., Okamoto, I. H., Brant, C. Q., & Bertolucci, P. H. (2011). A prospective study of nutrition education and oral nutritional supplementation in patients with Alzheimer's disease. *Nutrition Journal*, *10*(98), 1–6. PMID:21943331

Plisier, M. A., Tiest, W. M. B., & Kappers, A. M. L. (2009). Salient features in 3-D haptic shape perception. *Attention, Perception & Psychophysics*, *71*(2), 421–430. doi:10.3758/APP.71.2.421 PMID:19304631

Portocarrero, J. S., Burright, R. G., & Donovick, P. J. (2007). Vocabulary and verbal fluency of bilingual and monolingual college students. *Archives of Clinical Neuropsychology the Official Journal of the National Academy of Neuropsychologists*, *22*(3), 415–422. doi:10.1016/j.acn.2007.01.015 PMID:17336036

Pratt, J., Carff, J., Drakunov, S., & Goswami, A. (2007). Capture Point: A Step toward Humanoid Push Recovery. *Humanoid Robots, IEEE-RAS International Conference on*, (pp. 200-207).

Pratt, J., Koolen, T., De Boer, T., Rebula, J., Cotton, S., Carff, J., & Neuhaus, P. et al. (2012). Capturability-based analysis and control of legged locomotion, part 2: Application to m2v2, *a lower-body humanoid. The International Journal of Robotics Research*, *31*(10), 1117–1133. doi:10.1177/0278364912452762

Pratt, J., & Krupp, B. (2008). Design of a bipedal walking robot.*SPIE Defense and Security Symposium* (Vol. 6962). International Society for Optics and Photonics.

Prince, M., Albanese, E., Guerchet, M., & Prina, M. (2014). Nutrition and dementia. A review of available research. London: Alzheimer's Disease International (ADI).

Prior, A., & Macwhinney, B. (2010). A bilingual advantage in task switching. *Bilingualism: Language and Cognition*, *13*(2), 253–262. doi:10.1017/S1366728909990526

Quax, R., Apolloni, A., & Sloot, P. M. A. (2013). Towards understanding the behavior of physical systems using information theory. *The European Physical Journal. Special Topics*, *222*(6), 1389–1401. doi:10.1140/epjst/e2013-01933-9

Quax, R., Kandhai, D., & Sloot, P. M. A. (2013). Information dissipation as an early-warning signal for the Lehman Brothers collapse in financial time series. *Scientific Reports*, *3*, 1898. doi:10.1038/srep01898 PMID:23719567

Quigley, M., Conley, K., Gerkey, B., Faust, J., Foote, T., Leibs, J., & Ng, A. Y. et al. (2009). ROS: an open-source Robot Operating System.*In IEEE International Conference on Robotics & Automation workshop on open source software.*

Rach, S., Diederich, A., & Colonius, H. (2011). On quantifying multisensory interaction effects in reaction time and detection rate. *Psychological Research*, *75*(2), 77–94. doi:10.1007/s00426-010-0289-0 PMID:20512352

Raichle, M. E., Toga, A. W., & Mazziotta, J. C. (2000). *Brain mapping: the systems.* London: Academic Press.

Raichle, M. E., MacLeod, A. M., Snyder, A. Z., Powers, W. J., Gusnard, D. A., & Shulman, G. L. (2001). A default mode of brain function. *Proceedings of the National Academy of Sciences of the United States of America*, *98*(2), 676–682. doi:10.1073/pnas.98.2.676 PMID:11209064

Rakıcıoglu, N., Tek, N., Ayaz, A., & Pekcan, G. (2009). Yemek ve besin fotoğraf kataloğu: Ölçü ve miktarlar. Ankara: Ata Ofset Matbaacılık. (in Turkish)

Rämä, P., Sala, J. B., Gillen, J. S., Pekar, J. J., & Courtney, S. M. (2001). Dissociation of the neural systems for working memory maintenance of verbal and nonspatial visual information. *Cognitive, Affective & Behavioral Neuroscience*, *1*(2), 161–171. doi:10.3758/CABN.1.2.161 PMID:12467111

Rammsayer, T. H., & Vogel, W. H. (1992). Pharmacologic properties of the internal clock underlying time perception in humans. *Neuropsychobiology, 26*(1-2), 71-80.

Rammsayer, T. H. (1994). Effects of practice and signal energy on duration discrimination of brief auditory intervals. *Perception & Psychophysics*, *55*(4), 454–464. doi:10.3758/BF03205302 PMID:8036124

Rammsayer, T. H. (1997). Are there dissociable roles of the mesostriatal and mesolimbocortical dopamine systems on temporal information processing in humans? *Neuropsychobiology*, *35*(1), 36–45. doi:10.1159/000119328 PMID:9018022

Rammsayer, T. H. (1999). Neuropharmacological evidence for different timing mechanisms in humans. *The Quarterly Journal of Experimental Psychology. B, Comparative and Physiological Psychology*, *52*(3), 273–286. doi:10.1080/713932708 PMID:10467900

Randall, P., Burkhardt, S. J., & Kutcher, J. (1990). Exterior space for patients with Alzheimer's disease and related disorders. *American Journal of Alzheimer's Care and Related Disorders & Research*, *5*(4), 31–37. doi:10.1177/153331759000500408

Rappe, E. (2005). *The Influence of a Green Environment and Horticultural Activities on the Subjective Well-Being of the Elderly Living in Long-Term Care*. University of Helsinki, Department of Applied Biology.

Rashidi, P., & Mihailidis, A. (2013). A Survey on Ambient-Assisted Living Tools for Older Adults. *IEEE Journal of Biomedical and Health Informatics*, *17*(3), 579–590. doi:10.1109/JBHI.2012.2234129 PMID:24592460

Rasmussen, R. G., Acharya, S., & Thakor, N. V. (2006). Accuracy of a Brain-Computer Interface in Subjects with Minimal Training.*Proceedings of the IEEE 32nd Annual Northeast Bioengineering Conference* (pp. 167-168). IEEE. doi:10.1109/NEBC.2006.1629805

Ravizza, S. M., Delgado, M. R., Chein, J. M., Becker, J. T., & Fiez, J. A. (2004). Functional dissociations within the inferior parietal cortex in verbal working memory. *NeuroImage*, *22*(2), 562–573. doi:10.1016/j.neuroimage.2004.01.039 PMID:15193584

RDA/Recommended Dietary Allowances. (1989). Subcommittee on the tenth edition of the RDAs food and nutrition board commission on life sciences.Washington, DC: National Academy Press.

Reiman, E. M., Quiroz, Y. T., Fleisher, A. S., Chen, K., Velez-Pardo, C., Jimenez-Del-Rio, M., & Lopera, F. et al. (2012). Brain imaging and fluid biomarker analysis in young adults at genetic risk for autosomal dominant Alzheimer's disease in the presenilin 1 E280A kindred: A case-control study. *Lancet Neurology*, *11*(12), 1048–1056. doi:10.1016/S1474-4422(12)70228-4 PMID:23137948

Remig, V. M., & Weeden, A. (2008). Medical nutrition therapy for neurologic disorders. In L. K. Mahan & S. E. Stump (Eds.), *Krause's food and nutrition therapy* (pp. 923–955). Toronto: Saunders Elsevier.

Ren, Y.-N., Yang, W., & Wu, J. (2014). Book Review: The New Handbook of Multisensory Processing. Barry E. Stein, ed. June 2012. The MIT Press. No. of pages 823. ISBN: 987-0-262-01712-1. Neuroscience and Biomedical Engineering, 2, 105-108.

Richlan, F., Gagl, B., Schuster, S., Hawelka, S., Humenberger, J., & Hutzler, F. (2013). A new high-speed visual stimulation method for gaze-contingent eye movement and brain activity studies. *Frontiers in Systems Neuroscience*, *7*, 24. doi:10.3389/fnsys.2013.00024 PMID:23847475

Ripich, D. N., & Terrell, B. Y. (1988). Patterns of discourse cohesion and coherence in Alzheimer's disease. *The Journal of Speech and Hearing Disorders*, *53*(1), 8–15. doi:10.1044/jshd.5301.08 PMID:3339870

Risacher, S. L., Saykin, A. J., West, J. D., Shen, L., Firpi, H. A., & McDonald, B. C. (2009). Baseline MRI predictors of conversion from MCI to probable AD in the ADNI cohort. *Current Alzheimer Research*, *6*(4), 347–361. doi:10.2174/156720509788929273 PMID:19689234

Riviere, S., Gillette-Guvonnet, S., Voisin, T., Reynish, E., Andrieu, S., Lauque, S., & Micas, M. (2001). A nutritional education program could prevent weight loss and slow cognitive decline in Alzheimer's disease. *The Journal of Nutrition, Health & Aging*, *5*(4), 295–299. PMID:11753499

Rizzolatti, G., & Sinigaglia, C. (2008). Further reflections on how we interpret the actions of others. *Nature*, *455*(7213), 589. doi:10.1038/455589b PMID:18833249

Robert, P. H., König, A., Amieva, H., Andrieu, S., Bremond, F., Bullock, R., & Manera, V. et al. (2014). Recommendations for the use of Serious Games in people with Alzheimer's Disease, related disorders and frailty. *Frontiers in Aging Neuroscience*, *6*, 54. doi:10.3389/fnagi.2014.00054 PMID:24715864

Robinson, D. A. (1963). *A method of measuring eye movements using a scleral search coil in a magnetic field. In Transactions on Biomedical Engineering* (pp. 137–145). IEEE.

Robinson, K. M., Grossman, M., White-Devine, T., & D' Esposito, M. (1996). Category-specific difficulty naming with verbs in Alzheimer's disease. *Neurology*, *47*(1), 178–182. doi:10.1212/WNL.47.1.178 PMID:8710073

Roby, J. W., Gao, J. H., & Fox, P. T. (2000). A versatile, low-cost method for presenting visual stimuli during MRI. *Journal of Magnetic Resonance Imaging*, *11*(2), 223–227. doi:10.1002/(SICI)1522-2586(200002)11:2<223::AID-JMRI22>3.0.CO;2-G PMID:10713958

Röcker, C., Hinske, S., & Magerkurth, C. (2007). Universal Access in Human-Computer Interaction. Ambient Interaction (Vol. 4555). Berlin: Springer Berlin Heidelberg. http://doi.org/doi:<ALIGNMENT.qj></ALIGNMENT>10.1007/978-3-540-73281-5

Rogalski, E., Stebbins, G. T., Barnes, C. A., Murphy, C. M., Stoub, T. R., George, S., & deToledo-Morrell, L. et al. (2012). Age-related changes in parahippocampal white matter integrity: A diffusion tensor imaging study. *Neuropsychologia*, *50*(8), 1759–1765. doi:10.1016/j.neuropsychologia.2012.03.033 PMID:22561887

Rolland, Y., Abellan van Kan, G., & Vellas, B. (2008). Physical activity and Alzheimer's disease: From prevention to therapeutic perspectives. *Journal of the American Medical Directors Association*, *9*(6), 390–405. doi:10.1016/j.jamda.2008.02.007 PMID:18585641

Rolls, E. T., O' Doherty, J., Kringelbach, M. L., Francis, S., Bowtell, R., & McGlone, F. (2003). Representations of pleasant and painful touch in the human orbitofrontal and cingulate cortices. *Cerebral Cortex*, *13*(3), 308–317. doi:10.1093/cercor/13.3.308 PMID:12571120

Rosario Rueda, M., Pozuelos, J., & Cómbita, L. (2015). Cognitive Neuroscience of Attention From brain mechanisms to individual differences in efficiency. *AIMS Neuroscience, 2*(4), 183-202. doi: 10.3934/Neuroscience.2015.4.183

Ross, L. A., Saint-Amour, D., Leavitt, V. M., Javitt, D. C., & Foxe, J. J. (2007). Do you see what I am saying? Exploring visual enhancement of speech comprehension in noisy environments. *Cerebral Cortex, 17*(5), 1147–1153. doi:10.1093/cercor/bhl024 PMID:16785256

Rueda, M., Rothbart, M. K., McCandliss, B. D., Saccomanno, L., & Posner, M. I. (2005). Training, maturation, and genetic influences on the development of executive attention. *Proceedings of the national Academy of Sciences of the United States of America, 102*(41), 14931-14936.

Ruiz-Del-Solar, J., Palma-Amestoy, R., Marchant, R., Parra-Tsunekawa, I., & Zegers, P. (2009). Learning to fall: Designing low damage fall sequences for humanoid soccer robots. *Robotics and Autonomous Systems, 57*(8), 796–807. doi:10.1016/j.robot.2009.03.011

Rupp, R., & Cemer, H. J. (2004). NeuroProstheties of the upper extremity-elinieal applieation in spinal cord injury and future perspectives. *Bio/Technology, 49*, 93–98. PMID:15171589

Sahyoun, C., Floyer-Lea, A., Johansen-Berg, H., & Matthews, P. M. (2004). Towards an understanding of gait control: Brain activation during the anticipation, preparation and execution of foot movements. *NeuroImage, 21*(2), 568–575. doi:10.1016/j.neuroimage.2003.09.065 PMID:14980558

Sakamoto, D., Kanda, T., Ono, T., Kamashima, M., Imai, M., & Ishiguro, H. (2005). Cooperative embodied communication emerged by interactive humanoid robots. *International Journal of Human-Computer Studies, 62*(2), 247–265. doi:10.1016/j.ijhcs.2004.11.001

Salthouse, T. A., & Czaja, S. J. (2000). Structural constraints on process explanations in cognitive aging. *Psychology and Aging, 15*(1), 44–55. doi:10.1037/0882-7974.15.1.44 PMID:10755288

Salthouse, T. A., Hancock, H. E., Meinz, E. J., & Hambrick, D. Z. (1996). Interrelations of age, visual acuity, and cognitive functioning. *The Journals of Gerontology. Series B, Psychological Sciences and Social Sciences, 51*(6), 317–330. doi:10.1093/geronb/51B.6.P317 PMID:8931619

Salthouse, T. A., & Lichty, W. (1985). Tests of the neural noise hypothesis of age-related cognitive change. *Journal of Gerontology, 40*(4), 443–450. doi:10.1093/geronj/40.4.443 PMID:4008879

Salva, A., Andrieu, S., Fernandez, E., Schiffrin, E. J., Moulin, J., Decarli, B., & Vellas, B. (2011). Health and nutrition promotion program for patients with dementia (NutriAlz): Cluster randomized trial. *The Journal of Nutrition, Health & Aging, 15*(10), 822–830. doi:10.1007/s12603-011-0363-3 PMID:22159768

Sandro, M. I. (2000). Neural engineering: Real brains for real robots. *Nature, 408*, 305–306. PMID:11099027

Sandrone, S., Bacigaluppi, M., Galloni, M. R., Cappa, S. F., Moro, A., Catani, M., & Martino, G. et al. (2014). Weighing brain activity with the balance: Angelo Mosso's original manuscripts come to light. *Brain, 137*(Pt 2), 621–633. doi:10.1093/brain/awt091 PMID:23687118

Sandrone, S., Bacigaluppi, M., Galloni, M. R., & Martino, G. (2012). Angelo Mosso (1846–1910). *Journal of Neurology*, *259*(11), 2513–2514. doi:10.1007/s00415-012-6632-1 PMID:23010944

Sanlier, N., & Yabanci, N. (2006). Mini nutritional assessment in the elderly: Living alone, with family, a nursing home in Turkey. *Nutrition & Food Science*, *36*(1), 50–58. doi:10.1108/00346650610642197

Saragat, B., Buffa, R., Mereu, E., Succa, V., Cabras, S., Mereu, R. M., & Marini, E. (2012). Nutritional and psycho-functional status in elderly patients with Alzheimer's disease. *The Journal of Nutrition, Health & Aging*, *16*(3), 231–236. doi:10.1007/s12603-011-0347-3 and PubMed

Savini, N., Babilonib, C., Brunetti, M., Caulo, M., Gratta, C. D., & Ferretti, A. et al.. (2010). Passive tactile recognition of geometrical shape in humans: An fMRI study. *Brain Research Bulletin*, *83*(5), 223–231. doi:10.1016/j.brainresbull.2010.08.001 PMID:20696217

Savini, N., Brunetti, M., Babilonib, C., & Ferretti, A. (2012). Working memory of somatosensory stimuli: An fMRI study. *International Journal of Psychophysiology*, *86*(3), 220–228. doi:10.1016/j.ijpsycho.2012.09.007 PMID:23044088

Scarmeas, N., Levy, G., Tang, M.-X., Manly, J., & Stern, Y. (2001). Influence of leisure activity on the incidence of Alzheimer's Disease. *Neurology*, *57*(12), 2236–2242. doi:10.1212/WNL.57.12.2236 PMID:11756603

Schellenberg, G. D., Bird, T. D., Wijsman, E. M., Orr, H. T., Anderson, L., Nemens, E., & Alonso, M. E. et al. (1992). Genetic linkage evidence for a familial Alzheimer's disease locus on chromosome 14. *Science*, *258*(5082), 668–671. doi:10.1126/science.1411576 PMID:1411576

Schwartz, M. F., Marin, O. S., & Saffran, E. M. (1979). Dissociations of language function in dementia: A case study. *Brain and Language*, *7*(3), 277–306. doi:10.1016/0093-934X(79)90024-5 PMID:455049

Schwarz, B., & Rodiek, S. (2007). Introduction: Outdoor Environments for People with Dementia. In Outdoor Environments for People with Dementia (pp. 3-13). Routledge.

Scoville, W. B., & Milner, B. (1957). Loss of recent memory after bilateral hippocampal lesions. *Journal of Neurology, Neurosurgery, and Psychiatry*, *20*(1), 11–21. doi:10.1136/jnnp.20.1.11 PMID:13406589

Seelye, A., Mattek, N., Howieson, D., Riley, T., Wild, K., & Kaye, J. (2015). The Impact of Sleep on Neuropsychological Performance in Cognitively Intact Older Adults Using a Novel In-Home Sensor-Based Sleep Assessment Approach. *The Clinical Neuropsychologist*, *29*(1), 53–66. doi:10.1080/13854046.2015.1005139 PMID:25642948

Senkowski, D., Saint-Amour, D., Hofle, M., & Foxe, J. J. (2011). Multisensory interactions in early evoked brain activity follow the principle of inverse effectiveness. *NeuroImage*, *56*(4), 2200–2208. doi:10.1016/j.neuroimage.2011.03.075 PMID:21497200

Serino, A., Farnè, A., Rinaldesi, M. L., Haggard, P., & Làdavas, E. (2007). Can vision of the body ameliorate impaired somatosensory function? *Neuropsychologia*, *45*(5), 1101–1107. doi:10.1016/j.neuropsychologia.2006.09.013 PMID:17101158

Seth, R. V. (1994). Review: Weight loss in Alzheimer's disease. *International Journal of Geriatric Psychiatry*, *9*(8), 605–610. doi:10.1002/gps.930090803

Severinson-Eklundh, K., Green, A., & Hüttenrauch, H. (2003). Social and collaborative aspects of interaction with a service robot. *Robotics and Autonomous Systems*, *42*(3-4), 223–234. doi:10.1016/S0921-8890(02)00377-9

Shatenstein, B., Kergoat, M. J., & Reid, I. (2007). Poor nutrient intakes during 1-year follow-up with community-dwelling older adults with early-stage Alzheimer dementia compared to cognitively intact matched controls. *Journal of the American Dietetic Association*, *107*(12), 2091–2099. doi:10.1016/j.jada.2007.09.008 PMID:18060894

Sheehan, B., Burton, E. J., & Mitchell, L. (2006). Outdoor wayfinding in dementia. *Dementia (London)*, *5*(2), 271–281. doi:10.1177/1471301206062254

Sheline, Y. I., Morris, J. C., Snyder, A. Z., Price, J. L., Yan, Z., D'Angelo, G., & Mintun, M. A. et al. (2010). APOE4 allele disrupts resting state fMRI connectivity in the absence of amyloid plaques or decreased CSF Aβ42. *The Journal of Neuroscience*, *30*(50), 17035–17040. doi:10.1523/JNEUROSCI.3987-10.2010 PMID:21159973

Shi, F., Liu, B., Zhou, Y., Yu, C., & Jiang, T. (2009). Hippocampal volume and asymmetry in mild cognitive impairment and Alzheimer's disease: Meta-analyses of MRI studies. *Hippocampus*, *19*(11), 1055–1064. doi:10.1002/hipo.20573 PMID:19309039

Siegelbaum, S. A., & Kandel, E. R. (1991). Learning-related synaptic plasticity: LTP and LTD. *Current Opinion in Neurobiology*, *1*(1), 113–120. doi:10.1016/0959-4388(91)90018-3 PMID:1822291

Silva, A., Restivo, M. T., & Gzbriel, J. (2013). Haptic device demo using temperature feedback. *International Conference IEEE, 2*, 172-173.

Silva, M. F., D'almeida, O. C., Oliveiros, B., Mateus, C., & Castelo-Branco, M. (2014). Development and aging of visual hemifield asymmetries in contrast sensitivity. *Journal of Vision (Charlottesville, Va.)*, 14. PMID:25326605

Simao, C., & Seibt, B. (2015). Friendly touch increases gratitude by inducing communal feelings. *Frontiers in Psychology*, *6*, 815. doi:10.3389/fpsyg.2015.00815 PMID:26124737

Simoes-Franklin, C., Whitaker, T. A., & Newell, F. N. (2011). Active and passive touch differentially activate somatosensory cortex in texture perception. *Human Brain Mapping*, *32*(7), 1067–1080. doi:10.1002/hbm.21091 PMID:20669167

Singh, H., Bauer, M., Chowanski, W., Sui, Y., Atkinson, D., Baurley, S., & Bianchi-Berthouze, N. et al. (2014). The brain's response to pleasant touch: An EEG investigation of tactile caressing. *Frontiers in Human Neuroscience*, *8*, 893. doi:10.3389/fnhum.2014.00893 PMID:25426047

Sitzer, D., Twamley, E., & Jeste, D. (2006). Cognitive training in Alzheimer's disease: A meta-analysis of the literature. *Acta Psychiatrica Scandinavica, 114*(2), 75–90. doi:10.1111/j.1600-0447.2006.00789.x PMID:16836595

Skeet, M. (1983). *Protecting the health of the elderly*. Retrieved 10 March, 2015, from http://whqlibdoc.who.int/euro/phie/WHO_PHIE_18_(part1).pdf

Small, G. W., Kepe, V., Ercoli, L. M., Siddarth, P., Bookheimer, S. Y., Miller, K. J., & Vinters, H. V. et al. (2006). PET of brain amyloid and tau in mild cognitive impairment. *The New England Journal of Medicine, 355*(25), 2652–2663. doi:10.1056/NEJMoa054625 PMID:17182990

Smith, E. E., & Jonides, J. (1999). Storage and Executive Processes in the Frontal Lobes. *Science, 283*(5408), 1657–1661. doi:10.1126/science.283.5408.1657 PMID:10073923

Smith, G. E., & Bondi, M. W. (2013). *Mild cognitive impairment and dementia: definitions, diagnosis, and treatment*. Oxford University Press.

So, E. S. (2014). Waist Circumference and health-related quality of life by sex in the Korean elderly. *Journal of Aging and Health, 26*(6), 887–899. doi:10.1177/0898264314531618 PMID:24788716

Sofia, K. O., Jones, L. A., & Member, S. (2013). Mechanical and psychophysical studies of surface wave propagation during vibrotactile stimulation. *IEEE Transactions On Haptics, 6*(3), 320–329. doi:10.1109/TOH.2013.1 PMID:24808328

Son, C., Ko, K., Lee, H. J., Na, K., Han, J., & Yun, K. S. et al.. (2015). A flexible multimodal tactile display array for virtual shape and texture. *Microsystem Technologies*, 1–8.

Southwick, P. C., Yamagata, S. K., Echols, C. L. Jr, Higson, G. J., Neynaber, S. A., Parson, R. E., & Munroe, W. A. (1996). Assessment of amyloid β protein in cerebrospinal fluid as an aid in the diagnosis of Alzheimer's disease. *Journal of Neurochemistry, 66*(1), 259–265. doi:10.1046/j.1471-4159.1996.66010259.x PMID:8522962

Spaccavento, S., Del Prete, M., Craca, A., & Fiore, P. (2009). Influence of nutritional status on cognitive, functional and neuropsychiatric deficits in Alzheimer's disease. *Archives of Gerontology and Geriatrics, 48*(3), 356–360. doi:10.1016/j.archger.2008.03.002 PMID:18448178

Spaulding, W. D., Fleming, S. K., Reed, D., Sullivan, M., Storzbach, D., & Lam, M. (1999). Cognitive functioning in schizophrenia: Implications for psychiatric rehabilitation. *Schizophrenia Bulletin, 25*(2), 275–289. doi:10.1093/oxfordjournals.schbul.a033378 PMID:10416731

Spyrou, T., & Darzentas, J. (1996). Intention Modelling: Approximating Computer User Intentions for Detection and Prediction of Intrusions. In *Information Systems Security* (pp. 319–335). London: Chapman & Hall, Ltd. doi:10.1007/978-1-5041-2919-0_28

Srinivasan, M. A., & Lamotte, R. H. (1995). Tactual discrimination of softness. *Journal of Neurophysiology, 73*, 88–105. PMID:7714593

Staiano, A. E., & Calvert, S. L. (2011). The promise of exergames as tools to measure physical health. *Entertainment Computing, 2*(1), 17–21. doi:10.1016/j.entcom.2011.03.008 PMID:23378860

Stein, B. E., & Meredith, M. A. (1993). *The merging of the senses*. The MIT Press.

Stein, B. E., & Stanford, T. R. (2008). Multisensory integration: Current issues from the perspective of the single neuron. *Nature Reviews. Neuroscience*, *9*(4), 255–266. doi:10.1038/nrn2331 PMID:18354398

Stern, Y. (2002). Stern y. what is cognitive reserve? Theory and research application of the reserve concept. *Journal of the International Neuropsychological Society*, *8*(3), 448–460. doi:10.1017/S1355617702813248 PMID:11939702

Steve, C., Andy, R., Russ, T., & Martijn, W. (2005). Efficient bipedal robots based on passive-dynamic walkers. *Science*, *307*(5712), 1082–1085. doi:10.1126/science.1107799 PMID:15718465

Stevenson, R. A., Bushmakin, M., Kim, S., Wallace, M. T., Puce, A., & James, T. W. (2012). Inverse effectiveness and multisensory interactions in visual event-related potentials with audiovisual speech. *Brain Topography*, *25*(3), 308–326. doi:10.1007/s10548-012-0220-7 PMID:22367585

Stevenson, R. A., & James, T. W. (2009). Audiovisual integration in human superior temporal sulcus: Inverse effectiveness and the neural processing of speech and object recognition. *NeuroImage*, *44*(3), 1210–1223. doi:10.1016/j.neuroimage.2008.09.034 PMID:18973818

Stine, E. A., Wingfield, A., & Myers, S. D. (1990). Age differences in processing information from television news: The effects of bisensory augmentation. *Journal of Gerontology*, *45*(1), 1–8. doi:10.1093/geronj/45.1.P1 PMID:2295777

Stippich, C., Hofmann, R., Kapfer, D., Hempel, E., Heiland, S., Jansen, O., & Sartor, K. (1999). Somatotopic mapping of the human primary somatosensory cortex by fully automated tactile stimulation using functional magnetic resonance imaging. *Neuroscience Letters*, *277*(1), 25–28. doi:10.1016/S0304-3940(99)00835-6 PMID:10643889

Storf, H., Becker, M., & Riedl, M. (2009). Rule-based activity recognition framework: Challenges, technique and learning. In *Proceedings of the 3d International ICST Conference on Pervasive Computing Technologies for Healthcare* (pp. 1–7). ICST. http://doi.org/ doi:10.4108/ICST.PERVASIVEHEALTH2009.6108

Strenziok, M., Parasuraman, R., Clarke, E., Cisler, D. S., Thompson, J. C., & Greenwood, P. M. (2014). Neurocognitive enhancement in older adults: Comparison of three cognitive training tasks to test a hypothesis of training transfer in brain connectivity. *NeuroImage*, *85*(Pt 3), 1027–1039. doi:10.1016/j.neuroimage.2013.07.069 PMID:23933474

Stringer, E. A., Chen, L. M., Friedman, B. M., Gatenby, C., & Gore, J. C. (2011). Differentiation of somatosensory cortices by high-resolution fMRI at 7T. *NeuroImage*, *54*(2), 1012–1020. doi:10.1016/j.neuroimage.2010.09.058 PMID:20887793

Stuss, D. T., & Levine, B. (1996). The dementias: Nosological and clinical factors related to diagnosis. *Brain and Cognition*, *31*(2), 99–113. doi:10.1006/brcg.1996.0036 PMID:8811985

Styliadis, C., Kartsidis, P., & Paraskevopoulos, E. (n.d.). *Neuroimaging Approaches for Elderly Studies*. IGI Global. Retrieved from http://www.igi-global.com/chapter/neuroimaging-approaches-for-elderly-studies/129268

Styliadis, C., Kartsidis, P., Paraskevopoulos, E., Ioannides, A. A., & Bamidis, P. D. (2015). Neuroplastic Effects of Combined Computerized Physical and Cognitive Training in Elderly Individuals at Risk for Dementia: An eLORETA Controlled Study on Resting States. *Neural Plasticity*, *12*(2). Retrieved from http://doi.org/doi:10.1155/2015/172192 PMID:25945260

Summers, I. R., Chanter, C. M., Southall, A. L., & Brady, A. C. (2011). Results from a tactile array on the fingertip. *Eurohaptics*, 26-28.

Suominen, M. H., Puranen, T. M., Jyväkorpi, S. K., Eloniemi-Sulkava, U., Kautiainen, H., Siljamäki-Ojansuu, U., & Pitkälä, K. H. (2015). Nutritional guidance improves nutrient intake and quality of life, and may prevent falls in aged persons with Alzheimer disease living with a spouse (NuAD Trial). *The Journal of Nutrition, Health & Aging*, 1–7. PMID:26482691

Suvarna, A., Bak, T. H., Vasanta, D., Bapiraju, S., Mekala, S., & Anuj Kumar, S. et al.. (2013). Bilingualism delays age at onset of dementia, independent of education and immigration status. *Neurology*, *81*(22). PMID:24198291

Talsma, D., Doty, T. J., & Woldorff, M. G. (2007). Selective attention and audiovisual integration: Is attending to both modalities a prerequisite for early integration? *Cerebral Cortex*, *17*(3), 679–690. doi:10.1093/cercor/bhk016 PMID:16707740

Tang, X., Wu, J., & Shen, Y. (2016). The interactions of multisensory integration with endogenous and exogenous attention. *Neuroscience and Biobehavioral Reviews*, *61*, 208–224. doi:10.1016/j.neubiorev.2015.11.002 PMID:26546734

Tang, Y.-Y., Ma, Y., Fan, Y., Feng, H., Wang, J., Feng, S., & Li, J. et al. (2009). Central and autonomic nervous system interaction is altered by short-term meditation. *Proceedings of the National Academy of Sciences of the United States of America*, *106*(22), 8865–8870. doi:10.1073/pnas.0904031106 PMID:19451642

Tang, Y.-Y., Ma, Y., Wang, J., Fan, Y., Feng, S., Lu, Q., & Fan, M. et al. (2007). Short-term meditation training improves attention and self-regulation. *Proceedings of the National Academy of Sciences of the United States of America*, *104*(43), 17152–17156. doi:10.1073/pnas.0707678104 PMID:17940025

Tang, Y.-Y., & Posner, M. I. (2009). Attention training and attention state training. *Trends in Cognitive Sciences*, *13*(5), 222–227. doi:10.1016/j.tics.2009.01.009 PMID:19375975

Tardif, S., & Simard, M. (2011). Cognitive stimulation programs in healthy elderly: A review. *International Journal of Alzheimer's Disease*, *378934*. doi:10.4061/2011/378934 PMID:21876829

Tariot, P. N., Farlow, M. R., Grossberg, G. T., Graham, S. M., Mcdonald, S., Gergel, I., & Group, M. S. (2004). Memantine treatment in patients with moderate to severe Alzheimer disease already receiving donepezil: A randomized controlled trial. *Journal of the American Medical Association, 291*(3), 317–324. doi:10.1001/jama.291.3.317 PMID:14734594

Tarnanas, I., Schlee, W., Tsolaki, M., Müri, R., Mosimann, U., & Nef, T. (2013). Ecological validity of virtual reality daily living activities screening for early dementia: Longitudinal study. *JMIR Serious Games, 1*(1), e1. doi:10.2196/games.2778 PMID:25658491

Tasoglu, O., & Ozgirgin, N. (2013). Sarkopeni[Sarcopenia]. *Türkiye Fiziksel Tıp ve Rehabilitasyon Dergisi, 6*(4), 9–15.

Taylor, C. L., Albanese, E., & Stewart, R. (2012). The association of dementia with upper arm and waist circumference in seven low-and middle-income countries: The 10/66 cross-sectional surveys. *The Journals of Gerontology. Series A, Biological Sciences and Medical Sciences, 67*(8), 897–904. doi:10.1093/gerona/glr244 PMID:22389465

Taylor, D. M., Tillery, S. I. H., & Schwartz, A. B. (2002). Direct cortical control of 3d neuroprosthetic devices. *Science, 296*(5574), 1829–1832. doi:10.1126/science.1070291 PMID:12052948

Terry, H. & Cooper Marcus, C. (2006). Healing Gardens – Places for Nature in Health Care. *The Lancet, 368.*

Thompson, E. H., & Hampton, J. A. (2011). The effect of relationship status on communicating emotions through touch. *Cognition and Emotion, 25*(2), 295–306. doi:10.1080/02699931.2010.492957 PMID:21432672

Thorell, L. B., Lindqvist, S., Nutley, B., & Sissela, B. (2009). Training and transfer effects of executive functions in preschool children. *Developmental Science, 12*(1), 106–113. doi:10.1111/j.1467-7687.2008.00745.x PMID:19120418

Todd, J., Fougnie, D., & Marois, R. (2005). Visual short-term memory load suppresses temporo-parietal junction activity and induces inattentional blindness. *Psychological Science, 16*(12), 965–972. doi:10.1111/j.1467-9280.2005.01645.x PMID:16313661

Todd, J., & Marois, R. (2004). Capacity limit of visual short-term memory in human posterior parietal cortex. *Nature, 428*(6984), 751–754. doi:10.1038/nature02466 PMID:15085133

Tong, R. K. Y., Leung, W. W. F., Hu, X. L., & Song, R. (2009). Interactive robot-assisted training system using continuous EMG signals for stroke rehabilitation.*Proceedings of the 3rd International Convention on Rehabilitation Engineering & Assistive Technology: No.* 20. New York: ACM. doi:10.1145/1592700.1592723

Tractenberg, R. E., Singer, C. M., & Kaye, J. (2005). Symptoms of sleep disturbance in persons with Alzheimer's disease and normal elderly. *Journal of Sleep Research, 14*(2), 177–185. doi:10.1111/j.1365-2869.2005.00445.x PMID:15910515

Trainor, L. J. (2012). Predictive information processing is a fundamental learning mechanism present in early development: Evidence from infants. *International Journal of Psychophysiology, 83*(2), 256–258. doi:10.1016/j.ijpsycho.2011.12.008 PMID:22226901

Traynor, V., Fernandez, R., & Caldwell, K. (2013). The effects of spending time outdoors in daylight on the psychosocial wellbeing of older people and family carers: a comprehensive systematic review protocol. *JBI Database of Systematic Reviews & Implementation Reports, 11*(9), 36-55. Retrieved June 2015, http://ro.uow.edu.au/cgi/viewcontent.cgi?article=2184&context=smhpapers

Tsai, A. C. H., Lai, M. C., & Chang, T. L. (2012). Mid-arm and calf circumferences (MAC and CC) are better than body mass index (BMI) in predicting health status and mortality risk in institutionalized elderly Taiwanese. *Archives of Gerontology and Geriatrics, 54*(3), 443–447. doi:10.1016/j.archger.2011.05.015 PMID:21663980

Ulrich, R. S. (2002). Health Benefits of Gardens in Hospitals. In *Plants for People,Proceedings of the International Exhibition Floriade.*

Ulrich, R. S., Bogren, L., & Lundin, S. (2012). Toward a design theory for reducing aggression in psychiatric facilities. In Conference Arch 12: Architecture, Research, Care, Health. Gothenburg: Chalmers Institute of Technology.

Ulrich, R., Zimring, C., Quan, X., Joseph, A., & Choudhary, R. (2004). *The Role of the Physical Environment in the Hospital of the 21st Century: A Once-in-a-Lifetime Opportunity.* Report to The Center for Health Design for the Designing the 21st Century Hospital Project. Retrieved June 2015 http://www.healthdesign.org/chd/research/role-physical-environment-hospital-21st-century

Ulrich, R. S., Simons, R. F., Losito, B. D., Fiorito, E., Miles, M. A., & Zelson, M. (1991). Stress recovery during exposure to natural and urban environments. *Journal of Environmental Psychology, 11*(3), 201–230. doi:10.1016/S0272-4944(05)80184-7

Ulrich, R., & Gilpin, L. (2003). Healing arts – nutrition for the soul. In P. M. Charmel, S. B. Frampton, & L. Gilpin (Eds.), *Putting Patients First—Designing and Practicing Patient-Centered Care* (pp. 117–146). San Francisco: Jossey-Bass.

Urata, J., Nshiwaki, K., Nakanishi, Y., Okada, K., Kagami, S., & Inaba, M. (2012). Online walking pattern generation for push recovery and minimum delay to commanded change of direction and speed. In *Intelligent Robots and Systems, 2012 IEEE/RSJ International Conference on,* (pp. 3411-3416).

Valk, P. E. (2003). *Positron emission tomography: Basic sciences.* Springer Science & Business Media.

Vallbo, A. B., Olausson, H., & Wessberg, J. (1999). Unmyelinated afferents constitute a second system coding tactile stimuli of the human hairy skin. *Journal of Neurophysiology, 81*(6), 2753–2763. PMID:10368395

Vellas, B., Guigoz, Y., Garry, P. J., Nourhashemi, F., Bennahum, D., Lauque, S., & Albarede, J. L. (1999). The Mini Nutritional Assessment (MNA) and its use in grading the nutritional state of elderly patients. *Nutrition (Burbank, Los Angeles County, Calif.)*, *15*(2), 116–122. doi:10.1016/S0899-9007(98)00171-3 PMID:9990575

Vellas, B., Lauque, S., Gillette-Guyonnet, S., Andrieu, S., Cortes, F., & Nourhashemi, F. et al.. (2005). Impact of nutritional status on the evolution of Alzheimer's disease and on response to acetylcholinesterase inhibitor treatment. *The Journal of Nutrition*, *9*(2), 75–80. PMID:15791349

Vermeulen, J., Lefeber, D., Verrelst, B., & Vanderborght, B. (2006). Trajectory planning for the walking biped "lucy". *The International Journal of Robotics Research*, *25*(9), 867–887. doi:10.1177/0278364906069343

Vickers, J. C., Dickson, T. C., Adlard, P. A., Saunders, H. L., King, C. E., & Mccormack, G. (2000). The cause of neuronal degeneration in Alzheimer's disease. *Progress in Neurobiology*, *60*(2), 139–165. doi:10.1016/S0301-0082(99)00023-4 PMID:10639052

Vidal, J. J. (1973). Toward direct brain-computer communication. *Annual Review of Biophysics and Bioengineering*, *2*(4), 157–180. doi:10.1146/annurev.bb.02.060173.001105 PMID:4583653

Volicer, L., & Charette, L. B. (1999). *Enhancing the Quality of Life in Advanced Dementia*. Routledge.

Volkert, D., & Sieber, C. C. (2011). Protein requirements in the elderly. *International Journal for Vitamin and Nutrition Research*, *81*(2), 109–119. doi:10.1024/0300-9831/a000061 PMID:22139561

Vora, J. Y., Allison, B. Z., & Moore, M. M. (2004). A P3 brain computer interface for robot arm control. *Society for Neuroscience Abstract 30*, Program No 421.19.

Walker, M. D., Salek, S. S., & Bayer, A. J. (1998). A review of quality of life in Alzheimer's disease. *PharmacoEconomics*, *14*(5), 499–530. doi:10.2165/00019053-199814050-00004 PMID:10344915

Wang, X. (2014). Subjective well-being associated with size of social network and social support of elderly. *Journal of Health Psychology*. http://doi.org/<ALIGNMENT.qj></ALIGNMENT>10.1177/1359105314544136

Wang, J. (2012). Humanoid push recovery with robust convex synthesis. *IEEE/RSJ International Conference on Intelligent Robots and Systems*, *57*, 4354-4359. doi:10.1109/IROS.2012.6386211

Wang, J., Whitman, E. C., & Stilman, M. (2012, June). Whole-body trajectory optimization for humanoid falling. In *American Control Conference*, (pp. 4837-4842).

Wang, L., Zang, Y., He, Y., Liang, M., Zhang, X., Tian, L., & Li, K. et al. (2006). Changes in hippocampal connectivity in the early stages of Alzheimer's disease: Evidence from resting state fMRI. *NeuroImage*, *31*(2), 496–504. doi:10.1016/j.neuroimage.2005.12.033 PMID:16473024

Wang, P. N., Yang, C. L., Lin, K. N., Chen, W. T., Chwang, L. C., & Liu, H. C. (2004). Weight loss, nutritional status and physical activity in patients with Alzheimer's disease. *Journal of Neurology, 251*(3), 314–320. doi:10.1007/s00415-004-0316-4 PMID:15015012

Wang, Y. W., Ling, C. D., Yuan, B., Huang, L., Zhang, W. X., & Shen, D. L. (2010). Person perception precedes theory of mind: An event related potential analysis. *Neuroscience, 170*(1), 238–246. doi:10.1016/j.neuroscience.2010.06.055 PMID:20603189

Wellman, N. S., & Kamp, B. J. (2008). Nutrition in aging. In L. K. Mahan & S. E. Stump (Eds.), *Krause's food and nutrition therapy* (pp. 286–297). Toronto: Saunders Elsevier.

Wells, S. E. (2014). Horticultural Therapy and the Older Adult Population. *Activities, Adaptation & Aging, 22*(1-3).

Wessberg, J., Olausson, H., Fernstrom, K. W., & Vallbo, A. B. (2003). Receptive field properties of unmyelinated tactile afferents in the human skin. *Journal of Neurophysiology, 89*(3), 1567–1575. doi:10.1152/jn.00256.2002 PMID:12626628

Whall, A. L., Black, M. E., Groh, C. J., Yankou, D. J., Kupferschmid, B. J. & Foster, N. L. (1997, September/October). The Effect of Natural Environments Upon Agitation and Aggression in Late Stage Dementia patients. *American Journal of Alzheimer Disease*, 216-220.

Whear, R., Coon, J. T., Bethel, A., Abbott, R., Stein, K., & Garside, R. (2014). What Is the Impact of Using Outdoor Spaces Such as Gardens on the Physical and Mental Well-Being of Those with Dementia? A Systematic Review of Quantitative and Qualitative Evidence. *Journal of the American Medical Directors Association.* Retrieved June 2015, http://www.sciencedirect.com/science/article/pii/S1525861014003399

Whitaker, H. (1976). 1–a case of the isolation of the language function. *Studies in Neurolinguistics,* 1-58.

White, H. K., McConnell, E. S., Bales, C. W., & Kuchibhatla, M. (2004). A 6-month observational study of the relationship between weight loss and behavioral symptoms in institutionalized Alzheimer's disease subjects. *Journal of the American Medical Directors Association, 5*(2), 89–97. doi:10.1016/S1525-8610(04)70061-4 PMID:14984619

White, H., Pieper, C., & Schmader, K. (1998). The association of weight change in Alzheimer's disease with severity of disease and mortality: A longitudinal analysis. *Journal of the American Geriatrics Society, 46*(10), 1223–1227. doi:10.1111/j.1532-5415.1998.tb04537.x PMID:9777903

Whitmer, R. A., Gunderson, E. P., Barrett-Connor, E., Quesenberry, C. P. Jr, & Yaffe, K. (2005). Obesity in middle age and future risk of dementia: A 27 year longitudinal population based study. *British Medical Journal, 330*(7504), 1360. doi:10.1136/bmj.38446.466238.E0 PMID:15863436

WHO. (2012). *Dementia: a public health priority.* Retrieved from http://www.who.int/mental_health/publications/dementia_report_2012/en/

Wiener, M., Turkeltaub, P. E., & Coslett, H. B. (2010). Implicit timing activates the left inferior parietal cortex. *Neuropsychologia*, *48*(13), 3967–3971. doi:10.1016/j.neuropsychologia.2010.09.014 PMID:20863842

Wiener, M., Turkeltaub, P., & Coslett, H. B. (2010). The image of time: A voxel-wise meta-analysis. *NeuroImage*, *49*(2), 1728–1740. doi:10.1016/j.neuroimage.2009.09.064 PMID:19800975

Willat, J. (2011). Design as Therapy: Facilitating the lives of those with Alzheimer's disease through environmental design, Revista AUS, núm. 9 (pp. 4–9). Valdivia, Chile: Universidad Austral de Chile. Retrieved from http://www.redalyc.org/articulo.oa?id=281722876002

Winograd, C. H., Jacobson, D. H., Butterfield, G. E., Cragen, E., Edler, L. A., Taylor, B. S., & Yesavage, J. A. (1991). Nutritional intake in patients with senile dementia of the Alzheimer type. *Alzheimer Disease and Associated Disorders*, *5*(3), 173–180. doi:10.1097/00002093-199100530-00003 PMID:1772637

Winter, Y., Korchounov, A., Zhukova, T. V., & Bertschi, N. E. (2011). Depression in elderly patients with Alzheimer dementia or vascular dementia and its influence on their quality of life. *Journal of Neurosciences in Rural Practice*, *2*(1), 27. doi:10.4103/0976-3147.80087 PMID:21716831

Witucki, J. M., & Twibell, R. S. (1997). The Effect of Sensory Stimulation Activities on the Psychological Well Being of Patients with Advanced Alzheimer's Disease. *American Journal of Alzheimer's Disease*, *2*(1), 10–15. doi:10.1177/153331759701200103

Wolff, P. H. (1961). Observations on the early development of smiling. *Determinants of Infant Behavior, 2,* 113-138.

Wolpaw, J. R., Birbaumer, N., Mc Farland, D. J., Pfurtscheller, G., & Vaughan, T. M. (2002). Brain–computer interfaces for communication and control. *Clinical Neurophysiology*, *113*(6), 767–791. doi:10.1016/S1388-2457(02)00057-3 PMID:12048038

Wolpaw, J. R., & Mcfarland, D. J. (2005). Control of a two-dimensional movement signal by a noninvasive brain-computer interface in humans. *Proceedings of the National Academy of Sciences of the United States of America*, *101*(51), 17849–17854. doi:10.1073/pnas.0403504101 PMID:15585584

Woods, B., Portnoy, S., Head, D., & Jones, G. (1992). Reminiscence and life review with persons with dementia: which way forward. *Care Giving in Dementia*, 137-161.

Woods, C. L., Cook, M., Orrell, M., & Spector, A. (2003). Cognitive rehabilitation and cognitive training for early-stage Alzheimer's disease and vascular dementia. Cochrane Database Syst Rev, 4.

World Health Organization & Alzheimer's Disease International. (2012). *Dementia: a public health priority.* Author.

Wright, J. (2014). *Garden therapy for those with special needs.* Retrieved June 2015, http://www.thegardener.co.za/kb/article.php?id=996

Wu, J. (2012). Delayed audiovisual integration of patients with mild cognitive impairment and Alzheimer's disease compared with normal aged controls. *Journal of Alzheimer's Disease, 32*(2), 317–328. PMID:22810093

Wu, J. L., Yang, J. J., & Ogasa, T. (2010). Raised-angle discrimination under passive finger movement. *Perception, 39*(7), 903–1006. doi:10.1068/p6264 PMID:20842975

Wu, J., Wang, B., Yang, J., Hikino, Y., Takahashi, S., Yan, T., & Kanazawa, S. et al. (2013). Development of a method to present wide-view visual stimuli in MRI for peripheral visual studies. *Journal of Neuroscience Methods, 214*(2), 126–136. doi:10.1016/j.jneumeth.2013.01.021 PMID:23376498

Wu, J., Yu, Y., & Yang, J. (2012). Neuropsychological Parameters as Potential Biomarkers for Alzheimer's Disease. *Current Translational Geriatrics and Experimental Gerontology Reports, 1*(2), 68–75. doi:10.1007/s13670-012-0007-4

Xefteris, S., Baboshin, A., Tserpes, K., Androulidakis, A., Glickman, Y., Varvarigou, T., … D'Andria, F. (2011). Enabling risk assessment and analysis by event detection in dementia patients using a reconfigurable rule set. In *Proceedings of the 4th International Conference on Pervasive Technologies Related to Assistive Environments - PETRA '11* (p. 1). New York: ACM Press. http://doi.org/ doi:10.1145/2141622.2141678

Xefteris, S., Andronikou, V., Tserpes, K., & Varvarigou, T. (2010). Case-based approach using behavioural biometrics aimed at Assisted Living. *Journal of Ambient Intelligence and Humanized Computing, 2*(2), 73–80. doi:10.1007/s12652-010-0029-8

Xiong, S., Goonetilleke, R. S., & Jiang, Z. H. (2011). Pressure thresholds of the human foot: Measurement reliability and effects of stimulus characteristics. *Ergonomics, 54*(4), 292–293. do i:10.1080/00140139.2011.571831 PMID:21390958

Yamaguchi Shuhei, O. K. (2014). Early diagnosis of dementia by resting-state functional MRI. Higher Brain Function Research (Japan Society for Higher Brain Dysfunction), 34, 9-16.

Yang, G., Xie, L., Mantysalo, M., Zhou, X., Pang, Z., Xu, L., … Zheng, L.-R. (2014). A Health-IoT Platform Based on the Integration of Intelligent Packaging, Unobtrusive Bio-Sensor, and Intelligent Medicine Box. *IEEE Transactions on Industrial Informatics, 10*(4), 2180–2191. http:// doi.org/<ALIGNMENT.qj></ALIGNMENT>10.1109/TII.2014.2307795

Yang, J. (n.d.). Decline of human tactile angle discrimination in patients with mild cognitive impairment and Alzheimer's disease. *Journal of Alzheimer's Disease, 22*(1), 225-234.

Yang, J. J., Ogasa, T., Ohta, Y., Abe, K., & Wu, J. L. (2010). Decline of human tactile angle discrimination in patients with mild cognitive impairment and alzheimer's disease. *Journal of Alzheimer's Disease, 22*, 225–234. PMID:20847416

Yang, J. J., Wu, J. L., & He, J. P. (2011). Programmable tactile pattern presentations operational under MRI to investigate neural mechanisms of tactile shape discrimination. *Journal of Neuroscience Methods, 201*(1), 17–26. doi:10.1016/j.jneumeth.2011.06.030 PMID:21763724

Yang, J., Usairy Syafiq, M., Yu, Y., Takahashi, S., Zhang, Z., & Wu, J. (2015). Development and Evaluation of a Tactile Cognitive Function Test Device for Alzheimer's Disease Early Detection. *Neuroscience and Biomedical Engineering*, *3*(2), 58–65. doi:10.2174/2213385203666150804001349

Yang, S. (2010). Defining Exergames & Exergaming. *Proceedings of Meaningful Play, 2010*, 1–17. Retrieved from http://meaningfulplay.msu.edu/proceedings2010/mp2010_paper_63.pdf

Yang, W. H., Liu, J. H., & Zhang, W. L. (2010). The study about human information processing in tactile recognition.*International Conference on Mechatronics and Automation* (pp. 905-997). Xi'an. doi:10.1109/ICMA.2010.5589960

Yan, L. L., Daviglus, M. L., Liu, K., Pirzada, A., Garside, D. B., Schiffer, L., & Greenland, P. (2004). BMI and health-related quality of life in adults 65 years and older. *Obesity Research*, *12*(1), 69–76. doi:10.1038/oby.2004.10 PMID:14742844

Yan, T., Jin, F., He, J., & Wu, J. (2011). Development of a wide-view visual presentation system for visual retinotopic mapping during functional MRI. *Journal of Magnetic Resonance Imaging*, *33*(2), 441–447. doi:10.1002/jmri.22404 PMID:21274987

Yarbus, A. L. (1967). *Eye movements and vision*. New York: Plenum Press. doi:10.1007/978-1-4899-5379-7

Yousefi, B.H., Manook, A., Drzezga, A., & Reutern, , B., Schwaiger, M., Wester, H.-J. R., & Henriksen, G. (2011). Synthesis and Evaluation of 11C-labeled Imidazo [2, 1-b] benzothiazoles (IBTs) as PET tracers for Imaging β-Amyloid Plaques in Alzheimer's Disease. *Journal of Medicinal Chemistry*, *54*, 949–956. doi:10.1021/jm101129a PMID:21275403

Yu, H. H., & Rosa, M. G. P. (2010). A simple method for creating wide-field visual stimulus for electrophysiology: Mapping and analyzing receptive fields using a hemispheric display. *Journal of Vision, 10*(14). doi:10.1167/10.14.15

Yun, S. K., & Goswami, A. (2014). Tripod fall: Concept and experiments of a novel approach to humanoid robot fall damage reduction. *Robotics and Automation, IEEE International Conference on*, (pp. 2799-2805).

Yu, Z., Huang, Q., Ma, G., Chen, X., Zhang, W., & Li, J. (2014). Design and development of the humanoid robot bhr-5. *Advances in Mechanical Engineering*, *11*, 1–11.

Zahodne, L. B., Schofield, P. W., Farrell, M. T., Stern, Y., & Manly, J. J. (2014). Bilingualism does not alter cognitive decline or dementia risk among Spanish-speaking immigrants. *Neuropsychology*, *28*(2), 238–246. doi:10.1037/neu0000014 PMID:24188113

Zanto, T. P., Pan, P., Liu, H., Bollinger, J., Nobre, A. C., & Gazzaley, A. (2011). Age-related changes in orienting attention in time. *The Journal of Neuroscience*, *31*(35), 12461–12470. doi:10.1523/JNEUROSCI.1149-11.2011 PMID:21880908

Zarrabi, N., Prosperi, M. C. F., Belleman, R. G., Di Giambenedetto, S., Fabbiani, M., De Luca, A., & Sloot, P. M. A. (2013). Combining social and genetic networks to study HIV transmission in mixing risk groups. *The European Physical Journal. Special Topics*, *222*(6), 1377–1387. doi:10.1140/epjst/e2013-01932-x

Zeisel, J. (2007). Creating a Therapeutic Garden That Works for People Living with Alzheimer's. *Journal of Housing for the Elderly, 21*(12), 13-33.

Zelanti, P. S., & Droit-Volet, S. (2011). Cognitive abilities explaining age-related changes in time perception of short and long durations. *Journal of Experimental Child Psychology*, *109*(2), 143–157. doi:10.1016/j.jecp.2011.01.003 PMID:21334637

Zhang, Q. Z., Xi, X. G., & Luo, Z. Z. (2014). A Pattern Recognition Method for Surface Electromyography Based on Nonlinear Features. *Journal of Electronics & Information Technology*, *35*(9), 2054–2058. doi:10.3724/SP.J.1146.2012.01325

Zhang, W., Oya, S., Kung, M.-P., Hou, C., Maier, D. L., & Kung, H. F. (2005). F-18 stilbenes as PET imaging agents for detecting β-amyloid plaques in the brain. *Journal of Medicinal Chemistry*, *48*(19), 5980–5988. doi:10.1021/jm050166g PMID:16162001

Ziesel, J. (2003). Marketing therapeutic environments for Alzheimer' s care. *Journal of Architectural and Planning Research*, *20*(1), 75–86.

About the Contributors

Jinglong Wu was born in Jiutai, China, on August 4, 1958. He received the B.S. degree from Jilin Vocational Teachers College, China, the M.S. degree from Kyoto University, Japan, both in electric engineering, in 1984 and 1991, respectively, and the doctorate in electric engineering from Kyoto University, Japan, in 1994. He was an Assistant Professor at Ritsumeikan University, Japan, from April 1994 to March 1997, a Lectuer in Department of Mechanical Engineering, Faculty of Engineering, Yamaguchi University from April 1997 to March 1999. Since April 1999, he is Professor in the Department of Intelligent Mechanical Systems, Faculty of Engineering, Kagawa University. His current research interests are virtual reality, ergonomics, cognitive neuroscience and human science. Dr.Wu received the Best Paper Award of IEEE Joint International Conference on Neural Network in 1993 and the SICE Best Paper Award in 2000. In 2003 he received the Gennai Grand Prize, Ozaki Foundation, Japan.

* * *

Panagiotis E. Antoniou is a postdoctoral research associate in the Lab of Medical Physics, department of Medicine, Aristotle University of Thessaloniki. He received a degree in Physics from Aristotle University of Thessaloniki in 1997, a M.Sc. degree in Medical Physics in 2001 from the Democritus University of Thrace and a Ph.D. degree in Medical Physics in 2004 from Democritus University of Thrace. His research interests are in the area of Medical Informatics, in the fields of virtual patients in medical education and in the field of the elderly exergaming interventions. He has authored more than 35 publications in peer reviewed journals and conferences.

Panagiotis Bamidis is currently an Ass. Prof. in the Medical School of the Aristotle University of Thessaloniki, Greece. He has founded and is leading three working groups, namely, one in Medical Education Informatics, one in Assistive Technologies and Silver Science and one in Applied and Affective Neuroscience. In the last 6 years, he has been the coordinator of five large European projects

(SmokeFreeBrain.org; www.meducator.net; www.longlastingmemories.eu, www.epblnet.eu, www.childrenhealth.eu) as well as the principal investigator for a number of national and international funded projects. His publication record consists of more than 85 international refereed journal papers, and over 300 international peer reviewed conference papers, as well as several book chapters / edited conference proceedings volumes and over some 470 citations (h-index>16). In addition, he has been acting as a referee in more than 30 journals, and as Guest Editor in more than 17 journal special issues. Finally, he is the President of the Hellenic Biomedical Technology Society (ELEBIT), a member of the Administration Boards of the Greek Federation of Alzheimer's Associations and Related Disorders, the Greek AeroSpace & Space Medicine Research Association, a member of the Life Sciences Division of the International Academy of Astronautics and past member of the Innovation Zone of Thessaloniki, Greece. He has been the Chairman/Organiser of seven international conferences (iSHIMR2001, iSHIMR2005, MEDICON2010, GASMA2010, SAN2011, MEI2012, MEI2015) and several national Biomedical Technology conferences and he is the Conference Producer of the Medical Education Informatics Conference and associated Spring/Summer School Series. He is a visiting scientist at Karolinska Institute, Sweden. He is a member of the Advisory Board of the Open Knowledge Foundation and a founding member of Chapter Greece. In 2009, he was awarded the Prize of the AUTH Research Committee for the Best Track Record in funded research projects among AUTH young academic staff. In 2015, he was awarded the title of the Honorary Professor of Karaganda State Medical University, Kazakhstan, as well as the Pospelov Medal for his contributions to Medical Education development by the same University. His research interests are within technology enhanced learning in Medical Education (web2.0, semantic web and open linked data, serious games, virtual patients, PBL, learning analytics), Affective and Applied Neuroscience, Affective and Physiological Computing, multimodal interaction and HCI, Health Information Management, Bio-medical Informatics with emphasis on neurophysiological sensing, signal analysis, and imaging of human emotions, as well as, Assistive Technologies for Active and Healthy Ageing, as well as, special education/developmental disorders, and silvergaming/exergaming/silver-science.

Antonis S. Billis received his diploma in Electrical and Computer Engineering in 2007 and MSc in Medical Informatics in 2011, both from Aristotle University of Thessaloniki, Greece. He also holds a Ptychio in Business Administration and Management from the University of Macedonia, Greece. He is currently working toward the Ph.D. degree in gerontechnology and works with the Laboratory of Medical Physics, Medical School, AUTH. Main research interests include: clinical decision support systems, personal informatics, biomedical sensors, machine learning and data analytics.

Christos A. Frantzidis received the Diploma degree in electrical and computer engineering, in 2006, and the M.Sc. degree in medical informatics, in 2008, both from Aristotle University of Thessaloniki (AUTH), Thessaloniki, Greece. He recently received from the same university (November 2014) his Ph.D. degree in the neurophysiological evaluation of non-pharmaceutical cognitive and/or physical interventions aiming to promote healthy aging. He is also collaborating with the Greek Association of Alzheimer Disease and Related Disorders and the Laboratory of Medical Physics, School of Health Sciences, Aristotle University of Thessaloniki towards the early detection of dementia-related neurophysiological patterns based on synchronization and brain-network analysis. He is also studying the effects of both physiological and pathological aging on emotional processing. His involvement in the FP7 EU funded project Long Lasting Memories / LLM (http://www.longlastingmemories.eu/) and the PharmaCog project (http://www.alzheimer-europe.org/Research/PharmaCog) lied on the data acquisition of EEG recordings and particularly for the LLM project on the neuro-physiological estimation of the cognitive decline of the elderly. He is the first author of the paper entitled as "What are the symbols of Alzheimer? A Permutation Entropy based symbolic analysis for the detection of early changes of the electroencephalographic complexity due to mild Alzheimer" gained the 3rd prize in the best student paper competition on the 12th IEEE Conference on BioInformatics and BioEngineering (BIBE 2012) held in Larnaca, Cyprus, 11-13 November, 2012.

Panagiotis Emmanouil Kartsidis holds a Mathematics BSc and Medical Informatics MSc from Aristotle University of Thessaloniki. Working as research assistant at the Medical Physics Lab, School of Medicine of A.U.Th.

Alev Keser is an associate professor at Ankara University (Turkey), Faculty of Health Sciences, Department of Nutrition and Dietetics. She received her master's and doctorate degrees from the Department of Nutrition and Dietetics at Hacettepe University. Dr. Keser worked as dietician eight years at Kocaeli University Medical Faculty Training and Research Hospital, Division of Pediatrics Endocrinology and Diabetes. Her main research interests include childhood obesity, diabetes, metabolic syndrome and elderly nutrition.

Evdokimos Konstantinidis received the Diploma in electronic engineering from the Technological Educational Institute of Thessaloniki, in 2004 and the M.Sc. degree in medical informatics in 2008 from the Aristotle University of Thessaloniki,

Greece. He has just completed his Ph.D. degree in the Laboratory of Medical Physics of Medicine, School of Health Sciences, Aristotle University of Thessaloniki, Greece. His current research interests lie predominately in the area of Medical Informatics, particularly with respect to people with special needs and especially elderly. Recent research interests focus on intervention for elderly in the field of exergaming. He has authored more than 30 publications in various international peer-reviewed journals and conferences.

Evangelos Paraskevopoulos completed his bachelor and master studies in the psychology department of Aristotle University of Thessaloniki (A.U.TH.). At the same time he studied music theory and received a music diploma in Harmony, Counterpoint and Fugue. He then moved in Muenster, Germany to perform his PhD in cognitive neurosciences and Magnetoencephalography in the Institute for Biomagnetism and Biosignalanalysis with Prof. Dr. Christo Pantev as supervisor. He completed his PhD in 2013 receiving a Summa Cum Laude graduate. In 2011 he received an award in the young neuroscientist poster competition "NeuroVisionen 8" by the NeuroNRW - Ministry of Innovation, Science and Research of the State of North Rhine-Westphalia, Germany and a postdoctoral research fellowship from A.U.TH. (Excellence). His research interests focus on cortical plasticity, music perception (disorders) and multisensory integration. He has 15 published papers in international refereed journals, one in the scientific annals of the Department of Psychology, of A.U.TH., 2 book chapters and more than 20 contributions in international conferences with posters and talks.

Stefanos Xefteris holds a bachelor degree in mathematics from the Aristotle University of Thessaloniki. From 2001 to 2006 he has worked in the telecoms industry as researcher and later in the university of Patras as assistant researcher. He is now close to defending his Ph.d thesis in the school of Electrical and Computer Engineering of the National Technical University of Athens, with title "Behavioral biometrics and emotion recognition in Ambient Assisted Living Applications". Right now he is a research associate of the medical physics lab in the school of Medicine of Aristotle University of Thessaloniki. His research interests include pattern recognition, computational geometry, machine learning and behavioral biometrics and he has participated both as researcher and project manager in numerous research projects.

Filiz Yildirim is an associate professor at Ankara University (Turkey), Faculty of Health Sciences, Department of Social Work. She received her master's and doctorate degrees from the Department of Family and Consumer Sciences. She was awarded a "Doctorate Research Scholarship" from TUBITAK to carry out a part of her doctorate research at the Department of Sociology, Criminology & Law at the University of Florida, the USA in 2011. She received the "International Young Scholar Award" from the Society for Research on Adolescence in Canada in 2012. She worked as a "Visiting Research Associate" at London University, Institute of Education, Department of Childhood, Families & Health in 2014. Her main research interests include aging & youth sociology, love, early (child) marriage, social justice and health literacy. She is also a post-doctoral fellow at Hacettepe University (Turkey), Department of Sociology.

Jiabin Yu was born in Anhui Province, China, in 1987. He received a Master of Engineering degree from Changchun University of Science and Technology, China, in 2014. He is a second year doctor's student in the Biomedical Engineering Laboratory, Graduate school of Natural Science and Technology, Okayama University, Japan. Recently, he has been studying in the human brain mechanism of haptic Braille perception by fMRI.

Gökçen Firdevs Yücel received her BArch from Istanbul University, Landscape Architecture Department and MSc in Landscape Planning Program from Istanbul Technical University. She earned her PhD degree in Landscape Planning Program from Istanbul Technical University. Currently, she works as an Assistant Professor at Istanbul Aydın University, Landscape Architecture and Urban Design Department. Her major research interests include landscape design. Dr. Yücel has published in her areas of expertise in national and international congresses, national journals, and international book chapters.

Zhilin Zhang was born in Jingzhou City, Hubei Province, China, 1987. In 2014, he received the master's degree in biology from Liaoning Normal University. From 2014 until now, he was currently working toward the Ph.D. degree, in mechanical engineering, from Beijing Institute of Technology, China. His research interests include active touch, passive touch and intra-active touch.

Index

A

B

C

D

E

Q

R

S

T

U

V

W

X

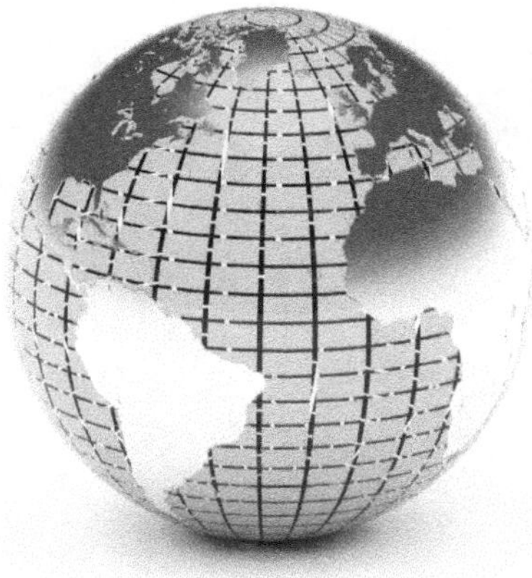

www.ingramcontent.com/pod-product-compliance
Lightning Source LLC
LaVergne TN
LVHW080601300926
849162LV00005B/1013